THE BIKINI BODY
28-DAY
HEALTHY EATING & LIFESTYLE GUIDE

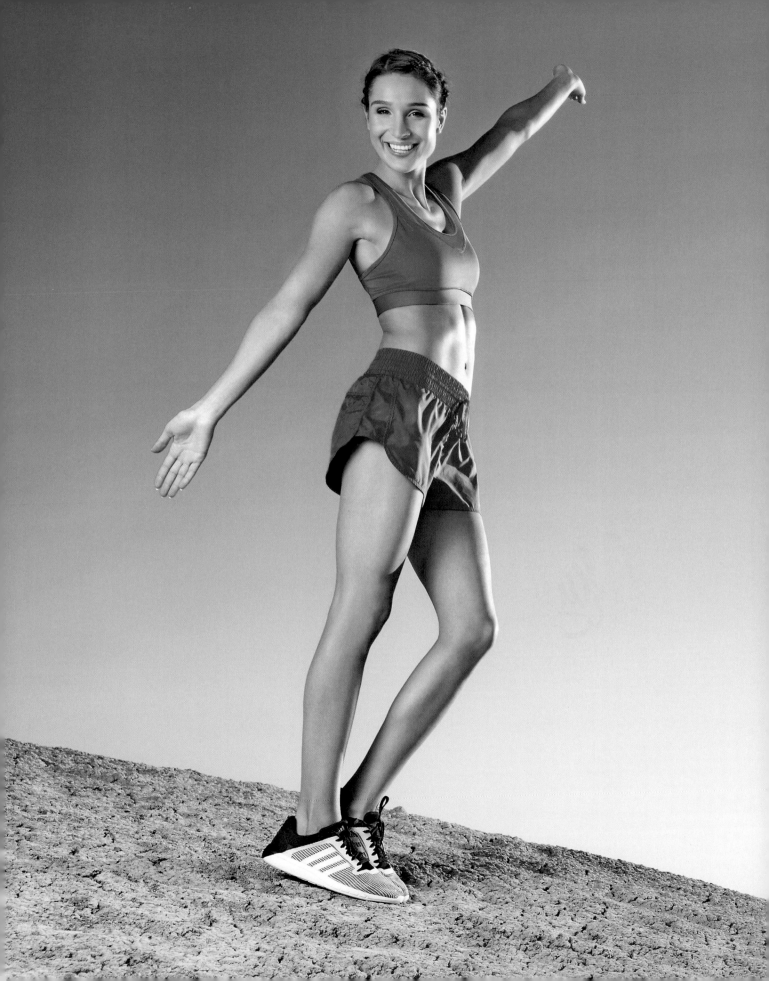

THE BIKINI BODY 28-DAY HEALTHY EATING & LIFESTYLE GUIDE

Kayla Itsines

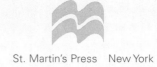

St. Martin's Press   New York

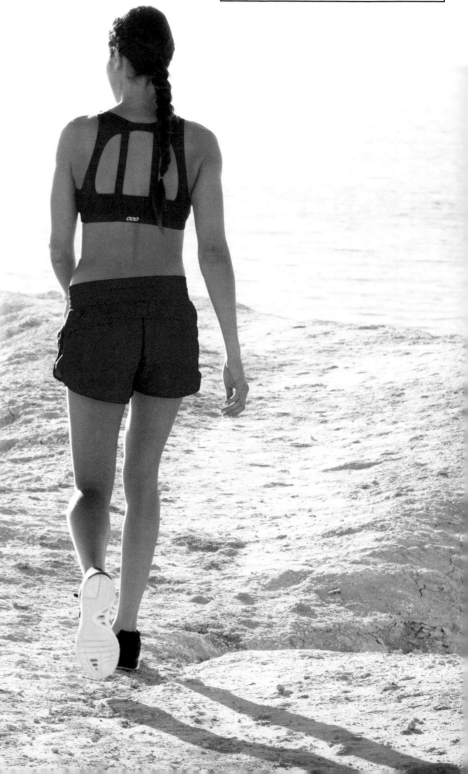

The Bikini Body 28-Day Healthy Eating & Lifestyle Guide. Text copyright © 2016 by Kayla Itsines. Photographs copyright © 2016 by Jeremy Simons. Illustrations copyright © 2016 by Anthony Calvert. All rights reserved. Printed in the United States of America. For information, address St. Martin's Press, 175 Fifth Avenue, New York, N.Y. 10010

www.stmartins.com

Design by Trisha Garner at DesignPatsy
Additional design by Elissa Webb
Photography by Jeremy Simons
Prop and food styling by Michelle Noerianto
Illustrations by Anthony Calvert
Food preparation by Tammi Kwok and Angela Devlin
Editing by Miriam Cannell, Rachel Carter, and Kathleen Gandy
Production Manager: Adriana Coada

The Library of Congress Cataloging-in-Publication Data is available upon request.

ISBN 978-1-250-12147-9 (hardcover)
ISBN 978-1-250-12148-6 (e-book)

Our books may be purchased in bulk for promotional, educational, or business use. Please contact your local bookseller or the Macmillan Corporate and Premium Sales Department at 1-800-221-7945, extension 5442, or by e-mail at MacmillanSpecialMarkets@macmillan.com.

First published 2016 by Pan Macmillan Australia Pty Limited
1 Market Street, Sydney, New South Wales, Australia 2000

First U.S. Edition: December 2016

10 9 8 7 6 5 4 3 2 1

CONTENTS

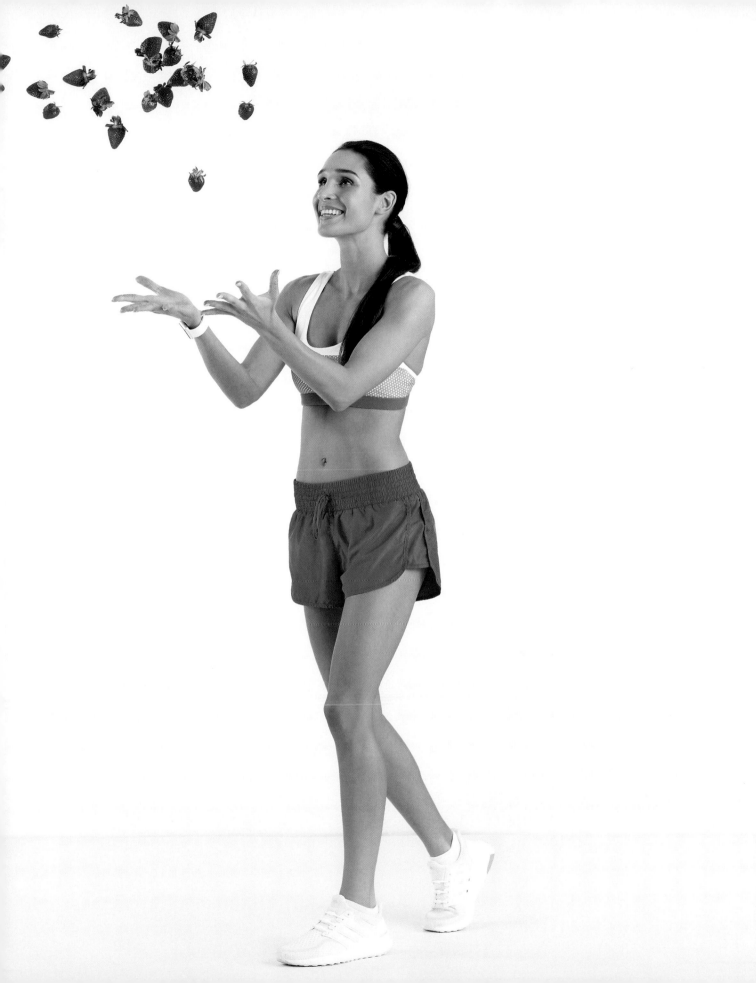

WHO AM I?

Dear Reader,

My name is Kayla Itsines and I am a personal trainer. I have been in the fitness industry for almost 10 years and chose personal training as my career because I am passionate about making people, especially women, feel better about themselves. As a child, I wanted to be a beauty therapist because I liked the way makeup makes women feel (at one point when I was really young, I even wanted to be a lawn mower, because I loved the way freshly cut grass made people smile—my dad still thinks this is funny!) As I matured, I discovered makeup is only skin deep, and therefore, a very temporary change. I realised I wanted to make a *permanent* change to women's lifestyles and mindsets. Something like this is only achievable through a comprehensive health and lifestyle change, not just a layer of concealer.

MY MISSION? I WANT TO HELP AS MANY WOMEN AS POSSIBLE ACHIEVE THEIR IDEAL BODY, CONFIDENCE, AND HAPPINESS.

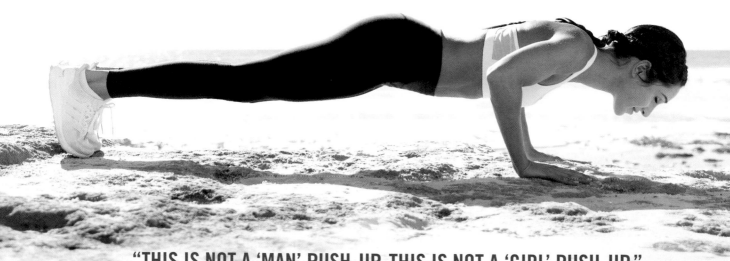

"THIS IS NOT A 'MAN' PUSH-UP. THIS IS NOT A 'GIRL' PUSH-UP."

Not only am I passionate about helping women change their lives, but I am passionate about exercise in general. I *love* training women. I love seeing them work hard and sweat, finishing their session with a big exhale as they look at me, exhausted, but with a huge grin of success. Exercise can be very empowering for women of any age, shape, or size.

Since 2009, I have trained women in a female-only studio and on the road with a portable training franchise. In 2014, I decided to take my workout advice away from what had become my very own personal training studio and into the online world, and this is when #bbg, or the Bikini Body Guide, was born. But the name Bikini Body Guide has nothing to do with the way you *look*; instead it represents an ideology that my partner Tobi and I created (see overleaf). The global fitness community we have established is now over 13 million women strong, and it's growing daily. Our mission is that this community of amazing women is going to change the world for the better through health and fitness, and now you're a part of it too.

Kayla xo

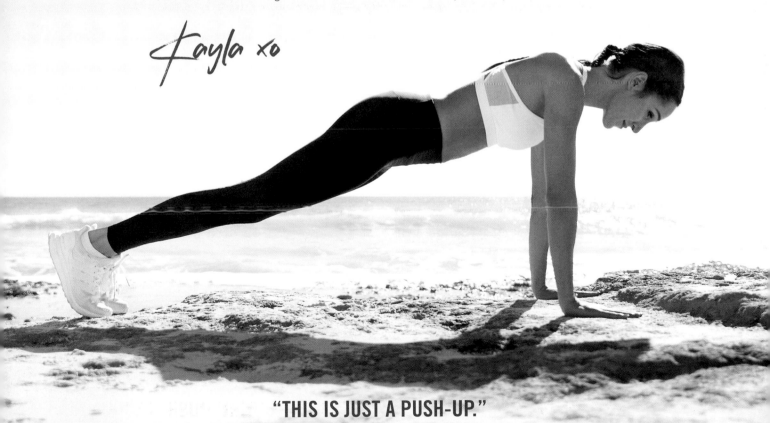

"THIS IS JUST A PUSH-UP."

BECOMING HEALTHY, CONFIDENT & STRONG

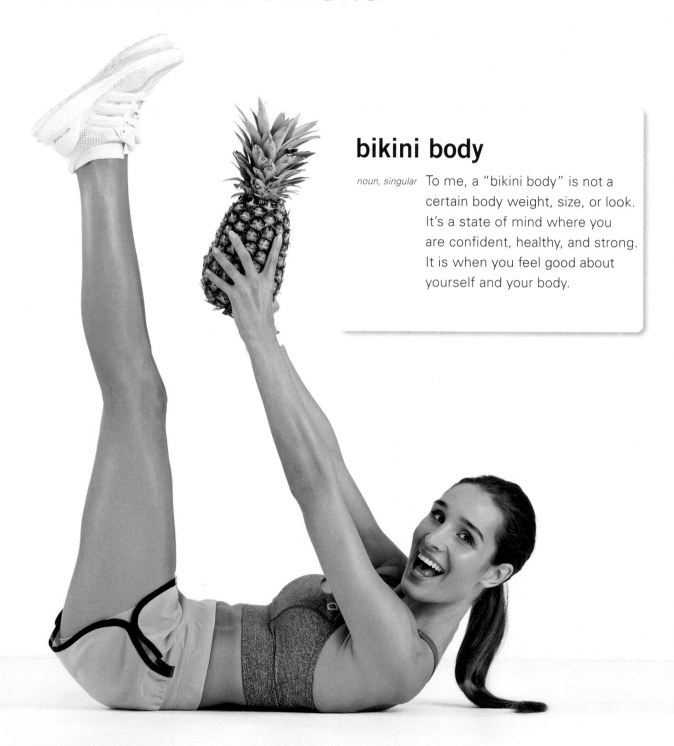

bikini body

noun, singular To me, a "bikini body" is not a certain body weight, size, or look. It's a state of mind where you are confident, healthy, and strong. It is when you feel good about yourself and your body.

I am a woman who has grown up in the age of mobile phones, social media, and apps. What this means is that conversation is everywhere, and both good and bad messages can be spread far and wide. The way social media is rapidly able to distribute messages to the world is phenomenal. Unfortunately, it is often the wrong messages that we see trending in our news feeds.

How is it anyone's right to set the standard? Why should a celebrity's appearance be the "body goal" for our society, when often it is their job to look a certain way? It's fine to idolise the *person*, but often young, impressionable girls idolise the *body* because of the way media pitches imagery.

Along with this altered perception of beauty, I now, more than ever, see people being publicly abused and shamed on social media, not even just for their appearance, but for their desire to change, their desire to do better and feel better. No one should be shamed for trying to improve themselves.

THE EXPECTATIONS WE HAVE OF OURSELVES ARE HIGHLY DRIVEN BY WHAT WE SEE, TYPICALLY IN THE MEDIA AND ON SOCIAL NETWORKS. THAT'S THE PROBLEM—OUR EXPECTATIONS AND GOALS SHOULD BE BASED ON WHAT WE *FEEL*, NOT ON WHAT WE *SEE*.

Because people's perception and expectation of "normal" has changed so dramatically, it alters their view of what truly is normal. Now, some people are attacked for being what should be acceptable, but instead they are shamed for not looking like what our manipulated perception of reality shows us.

MY CLIENTS ALL HAVE INDIVIDUAL GOALS AND THEIR TRANSFORMATION JOURNEYS ARE UNIQUE TO THEM.

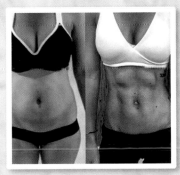

@kim_fairley
32 years old, mum of 2,
Gold Coast, Queensland

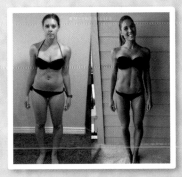

@mysweatlife
26 years old, mum of 1,
Texas, USA

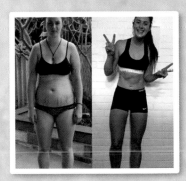

@danipguy
25 years old, mum of 1,
Mandurah, Western Australia

WE AS WOMEN are being attacked by a new breed of soldier. We are becoming victims of so-called "keyboard warriors," who are playing directly into the poor messaging of mass media. The worst part? These keyboard warriors can often be women.

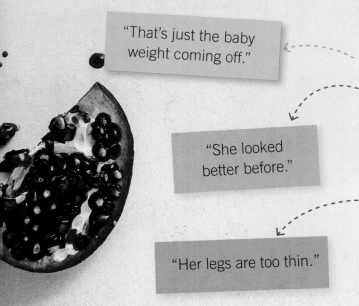

"That's just the baby weight coming off."

"She looked better before."

"Her legs are too thin."

keyboard warrior

noun, singular A person who believes their opinion in relation to your life choices and appearance matters. They often write rude, hateful, and disheartening comments about you on social media, thinking that it doesn't affect you.

So, in this generation of keyboard warriors and mass media trends, what effect is all this having on body image and the associated issues of anxiety, depression, and body dysmorphia for women of all ages? We have men degrading and body-shaming women, but we also have women doing the same to other women. This needs to stop.

I believe that one of the main reasons women suffer from anxiety and depression is because of the way they look or, more accurately, the way they *feel* about their appearance. In my opinion, a huge amount of this negative emotion can be caused by messages about women in the media and society. More specifically, the way women speak about each other's bodies, as well as their own.

After continually seeing huge amounts of negativity in the media, I wanted to make a stand and help create change in the way women see their bodies. There is so much negativity surrounding women and the supposed "benchmarks" for their appearance that it is easy to understand why so many women who would like to wear a bikini are uneasy about it.

"WHY SHOULD WE BE REQUIRED TO LOOK, ACT, OR DRESS A CERTAIN WAY, OR HAVE A CERTAIN BODY SHAPE, TO FIT INTO SOCIETY'S DEFINITION OF BEAUTIFUL? BEAUTY IS NOT CONFORMITY, IT IS NOT FINITE OR SINGULAR. BEAUTY IS UNIQUE."

Nothing is more disheartening than being unnecessarily ashamed or worried about your appearance. It is a very hard thing to assess objectively on your own, especially when we all know that we are often our biggest critics (and often you are your *only* critic).

Only you notice that one little freckle on your cheek that you hate. Everyone else loves it and thinks it's cute. **Only you** notice your "bad hair day"—no one else can see it because they're too busy staring at your beautiful eyes. **Only you** think that your bum is too flat or too big, your abs aren't good enough or your triceps are too "flabby."

The worst part is, the more you think these things in your own mind, the more they become a visual reality for you when you look in the mirror. This doesn't necessarily mean they *are* real, but the more you think and feel it, the more you see it.

No matter how much negative media you see, or how often you think about yourself critically or negatively, it doesn't matter—you can overcome all of this. The first step is becoming really clear about what you actually want, and often it isn't just the six-pack abs or a lifted bum.

Throughout my years of experience, the more I talked to my female clients it became obvious that many girls aspire to a specific yet common goal, and it's not necessarily just a certain body shape or a toned body. The body type they aspire to is a far cry from the overly muscular look that a lot of women often obtain through training. I found that some trainers in this industry either don't understand, or don't listen to their client's goals, and are therefore unable to advise women in a way that will help them attain these goals. I think trainers and coaches alike often aim for only physical changes in terms of your abs or body fat percentage, which are not one of the three measures I like to use to grade health and/or happiness.

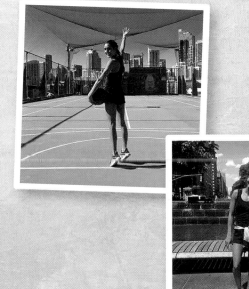

WHAT WOMEN REALLY WANT IS THE **CONFIDENCE**, **STRENGTH**, AND POSITIVE PHYSICAL CHANGE THAT COME AS A RESULT OF A **HEALTHY LIFESTYLE**.

WHAT IS HEALTH, CONFIDENCE & STRENGTH?

Through my experience, I have learnt that health, confidence, and strength are three key aspirations for most, if not all, women. To clearly understand what this means, I have defined them below in a way that is relevant and relatable to each of our lives.

Health—relates to your **physical state**. It's not necessarily just about having strong abs, but do you look healthy, is your skin clear, do you have good posture, are you "glowing"?

Confidence—relates to your **emotional state**. Not necessarily just being confident wearing a bikini, but when you look at yourself in the mirror, do you feel powerful, do you feel happy in your own body? Can you walk down the street with your head held high, empowered that you can do anything in the world?

Strength—relates to your **mental state**. Not just about how much weight you can lift, but how much you can endure. When you have a bad day, can you lift yourself up? How strong and sound are your internal thoughts about your health, your mind, and your body?

} *I BELIEVE THAT THROUGH THESE THREE WORDS, WE CAN ACHIEVE HAPPINESS THROUGH DIVERSITY.*

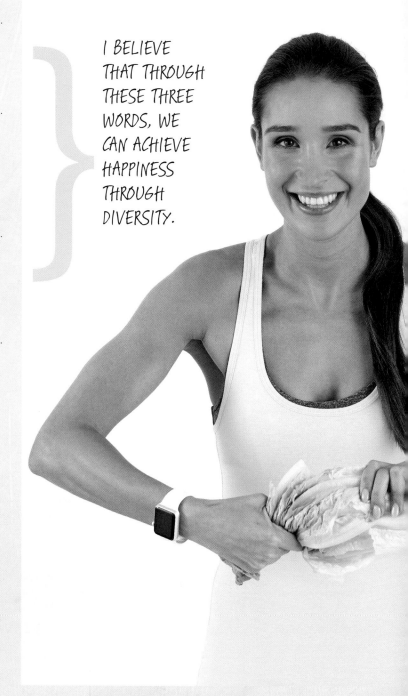

> # Confidence is knowing your worth and loving yourself…
>
> ## …DESPITE WHAT ANYONE ELSE THINKS OR SAYS.

My work is, and has always been, entirely about making women feel comfortable in their bodies, confident in life and strong enough to keep going each day. The journey of life, health, and happiness is much more comprehensive than just losing a few pounds. I don't believe everyone has to do the **same thing**, but I do believe everyone should do **something** each day to feel better about themselves, whether it be physically or emotionally. The biggest problem some women have is knowing where to start and what is right for them.

I have heard many trainers, fitness professionals, and individuals say lots of different things about how to get "results," such as what IS required, what is NOT required, shortcuts you can take, and things to avoid. Everyone has probably heard the following mantras: "Life is all about 80% diet plus 20% training" and "Eat whatever you want, just train at 120%." I firmly believe neither of these are the answer. *My* answer is being 100% committed to a healthy lifestyle and fully understanding the flexibility, simplicity, and balance you can have.

While we are all entitled to our own opinion, in this book I am hoping to clear up some of this confusion for you. This will allow you to focus on your goals and get better results by implementing real-world habits for good health into your lifestyle using a simple, flexible method.

Your lifestyle includes a range of things, from the foods you eat to the beverages you drink, how much exercise you do, how much sleep you get, how much work/study you do, and so much more! There is much to consider when accommodating your life, the world and the way it rapidly changes, and your health.

I want to help educate girls from all over the world, and help them understand that exclusionary diets or stringent training styles are not necessarily the best or only way to go. Rather, a well-rounded, healthy lifestyle can be far more flexible, beneficial, and enjoyable.

I always say that with a more educated mind, you will find it easier to obtain the things you want in life by wasting less time, energy, and emotion.

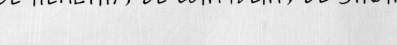

BE HEALTHY, BE CONFIDENT, BE STRONG.

So, how do we get healthy, confident, and strong?
And how do we stay that way?

I believe that to be healthy, confident, and strong, not only now but in the long term, your lifestyle should reflect your physical, emotional, and mental appearance.

In order to maintain this over a long period, three key points need to be practised daily.

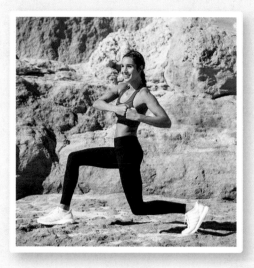

1 BALANCE

If you do not have balance, you cannot be steady. A lack of balance makes it easier for you to "fall over" and lose track of your health.

2 FLEXIBILITY

In order to have a balanced lifestyle, your choices need to be flexible to accommodate the real world. Your life and the world change every day, so you need to adapt to your environment and make the best choices possible in real time. No one can be perfect, because the world is not perfect or consistent.

3 SIMPLICITY

In order to have a flexible lifestyle, you need to lead a simple one. If your nutrition, training, or social regime is too complex, it limits your ability to adapt as necessary.

I BELIEVE THESE THREE QUALITIES PROVIDE THE FOUNDATION FOR SUCCESS, MUCH LIKE A WELL-BUILT BRIDGE. A BRIDGE IS WELL BALANCED, FLEXIBLE TO ALLOW FOR SOME MOVEMENT, AND USES SIMPLE TECHNOLOGY TO MINIMISE RISK AND ALLOW FOR CHANGE IN THE FUTURE.

"WITHOUT SIMPLICITY, WE CANNOT LEAD A FLEXIBLE LIFE. WITHOUT THE FLEXIBILITY TO ACCOMMODATE REAL-WORLD SCENARIOS, WE CANNOT BE BALANCED. IF WE ARE NOT BALANCED, WE WILL ULTIMATELY FALL OVER."

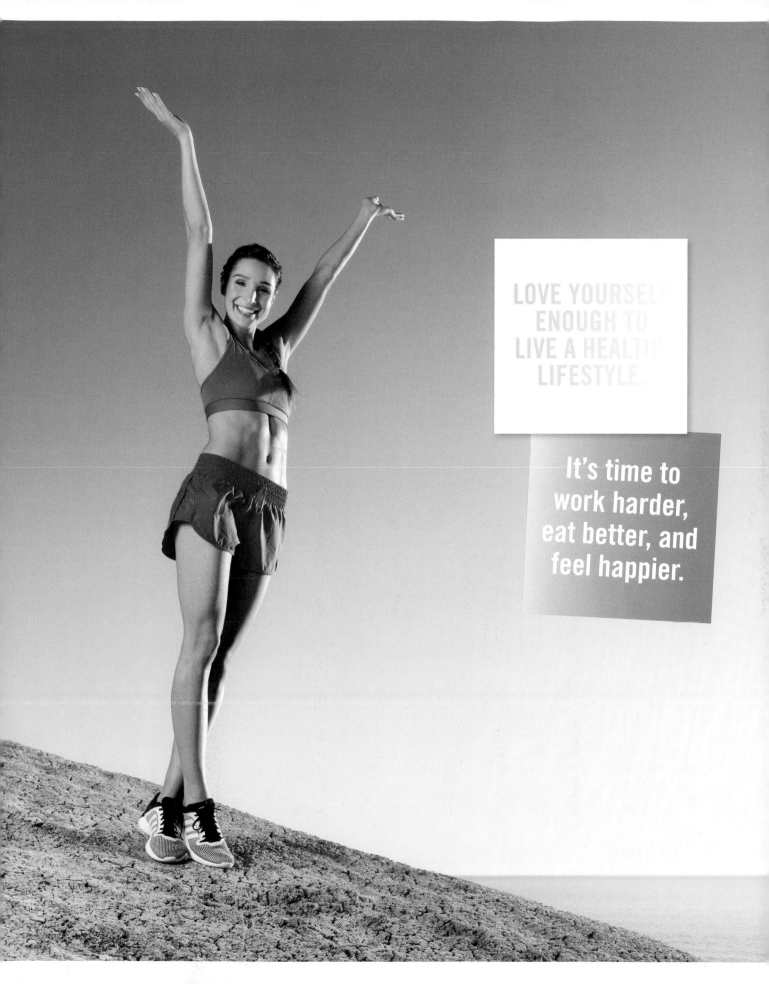

LOVE YOURSELF
ENOUGH TO
LIVE A HEALTHY
LIFESTYLE.

It's time to
work harder,
eat better, and
feel happier.

MY METHOD

BALANCE, FLEXIBILITY, SIMPLICITY

My experience tells me that these three principles, applied to all aspects of your lifestyle (including your diet, training, socialising, resting, and rehabilitation), are the best way to achieve health and happiness.

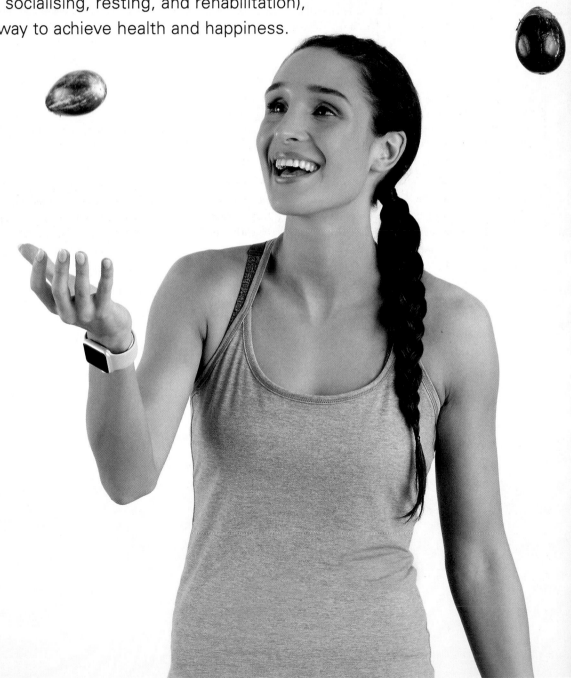

Nutrition

Healthy eating is essential for everyone. I am not in the business of promoting exclusionary diets ("no carbs" or "no fats"), but I am in the business of advocating balanced, healthy eating.

Rather than counting calories to control food intake, I prefer to use a simpler method based on food groups and serving sizes. While I understand that monitoring food intake is important, I do not believe that calorie counting is always the best or only way to do this. This is because, for many people, it can be a very tedious process, especially if not understood properly.

Sometimes when we delve into calorie counting and macronutrient distribution too much, we can get lost, confused, and make mistakes. This is typically the sort of nutrition profiling that an elite athlete would use, but I don't believe that it is mandatory in order for everyone to maintain good health. Further, I don't believe that it provides the same level of flexibility, balance, or simplicity that the food group distribution method does for most individuals.

In my opinion, the well-planned food group distribution method that I have devised in collaboration with dietitians is much simpler because it involves adding and subtracting easily manageable numbers. This can be a huge timesaver when planning meals!

As well as helping you meet the recommended calorie and nutrient requirements each day, it also allows you to easily substitute one food for another, while managing the calories and macronutrient content is done behind the scenes for you.

So, instead of endless analysis or breakdown of the amounts of calories, carbs, protein, fats, or vitamins, in my method you'll just see "exchange 2 slices of bread for 1 wrap." I've done the work for you. Less to think about means less stress for you!

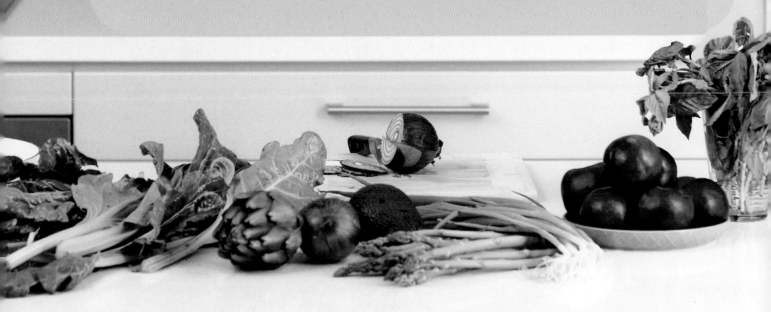

Training

Healthy eating alone is not the solution to sustaining comprehensive, long-term health. It is of primary importance that we also engage in regular physical activity with some form of resistance in order to stimulate our muscles. This resistance could be the weight of your body while you walk or jog, or using weights while you work out.

This physical activity benefits your body by:
- strengthening your muscles
- increasing your bone density
- improving your cardiovascular health
- decreasing your risk of lifestyle diseases
- reducing your risk of injury from a sedentary (inactive) lifestyle.

It is important to remember that in order for any positive change to occur, there must be a stimulus (activity) of some sort. It doesn't necessarily need to be a lot—as few as two to three 30-minute walks during the week will be beneficial to someone who lives a sedentary lifestyle. I always recommend, when possible, getting a good balance of and variation between cardio and resistance workouts to stimulate your muscles in multiple ways for maximum benefit.

> My training plans generally consist of two to four cardio sessions (of varying intensity) and three resistance circuit training sessions per week.

What is resistance training?

Resistance training involves using some form of resistance to increase the difficulty of different types of muscle movements. The resistance can come from your own body weight (as with squats or push-ups), or external weights such as dumbbells.

My resistance workouts include a mix of plyometric (jump), body-weight and strength-building exercises, which have been incorporated into high-intensity circuits.

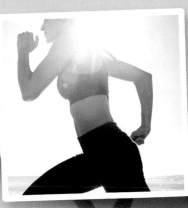

What is cardio training?

The word *cardio* is short for cardiovascular exercise, which is essentially any form of aerobic exercise, such as walking, running, swimming, or cycling. Aerobic means "in the presence of oxygen" (think "AIRobic.")

The two types of cardio that I recommend are:

- **Low-Intensity Steady State (or "LISS")**, which is equivalent to 30–45 minutes of walking or any other form of low-intensity cardio.

- **High-Intensity Interval Training (or "HIIT")**, which is equivalent to a 30-second sprint (defined as "work"), followed by a 30-second walk (defined as "rest"). These "work" and "rest" periods are then repeated for a designated amount of time, usually 10–15 minutes.

Lifestyle

In the same way it is important for us to have a good balance of nutrients in our diet and a variety of types of exercise in our training, it is also very important to have a balance of work and play in our lives. This can be the most difficult balance to achieve, because it doesn't just involve managing your own needs, but also how your needs integrate with those of others.

As funny as it may sound, we all need a little stress to operate at our best. Living with a positive amount of stress and stimulation means you continue to develop emotionally and intellectually, in the same way that exercising regularly develops you physically. This development helps us appreciate the "rest and recovery" time in our life better and helps us grow as people. Without any stimulation, we can become bored and complacent, in the same way that without rest we become tired and irritable. This can often lead us to make bad decisions in one area of our life or another.

Having a healthy balance of social life and work life is hugely important. Part of this is choosing the people who are around you most, like your best friends. Being a Greek Australian, my family is huge, and I definitely understand you can't choose your family. However, your best and closest friends, the people you choose to associate with most, are often the people who will help shape your life, and you can definitely choose them! This is your own personal community. The support that this personal community can provide is something that has helped many of my clients be successful at changing their life. This sometimes means you need to choose that friend who will say, "Hey, okay, I'll join you at the gym" rather than "Go to the gym by yourself later, because I want coffee now." A good friend doesn't just look out for themselves—they'll respect your lifestyle, your needs, and your choices, regardless of whether or not they share the same priorities.

CHECK OUT THE HASHTAGS **#SWEATWITHKAYLA #BBGCOMMUNITY** AND **#KAYLAITSINES** TO CONNECT WITH MILLIONS OF WOMEN WHO ARE UNITING THROUGH HEALTH AND FITNESS AND WILL SUPPORT YOU ALL THE WAY.

The importance of sleep

One aspect of a healthy lifestyle that is commonly overlooked is getting enough sleep. Although many might view sleep as just lying for hours with your eyes closed, it is so much more than that! It gives our brain the chance to process everything we've learnt or experienced that day, as well as to prepare for tomorrow. Sleep helps you stay focused and make decisions, and it regulates your mood. When we sleep, it gives our body the chance to repair itself (hence the term "beauty sleep") and ensure our regulatory hormones stay in check.

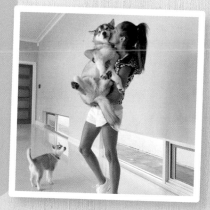

> **Kayla, this seems like a LOT of information to remember. What if I can't do it all?**

HOW NOT TO FAIL
Be realistic, expect change, and be educated.

Be realistic

QUICK FIXES DO NOT EXIST. There is no shortcut to good long-term health, because you can't rush to the end of a lifelong journey. As I always say, you can't fake fitness, and fitness is dedication and consistency.

Expect and welcome change

The world is a constantly changing place. Your work hours might change, your location might change, or there might suddenly be a worldwide avocado shortage! When the world changes around you, you need to change with it, so be prepared to adapt and be flexible (but seriously, I hope there is never an avocado shortage—haha!).

Educate yourself

Really learn what it is you're doing and what the actual commitment is that you're making. You wouldn't sign an important contract without reading it, so why would you just believe what's in the diet pages of a book without understanding all the principles that back up this information? Having trust in an author or your trainer is one thing, being naive is another. With a fuller understanding of what you're doing, you'll do it better, make fewer mistakes, and have fewer questions to ask during the process. You should be more concerned with sticking to the plan (and how it suits your life) and succeeding, than with second-guessing whether you're doing everything right.

END YOUR NIGHT WITH A QUIET REFLECTION OF YOUR DAY.

THINK ABOUT ALL YOU HAVE ACHIEVED THROUGHOUT THE DAY AND SET SOME GOALS FOR TOMORROW.

FAILING TO PLAN IS PLANNING TO FAIL.

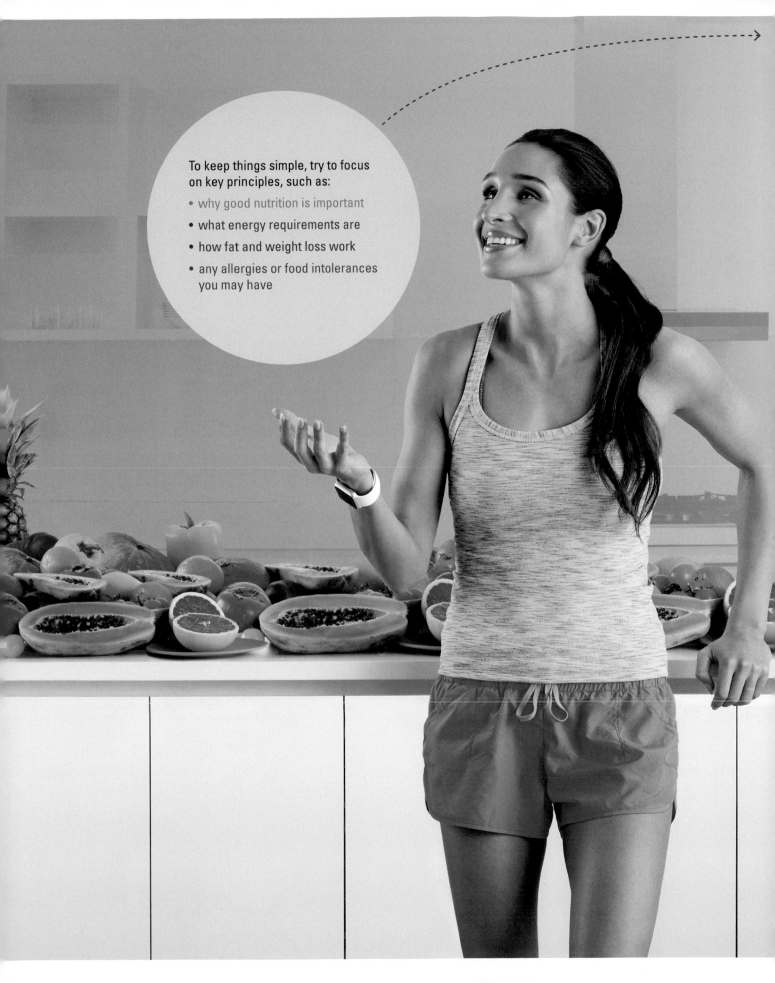

To keep things simple, try to focus on key principles, such as:

- why good nutrition is important
- what energy requirements are
- how fat and weight loss work
- any allergies or food intolerances you may have

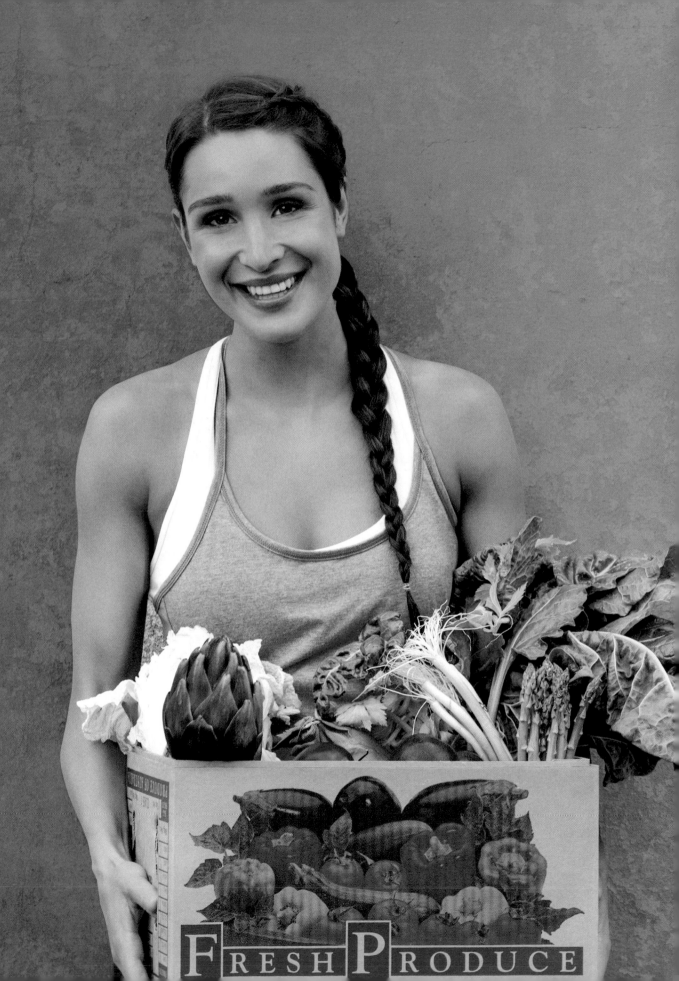

FRESHPRODUCE

PART 1 UNDERSTANDING THE 28-DAY MEAL PLAN

WHY EDUCATION IS IMPORTANT

I personally think that the most important thing to have when embarking on your healthy lifestyle journey is a sound education that is relevant to your goals.

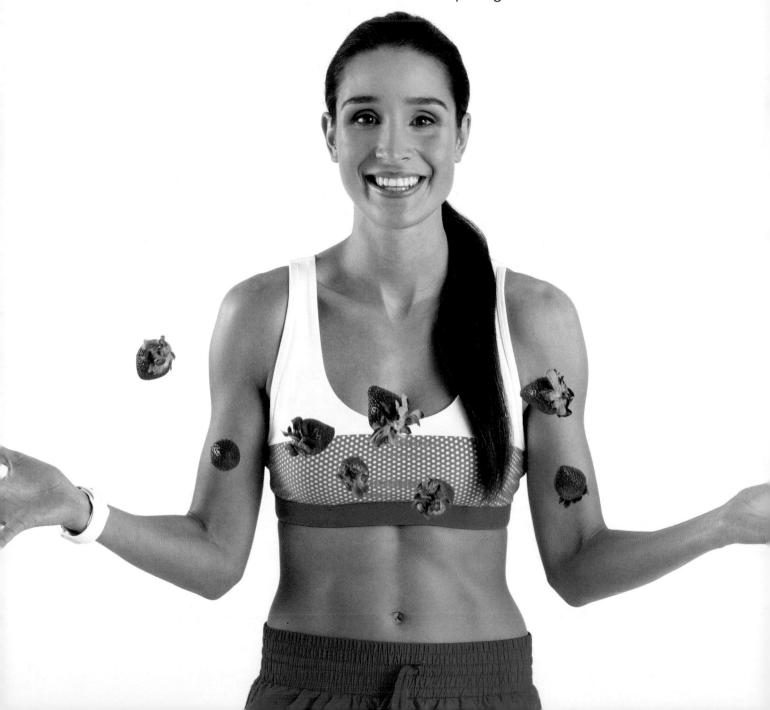

Consider this: if you are a first-year mechanical apprentice and you pop a tyre on a car, you'll have the knowledge to fix it. Unfortunately, this is not always the case with your body! For example, if you've never lifted weights above your head before, and you lean too far back when doing an overhead press, you could badly hurt your shoulder and it could take months to heal. Similarly, if you eat too many or not enough calories, or food that lacks nutritional variety, you could end up deficient in a particular nutrient and potentially experience hormonal, weight, or digestive problems. Without sounding too scary, the potential damage done to your body can be long term, and sometimes irreversible.

I understand that many of us learn best from our mistakes, but I think that with the amount of information available to us today and how easy it is to access, people can educate themselves before beginning any new journey to avoid basic mistakes.

In saying that, it is important to understand that there are many different views about what constitutes "good health," such as what you should and shouldn't eat, the type of training that you should do, and at what times of the day, and so on. In today's society, social media and clever marketing have led to a saturation of health advice: it is everywhere! And I believe this has severely damaged the general quality of the advice. So rather than taking as gospel what's written by a journalist in a magazine or on a website, it is important that you do your research. And I'm not talking about a simple Google search—I mean reading books and articles by reputable authors, chatting to individuals experienced in the area, and much more. Together, this research can help you make an educated decision when it comes to determining what is factually correct and what is not, and ultimately what goes into your body.

In addition to understanding the facts, it is important to recognise which of these facts are *relevant* to you. We are all individual—there are no two people alike. Factors such as your lifestyle, genetic makeup, and goals will have a significant impact on what works best for you. While it is great to have role models and people who inspire you, when it comes to making decisions about health and fitness, it is important that you recognise whether or not your lifestyle and goals are aligned with theirs and their knowledge base.

FOLLOWING THE SAME DIET AND TRAINING PLAN AS YOUR FAVOURITE OLYMPIC SPORTSPERSON MAY NOT BE SUITABLE FOR YOU, ESPECIALLY IF YOU'RE JUST LOOKING TO GET A LITTLE FITTER AND BE MORE CONFIDENT IN YOUR BODY.

Knowledge is such a powerful tool, and it can lead to growth in all aspects of our lives. Be aware of what you read and absorb, and look at it objectively. Understand your own body and your lifestyle and use what you read to complement this. It is all about using the tools you have to inform yourself and make the right decisions based on your personal choices.

So, if there's a healthy food you really can't stand or an exercise that doesn't work for you, making an *educated* decision to choose an alternative can create more flexibility and make sticking to your goal easier. For example, I love mango, but Tobi hates it! Even if mango was going to make Tobi a little healthier, I would recommend he find an alternative that he enjoys, such as an apple, as the result will likely be the same. Having an understanding of basic nutrition principles means you can make simple decisions like these on your own, which in turn leads to a happier, healthier, and more flexible lifestyle.

WHILE IT IS GREAT TO INCORPORATE ADVICE INTO YOUR LIFESTYLE TO IMPROVE YOUR HEALTH, IF IT MAKES YOU MISERABLE, THEN YOU SHOULD FIND AN ALTERNATIVE.

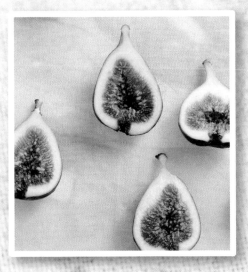

THE IMPORTANCE OF GOOD NUTRITION

What is good nutrition?

Good nutrition can simply be understood as balanced nutrition. This means you are getting a balanced range of vitamins and minerals, and that you're consuming enough energy from food to accommodate your lifestyle. This balance comes from consuming a wide variety of healthy foods from all six food groups (see page 57 for detailed information on food groups).

The method I use advocates a healthy, balanced diet by consuming these food groups in the amounts recommended by the *Australian Guide to Healthy Eating* (AGHE; eatforhealth.gov.au).* My weekly meal plans and variations are based around this approach, allowing you to eat a delicious range of foods knowing that you are comfortably meeting your energy and nutrient requirements.

What is malnourishment?

Malnourishment is a set of health problems that can be caused by a diet that contains too much or not enough of a particular nutrient or nutrients. *It is important to understand that there are many different types and possible causes of malnourishment and it is not just experienced by people living in developing countries.* For example, someone might have a medical issue where their digestive system is unable to absorb nutrients properly (such as celiac disease, see page 54). People living in remote areas may not have access to fresh foods that others do by living in the city. Or people might simply choose to rely on highly processed, packaged foods rather than eating whole foods.

While it may not be possible to change your genetics or where you live, you usually do have a choice when it comes to the foods you eat. Yes, processed and packaged foods might provide you with energy, but over time, it is unlikely that they will be able to provide you with all the nutrients you need and in the right amounts. As I mentioned earlier, all of the food groups provide us with their own unique set of nutrients and it is important that we eat foods from all food groups (and in the right amounts) to avoid deficiency and malnourishment.

EVERY TIME YOU EAT, IT IS AN OPPORTUNITY TO NOURISH YOUR BODY.

Fill your body with healthy food that is going to make you feel good on the inside and outside.

* *Different countries may have their own healthy eating guidelines that are similar, so the information provided here should be used as a guide only.*

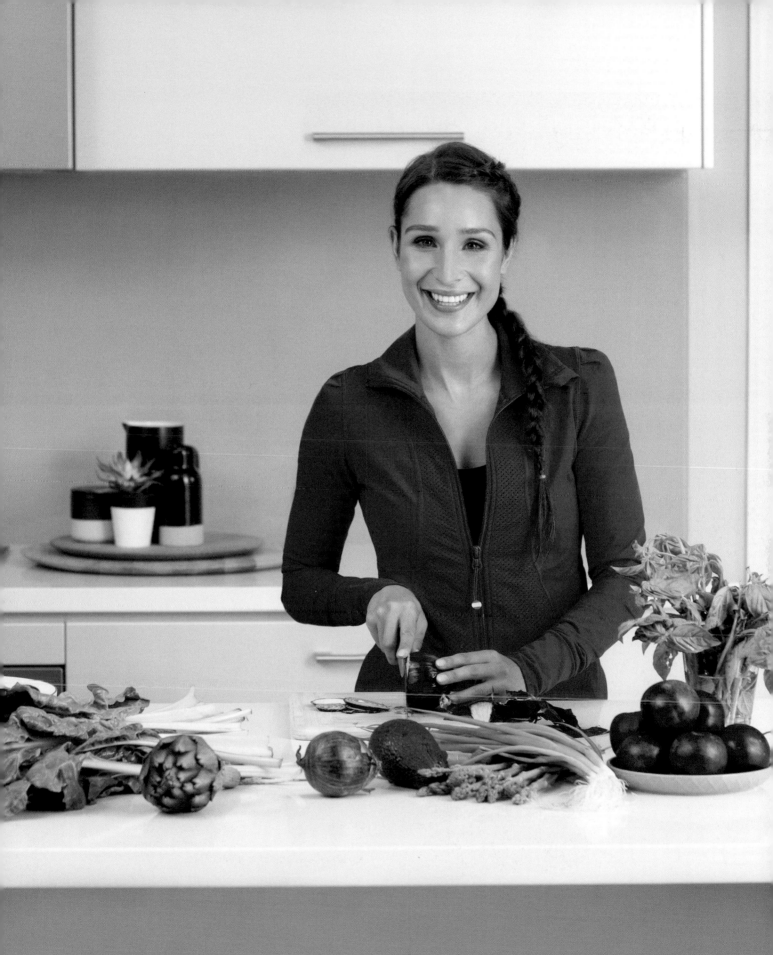

ENERGY REQUIREMENTS & FAT-LOSS FACTS

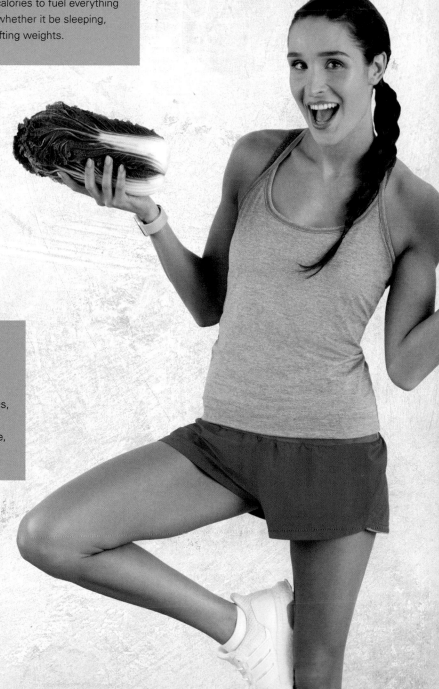

Why do we need energy?

In the same way that a car needs petrol, our bodies need energy in the form of calories to fuel everything that we do, whether it be sleeping, walking, or lifting weights.

Where do we get energy?

As well as providing our body with a number of nutrients, food also provides us with energy. The amount of energy found in food can be measured in either calories or kilojoules.

FACT: 1 CALORIE = 4.2 KILOJOULES

How much energy do we need?

The number of calories we need each day depends on several things, such as our age, height, weight, gender, how physically active we are, and our health and fitness goals.

SEE PAGE 28 FOR MORE INFORMATION ON WHERE OUR ENERGY COMES FROM.

How does energy intake influence our weight?

The effects of energy intake on body weight can be understood using the simple **"calories in–calories out"** concept. "Calories in" refers to all the energy that we *receive* from food each day, whereas "calories out" is the energy that is *used* by the body to fuel basic functions such as breathing and blinking, as well as physical activity.

Now, imagine that both "calories in" and "calories out" are sitting on a seesaw, as shown here.

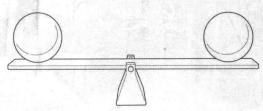

When we eat the same number of calories that we burn **(calories in = calories out)**, the seesaw will remain balanced. This is called **neutral energy balance** and generally means our weight will remain the same.

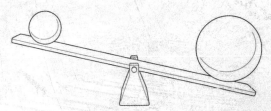

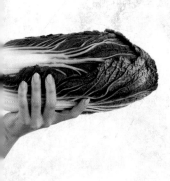

When we eat a lot more calories than we burn **(calories in > calories out)**, then the seesaw becomes unbalanced. This creates **positive energy balance**, and as a result the excess energy received from food can be stored within the body for use later and may result in weight or fat gain.

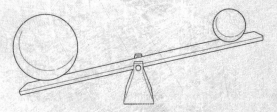

Eating fewer calories than we burn **(calories in < calories out)** will also cause the seesaw to become unbalanced, but in the other direction. This is called **negative energy balance** and can potentially result in weight or fat loss.

This highlights the importance of regulating both "calories in" and "calories out" to help achieve the energy balance (neutral, positive, or negative) best suited to your health and fitness goals. For example, if your goal is to maintain your weight (meaning that your weight is neither increasing or decreasing significantly), then you may get best results by consuming around the same number of calories that you burn. Alternatively, if your goal is to lose weight or fat, then you may need to burn more calories than you consume.

How do I achieve the right energy balance for fat or weight loss?

Generally speaking, women aged between 16 and 25 who do a moderate amount of exercise and weigh 121 pounds or more need to eat approximately 2100 calories per day in order to maintain their weight. This is called the **maintenance requirement**.

Eating fewer calories than we use creates a **calorie deficit**, meaning the body has to burn existing energy stores (usually fat) to meet its energy needs. Of course, weight/fat loss is quite a complex process and can be influenced by many other variables, but in general if you consume around 500 calories *less* than your maintenance requirement, and do a moderate amount of exercise, you can expect a 1 pound weight (or fat) loss per week. This is because 1 pound of human fat is equivalent to approximately 3500 calories. So, seven days of a 500-calorie deficit will result in a weekly deficit of 3500 calories. For this reason, the meal plans that I have provided for healthy weight loss are based on a daily calorie intake of approximately 1600–1800 calories.

One of the best ways to work out your recommended energy intake is to determine your basal metabolic rate or BMR. Without getting too technical, BMR is defined as the minimum amount of energy that your body needs in order to keep functioning if you are inactive, for example lying in bed all day. The reason this is important is that it allows us to calculate what increase or decrease in calories is appropriate to create a deliberate change in body weight.

After a lot of study, scientists created a formula that can approximate your BMR using personal information such as gender, weight, height, and physical activity level. A very common example used by most nutritionists and dietitians is the Harris–Benedict equation, which is the method I have used to determine the energy intake of my meal plans.

In simple terms, if you consume 1600 calories a day but burn 2100, your body needs to source energy in order to bridge this 500-calorie gap. This will generally come from energy stores that already exist in your body, such as fat.

As I mentioned earlier, our bodies require energy to fuel *all* of our body's functions. So even if your goal is to lose weight or fat, it is important to provide your body with enough food for it to function at its best and to meet all of your nutrient requirements.

FAQ

Q IF I EAT LESS AND TRAIN MORE, WILL I LOSE WEIGHT?

A It is a common misconception that if you eat less and train more you will be able to lose weight or fat faster. However, if you do not provide your body with the energy and nutrients it needs, then it may begin to direct these things to some processes at the expense of others. This can result in fatigue, an impaired immune system, and reduced hormone activity, which may actually make it harder for your body to lose weight or fat. Being fit and healthy long term requires a permanent lifestyle change, which includes a healthy balance of good nutrition and training.

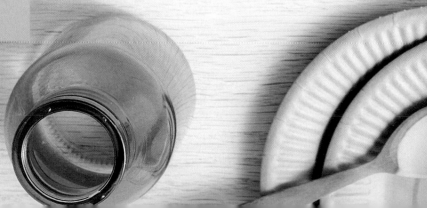

What is the difference between weight loss and fat loss?

It is important to understand that your weight is dynamic, not static. This means that you can jump on the scales first thing in the morning, in the middle of the day, and again at night and see three slightly different weight values. These small fluctuations can be caused by how much water you have had to drink, the foods you have eaten, and going to the bathroom—they are *not* a reflection of your eating and exercise habits that day.

When my clients are embarking on a new health and fitness journey, I always tell them not to get caught up with the number on the scales. This is because scales cannot distinguish between different masses in your body, such as water, muscle, and fat. For example, if the scales are showing that you have lost a pound, it is possible that this is from a combination of body masses. And as we know, our weight can also fluctuate slightly throughout the day.

Fat loss, on the other hand, generally leads to better muscle definition and tone. You've probably heard the phrase "muscle weighs more than fat," but it is important to understand that while muscle may be heavier than fat, it also takes up less space within the body. This explains why many girls begin to see noticeable changes in the mirror, but their weight on the scales is the same or even a little bit higher as a result of their training.

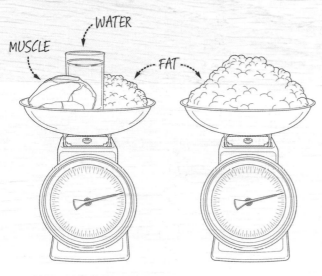

WATER

MUSCLE

FAT

THE WAY YOU FEEL WILL ALWAYS BE MORE IMPORTANT THAN THE NUMBER ON THE SCALES.

FAQ

Q I HAVE LOW ENERGY THROUGHOUT THE DAY. WHAT SHOULD I DO?

A If you maintain a healthy lifestyle, which includes eating foods from all of the food groups, exercising regularly, distributing your macronutrients throughout the day, including complex carbohydrates, drinking lots of water, and getting enough sleep, then your energy levels should be excellent. Depending on your health goals and lifestyle, some people may find that the recommendations within the meal plan may not be enough to meet their needs. If this is the case, I recommend increasing your food intake in small increments until you feel these needs are met. This can be as simple as adding extra servings of vegetables and/or protein to your meals. Do bear in mind that low energy levels can be caused by a number of factors. So if you are following all of these guidelines and are still feeling tired, then I recommend that you consult a health professional to investigate further.

The key is to listen to your body and adjust your diet accordingly.

MACRONUTRIENTS

What are macronutrients?

The term *macro* means large, and macronutrients are nutrients our bodies need in large amounts.

Carbohydrates, protein, and fats are the three macronutrients we cannot live without. We need to consume these every day in large amounts in order to stay alive and healthy.

If weight or fat loss is your health goal, you need to recognise that many of the diets we see advertised (for example, very low-carb or very low-fat diets) may not be the healthiest option for you. Each of these macronutrients plays an important role in the overall functioning of our body, therefore restricting one or more of these can have a number of negative effects, including fatigue and illness. This is particularly common for girls who follow extreme or "fad" diets. Although these diets may cause you to lose weight to begin with, this is not always sustainable (or enjoyable!) in the long term. In my experience, girls who follow these types of diets often end up giving up and eventually regain a lot (if not all) of the weight that they previously lost.

Why are they important?

Carbohydrates, protein, and fats provide our bodies with the building blocks we need for growth, metabolism, and body function. They also provide us with energy. However, it is important to note that each provides us with slightly different amounts of energy.

1 gram of carbohydrate provides 4 calories (17 kJ)
1 gram of protein provides 4 calories (17 kJ)
1 gram of fat provides 9 calories (38 kJ)

Each macronutrient has different effects on satiety (the feeling of "fullness" we get after a meal that causes us to stop eating). Simply speaking, protein has the strongest effect on satiety, followed by carbohydrates and fats respectively. In other words, protein makes you feel more full.

Both of these things are important to bear in mind if you want to lose weight or fat. For example, at 9 calories per gram, along with their lower effects on satiety, fats (such as peanut butter) can be easy to eat in excessive amounts. This may result in us eating more calories than we need without even realising it, and can potentially result in weight gain. We still need fats in our diet, but it is important to distinguish between "good" and "bad" fats, and to determine what an appropriate intake is. See page 31 for more on this.

It is essential for us to understand how each of these three macronutrients is used by the body and how eating too much of any one of them can cause health problems.

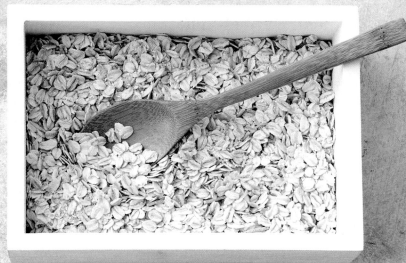

CARBOHYDRATES

What are carbohydrates?

Carbohydrates are vital because they provide us with the most essential nutrient for our survival—glucose. Glucose is the preferred source of energy for our brain and muscles. Therefore, very low intakes of carbohydrates may mean that we are not able to think properly or our muscles may not work at full strength. In my opinion, most "low carb" diets are not designed to help us lose weight healthily and, most importantly, to maintain this weight loss long term.

The best sources of carbohydrates are grain-based foods such as bread, oats, muesli, rice, and quinoa, particularly whole wheat or wholegrain versions. This is because they are broken down slowly by the body and provide us with long-lasting energy. Other sources of carbohydrates include fruits, vegetables, legumes, and low-fat dairy foods. Foods rich in carbohydrates also contain generous quantities of other essential vitamins and minerals.

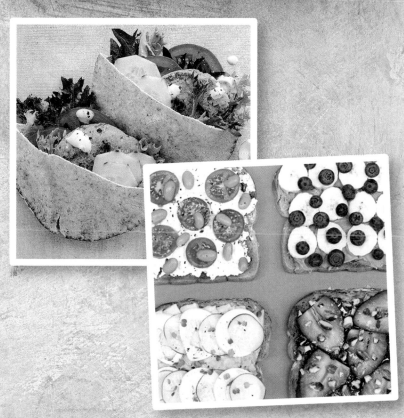

FUN FACT

Fuelling your body before your workout is SO important! I love eating tuna with a whole wheat roll or natural peanut butter on a slice of rye toast.

PROTEIN

What is protein?

Protein is important for the growth, maintenance, and repair of the body's cells. It also provides the building blocks for a number of structures within the human body, such as muscles, hormones, enzymes (which facilitate chemical reactions in the body), and antibodies (cells that help fight infection).

More specifically, proteins are made up of chains of smaller units called amino acids. There are 22 amino acids that make up most proteins. While our bodies are able to produce most of these, there are nine amino acids that can only be obtained from our diet. These are known as "essential" amino acids. Essential nutrients are ones that the body cannot make on its own and need to be obtained from the diet. Animal foods such as red meat, poultry, fish, milk, and eggs naturally contain all nine essential amino acids and are considered complete proteins. While plant foods such as beans, peas, and lentils also contain protein, they are considered incomplete proteins because individually they lack one or more essential amino acids.

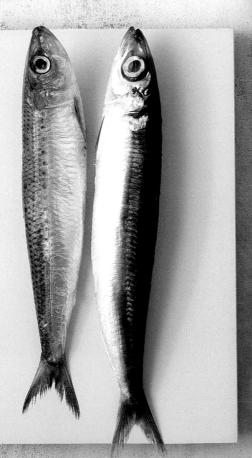

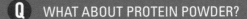

FAQ

Q WHAT ABOUT PROTEIN POWDER?

A You will see that I have included a small amount of protein powder in the meal plans. If you choose to incorporate protein powder into your diet, it should not be used to completely replace protein foods, but as an optional addition to some of your meals and snacks. Remember, supplements like protein powder are designed to boost an already healthy lifestyle.

As well as providing our bodies with amino acids, protein also helps us to feel full after meals. As mentioned previously, protein generally leaves us more satisfied than both carbohydrates and fats, which means that including protein foods in each of your main meals may help reduce hunger and unhealthy snacking. When choosing sources of protein to include in your meals, I recommend ones that are low in saturated and trans fats. While these can naturally occur in some foods, keeping your intake as low as possible is important in maintaining a healthy lifestyle.

FUN FACT

It's no surprise that eggs are one of my favourite sources of protein! I love them poached and served on rye toast with avocado, tomato, and balsamic glaze in the mornings.

FATS

What are fats?

Fats play a number of important roles in our body. They help cushion our organs, contribute to the structure of cells, promote growth and development, and allow us to absorb essential vitamins—namely vitamins A, D, E, and K.

In recent decades, fats have acquired a bad reputation, but they have an essential role to play in our diets. Not all fats are created equal though, so it is important that we consume the right types and in the right proportions.

What are "good" and "bad" fats?

"Good" fats are those derived from vegetables, nuts, seeds, and fish. These fats, called monounsaturated and polyunsaturated fats, are important for reducing LDL (bad) cholesterol, lowering the risk of heart disease and stroke, and promoting a healthy brain and joints. It is therefore recommended that we prioritise these for our daily fat servings. Trans fats and saturated fats are considered the "bad" fats, and it is recommended that we limit the intake of these in our diet. Trans fats are of particular concern because they elevate LDL (bad) cholesterol and reduce HDL (good) cholesterol levels, which together can increase our risk of heart attack or stroke. Trans fats do not naturally occur in many foods, but can be produced during processing. By eating a diet full of whole foods rather than highly processed foods, it is quite simple to avoid trans fats altogether. Saturated fats, on the other hand, are most commonly found in meat and dairy foods. These fats are also believed to increase our risk of heart disease by increasing our levels of LDL (bad) cholesterol, so it is recommended that we limit our intake by choosing lean cuts of meat and reduced-fat dairy products.

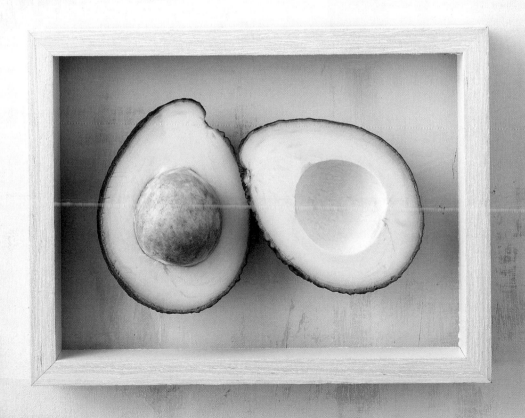

FIBRE

What is fibre?

Fibre is the part of plant food that is not able to be digested or absorbed within the small intestine, which is where a lot of our digestive processes occur. Instead, fibre is broken down in the large intestine. While it doesn't provide our body with a lot of energy in the same way as carbohydrates, fats, and proteins do, it does offer our bodies a number of other health benefits.

Why is fibre good for you?

There is a lot of research to suggest that a diet rich in fibre can help protect us against a number of lifestyle diseases (diseases associated with poor diet, a lack of physical activity, stress, and drug and alcohol use). Some examples of lifestyle diseases include cancer, heart disease, obesity, and type 2 diabetes.

While our food offers a lot of beneficial nutrients, it can also contain harmful substances. As fibre has a "cleansing" effect and helps food move through our digestive system, it helps prevent our gut wall from being exposed to these substances which can reduce our risk of digestive diseases, such as colon cancer. Fibre can also help us eliminate excess cholesterol via the digestive system, which can help reduce our risk of heart disease. As fibre has quite a complex structure, good bacteria (yes, bacteria can be good!) in our digestive system are needed to help break it down. By consuming fibre regularly, we can help to promote the growth of these good bacteria, which play an important role in maintaining digestive and overall health. It also helps regulate the release of insulin after we have eaten. This helps us feel full between meals, prevents overeating and unhealthy snacking, and helps us maintain a healthy weight.

How much fibre should you be eating?

The National Health and Medical Research Council (NHMRC) of Australia recommends that women eat a minimum of 25 grams of fibre every day. This can quite easily be achieved by eating a diet that is rich in fruits, vegetables, and cereal grains (particularly wholegrain versions), which is reflected in my meal plans. However, if you eat a high-fibre diet, it's also important that you drink lots of water too, as this will help the fibre work its magic within your digestive system!

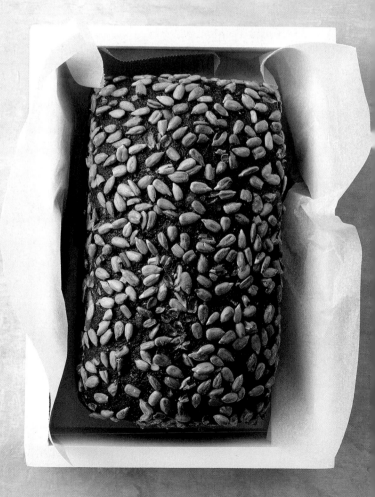

FUN FACT

Did you know that avocado is a source of fibre? I love spreading it on rice cakes with black pepper or having it smashed on rye toast—delish!

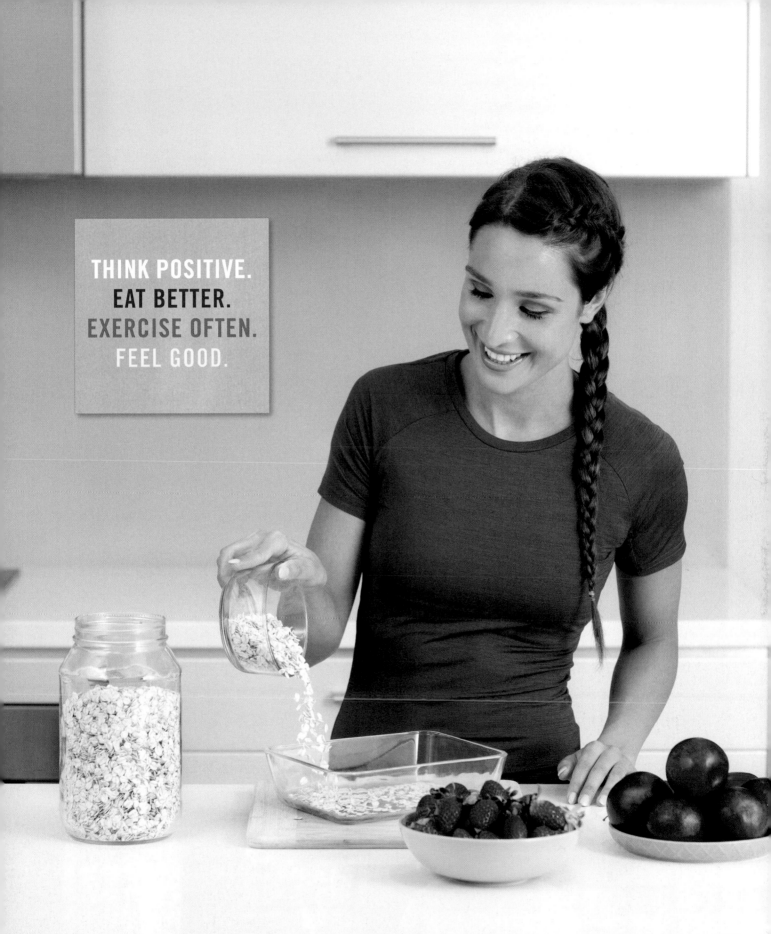

THINK POSITIVE.
EAT BETTER.
EXERCISE OFTEN.
FEEL GOOD.

MICRONUTRIENTS

What are micronutrients?

The term *micro* means small. When compared with macronutrients, micronutrients are only required in small amounts and are much smaller in size. But just because they're small doesn't mean they're not important!

There are two different types of micronutrients—vitamins and minerals—that our bodies need to function properly and to keep us healthy long term. It is very important that we obtain enough vitamins and minerals from the foods we eat.

As well as the different roles they play in our bodies, one of the main differences between vitamins and minerals is their origin. Simply speaking, vitamins are substances that are *produced* by plants or animals. Minerals, on the other hand, are substances found within the soil that are then *absorbed* by plants or eaten by animals.

Taking a multivitamin supplement does not make up for an unhealthy diet. As each food group provides certain macronutrients (carbohydrates, proteins, and fats) and micronutrients (vitamins and minerals), it is important that we eat foods from ALL foods groups in balanced amounts. If you exclude a food from a particular food group altogether, your diet may become imbalanced and unhealthy in the long term.

Make an effort today to create better habits;

think positive, eat a healthy, clean diet;

AND MOST IMPORTANTLY, **LOVE YOURSELF.**

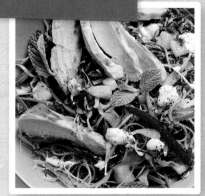

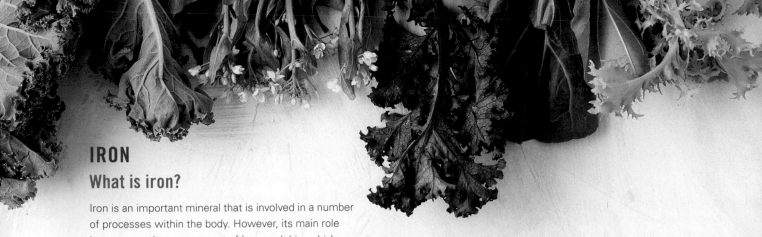

IRON

What is iron?

Iron is an important mineral that is involved in a number of processes within the body. However, its main role is to act as a key component of haemoglobin, which is a protein found in red blood cells. Not only does haemoglobin give red blood cells their colour, but it also carries oxygen to the rest of our body. The remainder of the body's iron can be found in iron-storage proteins, such as ferritin.

Unfortunately, iron deficiency is one of the most common deficiencies in young women. A lot of our body's iron is stored within the blood (via haemoglobin), and we do lose a small amount once a month with our period. So it is important that we provide our bodies with iron-rich food every day to ensure that we maintain healthy iron levels and avoid deficiency.

> AS IRON IS IMPORTANT FOR ENERGY AND DELIVERY OF OXYGEN, IT IS PARTICULARLY IMPORTANT FOR GIRLS WHO ARE ACTIVE AND GET HEAVY PERIODS TO HAVE A STEADY INTAKE OF IRON FROM FOOD SOURCES.

What happens when we don't get enough iron?

If you don't receive enough iron over long periods of time, it can result in the gradual depletion of the body's ferritin stores. Once these stores have run out, your body's ability to produce haemoglobin can begin to decrease. Low levels of haemoglobin are usually a sign of late-stage iron deficiency, which is also known as anaemia. The first signs of anaemia may include headaches, tiredness, lack of energy, poor concentration, and frequent infections.

As well as resulting from insufficent iron from food, anaemia can also be caused by loss of blood (for example, if you have heavy periods), which is why your health professional may look for both dietary and non-dietary causes of anaemia.

What foods do we get it from?

There are two types of iron found in foods, called haem iron and non-haem iron.

1. Haem iron can be found in animal foods, such as red meat and poultry. Of these, red meats contain the most haem iron, but they also tend to be higher in saturated fats, so it is important to select leaner cuts where possible. Meats such as liver or kidney are also rich in iron, but are not necessarily the most popular choices. If you don't mind the taste, you can spread pâté on crackers for a light lunch or snack.

2. Non-haem iron can be found in eggs and plant foods, such as breads and cereals, green leafy vegetables, legumes, nuts, and nut pastes.

Of these, haem iron is absorbed more readily, which is why we need to eat far more non-haem iron in order to reach the same recommended requirements. The amount of iron you absorb from your food will depend on your body's needs. For example, if you are lacking in iron, your body will generally absorb more.

When trying to incorporate foods that are rich in iron into your diet, it is important to be aware of the way other foods affect your body's ability to absorb it. For example, eating foods high in vitamin C in the same meal can increase absorption of non-haem iron. Some examples of vitamin C–rich foods include citrus fruits, berries, capsicums, and green vegetables such as broccoli and kale.

On the other hand, dairy foods and tannins naturally found in black tea may interfere with the absorption of iron. If you drink black tea regularly, I recommend that you avoid drinking it at meal times and, where possible, make weaker tea or replace with herbal teas. Once again, following the recommended number of servings from each food group can help ensure that you are receiving enough iron from your diet.

CALCIUM

Why is calcium important?
What foods do we get it from?

Calcium is an important mineral for the development of healthy bones and teeth. It also plays a role in blood clotting and allows our muscles and nerves to function. The best sources of calcium are dairy products such as milk, cheese, and yoghurt. Small amounts of calcium can also be found in plant foods such as broccoli, chickpeas, dried fruit, and nuts, such as almonds and brazil nuts. If you can't consume dairy products because of an allergy or intolerance, see page 51 for more information on how to select the best non-dairy alternatives.

MAGNESIUM

Why is magnesium important?
What foods do we get it from?

Magnesium is another essential mineral for healthy bones, muscles, and nerves. While calcium is needed to help muscles contract, magnesium helps them relax. This is why magnesium supplements are sometimes used to help reduce headaches that are caused by muscle tension. Magnesium can also help alleviate period symptoms, such as cramps. The best sources of magnesium include green leafy vegetables, legumes, cereals, and nuts. These foods are also high in fibre, so it's a win–win!

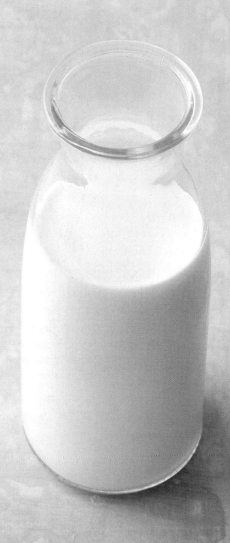

FUN FACT

Have bananas or figs for a serious (and tasty!) magnesium boost. My papou (grandpa) grows the best figs (we call them sika).

VITAMINS

While there are a number of individual vitamins, these can be grouped together based on the role they play in our bodies. For example:

A group vitamins can help maintain eyesight and strengthen our immune system. Some of the best food sources of A group vitamins include eggs and dairy foods, as well as yellow, orange, and green vegetables such as pumpkin, carrot, kale, and spinach. (Funnily enough, if you cut a carrot crossways, it actually looks like an eye! Coincidence? Maybe not!)

B group vitamins can help our body convert food into energy, which is why they tend to form a large part of most multivitamin supplements. They also help support our nervous and digestive systems, and the production of red blood cells. These vitamins are typically found in meat, fish, poultry, eggs, and dairy products, as well as legumes, leafy green vegetables, and some fruits.

Vitamin C is a very powerful antioxidant and can help to strengthen our immune system. However, it is also involved in a number of important processes, such as increasing iron absorption and the production of collagen, which keeps our skin feeling firm and youthful. Some examples of vitamin C–rich foods include citrus fruits, berries, capsicum, and green vegetables such as broccoli and kale.

Vitamin D can help our body absorb calcium and phosphorus, two minerals that are crucial in maintaining bone health. Vitamin D can also help strengthen our immune system and improve our mood. While you can get small amounts by eating oily fish and eggs, exposure to sunlight is the best natural source of vitamin D, which is why it is sometimes called the "sunshine vitamin."

Vitamin E is also a powerful antioxidant that helps reduce free-radical damage and inflammation within the body. It can also help promote healthy hair and skin. Some of the best food sources of vitamin E are nuts, seeds, and oils.

Vitamin K plays an important role in blood clotting and maintaining bone health. While the body can produce small amounts of vitamin K, it is important that we get enough of this vitamin from food. Some examples include leafy green vegetables and fermented foods (such as sauerkraut).

As you can see, eating foods from all food groups in balanced amounts is important to enable our bodies to function at their best.

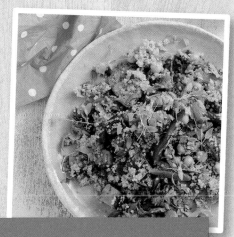

Typically, brightly coloured foods can have higher amounts of certain vitamins. To make sure you get a good range and balance of vitamins, a concept I like to use is called "eat a rainbow." See the next page!

EAT A RAINBOW

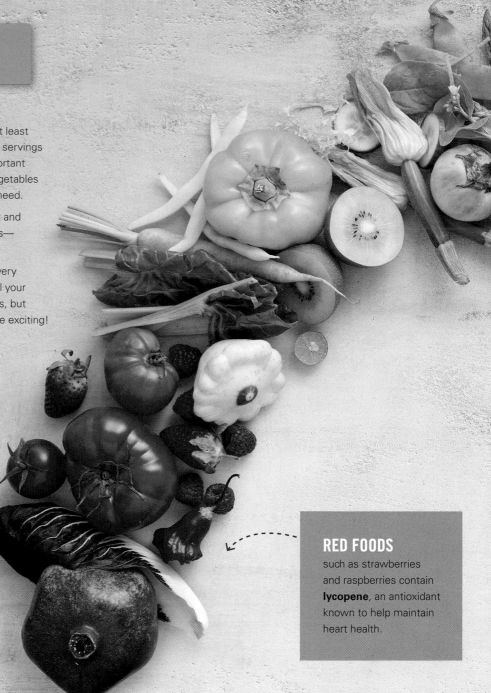

It is recommended that adults eat at least five servings of vegetables and two servings of fruit every day. However, it's important that you eat a variety of fruit and vegetables to get the balance of nutrients you need.

An easy way to do this is to eat fruit and vegetables of many different colours—"eat a rainbow!"

Aim to eat at least one food from every colour group every day. Not only will your body be getting a variety of nutrients, but your plate will look that little bit more exciting!

FUN FACT

Did you know that these colours indicate which phytochemicals, or "super powers," these foods contain?

RED FOODS

such as strawberries and raspberries contain **lycopene**, an antioxidant known to help maintain heart health.

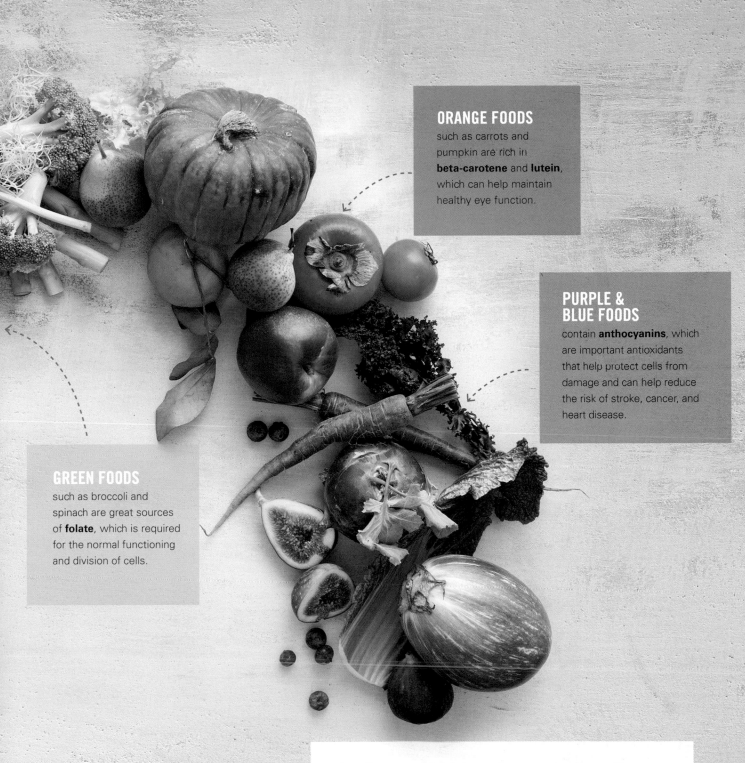

ORANGE FOODS
such as carrots and
pumpkin are rich in
beta-carotene and lutein,
which can help maintain
healthy eye function.

**PURPLE &
BLUE FOODS**
contain **anthocyanins**, which
are important antioxidants
that help protect cells from
damage and can help reduce
the risk of stroke, cancer, and
heart disease.

GREEN FOODS
such as broccoli and
spinach are great sources
of **folate**, which is required
for the normal functioning
and division of cells.

Another good trick to make sure you're getting
all your vitamins and minerals is to consume
superfoods, which often contain higher amounts
than other foods. Similar amount of food, only more
nutrients! See the following pages for examples.

SUPERFOOD BERRIES

Berries, such as blueberries, strawberries, raspberries, and goji and acai berries, are considered superfoods because of their naturally high antioxidant content. While these berries do have some differences in terms of the amounts and types of nutrients they provide, they do have a few things in common—for example, their vibrant colour can be attributed to high levels of anthocyanins, a group of antioxidants that protect our cells and DNA from damage. Berries are also high in vitamin C, which can help strengthen the immune system and give our skin a youthful glow. They also contain fibre, which is important to maintain a healthy digestive system and to keep you feeling full between meals.

Generally, blueberries, strawberries, and raspberries can be found in your local market, supermarket, or fruit and veg store. Unless you live in areas where these berries are grown, goji berries and acai berries are generally not available fresh—instead, they are often dried or pureed, or freeze-dried and ground into a powder.

RASPBERRIES

Raspberries have quite a sour taste with small amounts of underlying sweetness.

ACAI BERRIES

Acai berries have more of a "red wine" flavour with chocolatey undertones. They also contain essential fatty acids, which are important for a healthy heart and nervous system.

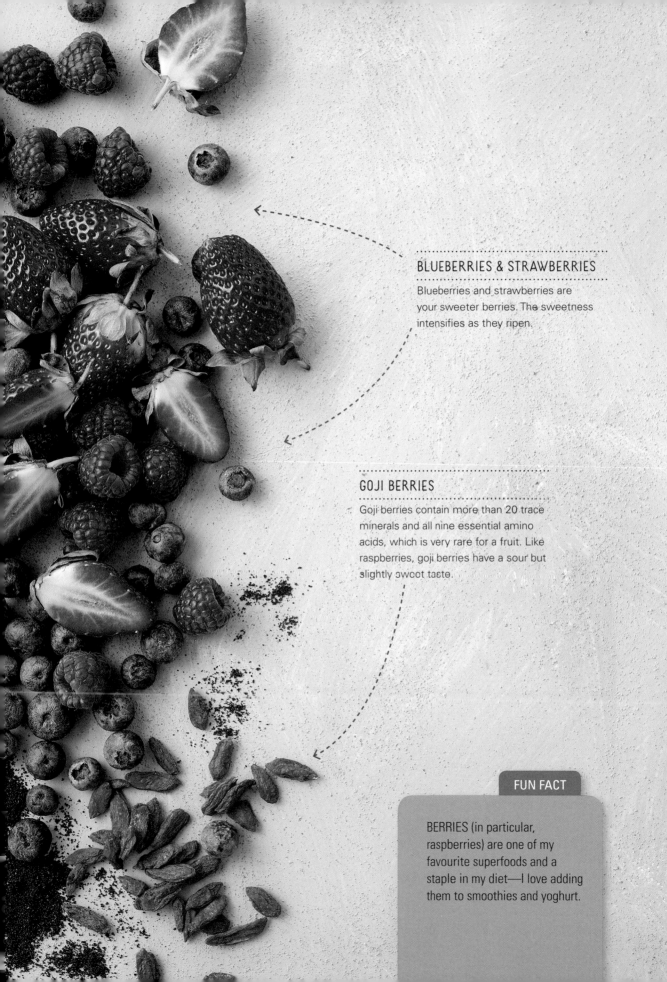

BLUEBERRIES & STRAWBERRIES

Blueberries and strawberries are your sweeter berries. The sweetness intensifies as they ripen.

GOJI BERRIES

Goji berries contain more than 20 trace minerals and all nine essential amino acids, which is very rare for a fruit. Like raspberries, goji berries have a sour but slightly sweet taste.

FUN FACT

BERRIES (in particular, raspberries) are one of my favourite superfoods and a staple in my diet—I love adding them to smoothies and yoghurt.

SUPERFOOD GREENS

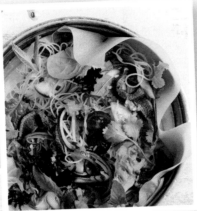

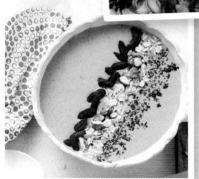

SPINACH

Popeye definitely knew what he was doing! Overall, spinach provides our bodies with similar nutrients to kale, but it does contain more **folate**, a B vitamin that can help our cells function and divide properly. Spinach, particularly baby spinach, can be quite mild in flavour and may be added to juices and smoothies without significantly changing the taste.

BARLEY GRASS

Like wheatgrass, this is the leafy part of the barley plant that is cut before the grain is formed. Although its vitamin and mineral content is quite similar to wheatgrass, it is known for its ability to help clear the body of toxins. It also contains **chlorophyll**, which is the green substance in plants and is believed to work as an "internal deodorant" within the body. Both wheatgrass and barley grass are available in powder form, making them an easy addition to your favourite green juice recipe.

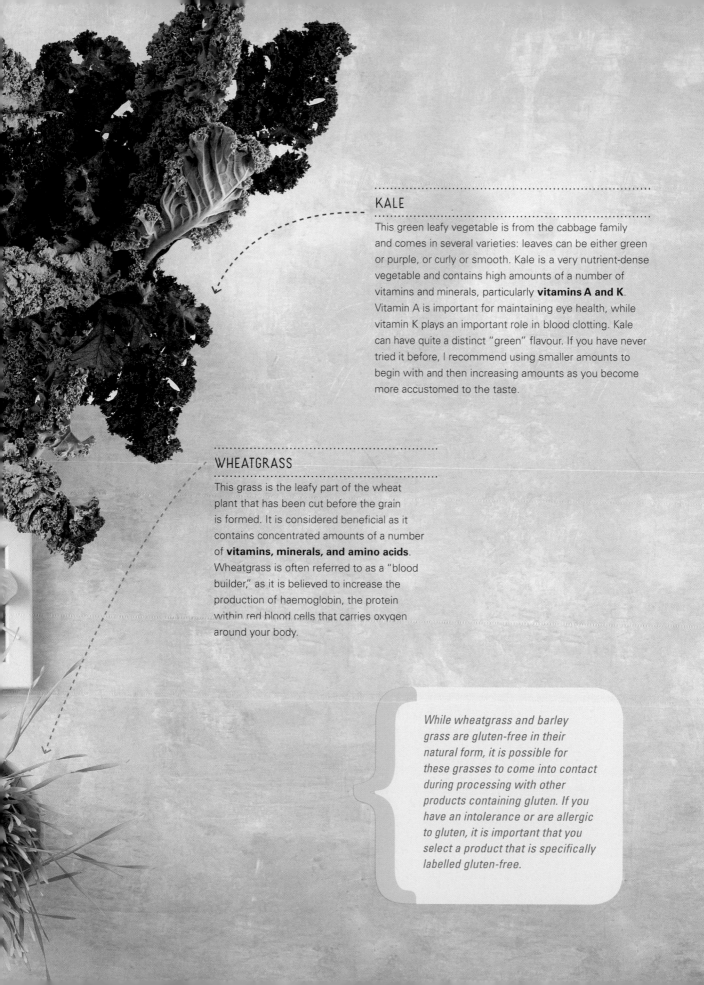

KALE

This green leafy vegetable is from the cabbage family and comes in several varieties: leaves can be either green or purple, or curly or smooth. Kale is a very nutrient-dense vegetable and contains high amounts of a number of vitamins and minerals, particularly **vitamins A and K**. Vitamin A is important for maintaining eye health, while vitamin K plays an important role in blood clotting. Kale can have quite a distinct "green" flavour. If you have never tried it before, I recommend using smaller amounts to begin with and then increasing amounts as you become more accustomed to the taste.

WHEATGRASS

This grass is the leafy part of the wheat plant that has been cut before the grain is formed. It is considered beneficial as it contains concentrated amounts of a number of **vitamins, minerals, and amino acids**. Wheatgrass is often referred to as a "blood builder," as it is believed to increase the production of haemoglobin, the protein within red blood cells that carries oxygen around your body.

While wheatgrass and barley grass are gluten-free in their natural form, it is possible for these grasses to come into contact during processing with other products containing gluten. If you have an intolerance or are allergic to gluten, it is important that you select a product that is specifically labelled gluten-free.

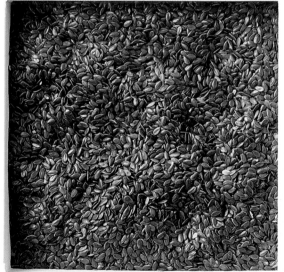

SUPERFOOD NUTS & SEEDS

CHIA SEEDS

Not only do chia seeds provide an irresistible texture to your juices and smoothies, but they also contain lots of **fibre**, which is really important for digestive health and increasing feelings of fullness after meals. They contain **all nine essential amino acids** plus **omega-3** (the good fat that is known to improve heart health). They are also jam-packed with a number of **vitamins and minerals**. Chia seeds can be either black or white, but this makes no difference to their nutritional value.

FLAXSEEDS

Also known as linseeds, flaxseeds contain **omega-3 fatty acids** and are high in **fibre**, which can help lower blood cholesterol, help you feel fuller for longer, and stabilise blood sugar levels. Flaxseeds can be either brown or golden, but as for chia seeds, this makes little difference to their nutritional value.

PUMPKIN SEEDS

Also known as pepitas, pumpkin seeds are a tasty way of obtaining protein, B vitamins, and minerals such as magnesium, iron, and zinc. These little beauties contain an amino acid called **tryptophan**, which can increase the production of hormones needed to help you sleep.

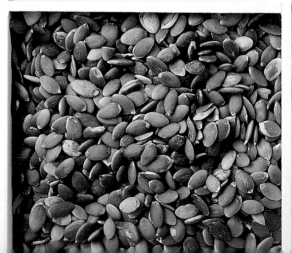

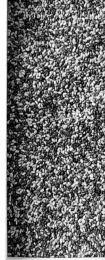

WHEATGERM

This grain food is the tiny, nutrient-dense centre of the wheat kernel. It may be small, but it is packed full of beneficial qualities! By adding wheatgerm to your diet, you can increase your intake of **B vitamins**, which are important in helping your body obtain energy from food. Wheatgerm is also high in **fibre**, which is good for keeping your appetite in check and maintaining a healthy digestive system.

FUN FACT

Making your own LSA at home is super-quick and easy! Just place 3½ ounces of raw almonds, 1¾ ounces of raw flaxseeds (linseeds), and 1¾ ounces of raw sunflower seeds in a food processor or blender and grind until the mixture looks like breadcrumbs. Store in an airtight container in the fridge for up to 2 months.

LSA

This mix is made from a combination of ground linseeds (flaxseeds), sunflower seeds, and almonds, which means that you can obtain the benefits of all three ingredients in one go! LSA is particularly rich in **protein**, which can help keep sugar cravings at bay by stabilising blood sugar levels. It also contains a number of minerals, including **calcium**, which is important for bone and muscle health.

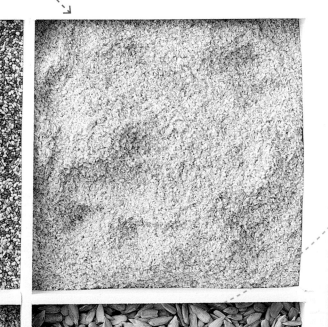

SUNFLOWER SEEDS

These contain **vitamin E**, which has anti-inflammatory properties and can help promote healthy skin and hair. These are also rich in **protein** and heart-healthy **fats**.

SUPERFOOD GRAINS

OATS

Grown all over the world, this popular grain is full of many vitamins and minerals that are necessary for a healthy functioning body. Oats contain six of the eight **B vitamins,** which help us convert food into fuel. They also naturally contain **beta-glucan**, a type of carbohydrate known to improve blood glucose control and cholesterol levels. These super grains can be quite filling due to their high fibre content. Oats are great as a breakfast cereal, porridge, overnight oats, or muesli, or added to smoothies and breakfast bowls.

FUN FACT

OATS, usually in muesli, are one of my staple breakfast dishes. Make sure to choose naturally processed oats.

QUINOA FLAKES

This highly nutritious ancient grain is native to South America. Quinoa flakes are made from pressed quinoa, and the benefits are the same as wholegrain versions. Quinoa is completely gluten-free and one of the few plant foods that contains **all nine essential amino acids**. The flakes can be used in similar ways to rolled oats: in muesli or porridge and in smoothies or smoothie bowls.

FUN FACT

QUINOA is definitely one of my favourite grains! I add it to my lunch salads with fresh grilled shrimp.

BUCKWHEAT

The edible grain-like seeds of the buckwheat plant are used in similar ways to oats, rice, and quinoa. These seeds contain **rutin**, which can help maintain normal blood flow and blood clotting; and **magnesium**, which can promote the relaxation of blood vessels and reduce blood pressure. Together, these nutrients may promote a healthy cardiovascular system. While its name might be deceiving, buckwheat does not contain gluten, meaning that it can be used as part of a gluten-free or gluten-sensitive diet.

RICE FLAKES

Similar to quinoa flakes, rice flakes are rice grains that have been steamed, then rolled and dried. Both white and brown rice can be used in this process, but I recommend using wholegrain or brown rice versions as they generally contain more **fibre, vitamins, and minerals** than more refined, white versions. Like regular rice, rice flakes are free from gluten and therefore can be used as another gluten-free alternative to rolled oats.

NEVER EAT INGREDIENTS YOU CAN'T PRONOUNCE.

EXCEPT QUINOA

YOU SHOULD EAT QUINOA

SUPERFOOD POWDERS

HEALTH IS NOT THE WEIGHT YOU LOSE, BUT THE LIFE YOU GAIN!

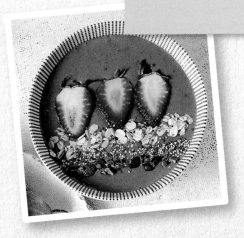

SPIRULINA

This dark green powder is made from blue-green algae. It is sometimes used as a natural multivitamin in vegetarian or vegan diets as it contains **all nine essential amino acids** and good amounts of **iron**. Spirulina can have quite a distinct earthy flavour, so it is best suited to your vegetable or green-based juices.

MACA

This root vegetable is native to Peru. As well as being jam-packed with **vitamins and minerals**, it also contains a number of unique **alkaloids** (natural plant-based chemicals) that may help improve the overall functioning of the body's hormonal systems. Native practitioners have used maca as a remedy for a number of hormone-related issues, including irregular periods, infertility, fatigue, and loss of libido. Maca has an earthy, nutty taste and can be added to smoothies to provide a caramel or malty flavour.

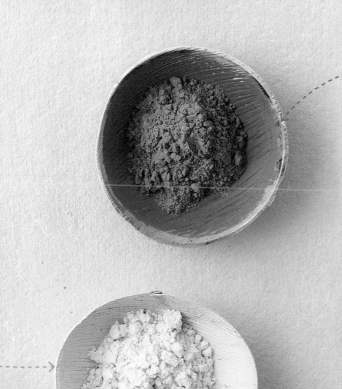

RAW CACAO

Raw cacao is chocolate in its rawest form. It contains a number of minerals, particularly **magnesium**, which is important for energy production and relaxation of muscles. It may also help to increase the body's production of serotonin and dopamine, which are two neurotransmitters (brain chemicals) that are known to improve mood and well-being. Cacao can be added to smoothies or shakes that need a chocolatey spin. However, it can have quite a bitter taste, so if you're not used to it, start with small amounts.

CAROB

This powder is made from the reddish-brown edible beans that grow on the carob tree. Carob contains a number of **minerals** as well as a substance called **gallic acid**, which is known for its antibacterial, antiviral, and antiseptic properties. Free from both gluten and caffeine, carob can be added to desserts and smoothies that need a chocolatey flavour, and is a great substitute for the slightly more bitter cocoa or cacao.

What is a food allergy or intolerance?

Food allergies and intolerances are negative reactions that occur after eating a certain food or nutrient. However, it is very important that we don't get the two confused!

A food **allergy** is an abnormal reaction to a food **that involves the immune system**. Symptoms of food allergies can include hives, rashes, and swelling, and can be life-threatening in some cases (for example, anaphylaxis). If you have a food allergy, then it is important that you strictly avoid the foods you react to.

A food **intolerance**, on the other hand, is a negative reaction to a food **that does not involve the immune system**. Symptoms of food intolerances can include bloating and altered bowel motions, which can be unpleasant and severe, but are generally not life-threatening. Because of these negative side effects, food intolerances can reduce the types of foods that a person can eat comfortably. They can also make it more difficult to get the full range of vitamins and minerals that our bodies need.

Let's take a look at some common allergies and intolerances ...

WHEN ADJUSTING YOUR DIET TO SUIT AN INTOLERANCE, IT IS IMPORTANT TO UNDERSTAND THAT THE SOLUTION IS NEVER AS SIMPLE AS CUTTING THAT FOOD (OR FOOD GROUP) OUT OF YOUR DIET ALTOGETHER.

Not everyone will understand your journey, and that's okay.

You are here to become a healthier, stronger, and happier person.

Focus on yourself!

LACTOSE INTOLERANCE

What is lactose?

Lactose is the carbohydrate (sugar) that can be found in dairy foods such as milk, cheese, and yoghurt. In our digestive system, lactose is broken down into smaller carbohydrate units by an enzyme called lactase.

What is lactose intolerance and how do we treat it?

Lactose intolerance occurs when the body cannot digest and absorb lactose well. The most common symptoms generally include bloating, diarrhoea, wind, and pain after eating foods that are high in lactose. Lactose intolerance can either be temporary (for example, after you have had a gastrointestinal illness or not had milk for a long period of time) or a longer lasting problem. After the age of five to seven years, people can lose their ability to digest lactose as the lactase enzyme (which breaks down lactose) is less active in their digestive system. These people may be able to have small amounts of lactose (such as a small glass of milk) without experiencing any negative effects, but larger intakes can result in symptoms such as abdominal pain and diarrhoea.

Lactose intolerance can be treated by reducing the amount of lactose you eat in your diet. Our main sources of lactose are dairy foods. It is important to remember that everyone is different and will tolerate different amounts of lactose in their diet. Some people can tolerate a small amount, while others can't tolerate any at all. Your symptoms will help you decide how strict you need to be.

When reducing your intake of dairy foods, it is important to realise that you are also removing one of your best sources of calcium. To ensure that your diet is balanced and that you are not deficient in any way, you'll need to find appropriate replacements.

So, what are appropriate dairy replacements and where can we find them?

1 MILK

In some countries, it is possible to buy lactose-free cow's milk. With these products, manufacturers have often added small amounts of lactase enzyme during processing. This saves your body from having to digest the lactose, which can reduce the negative side effects if you have an intolerance.

NOT ALL "MILKS" ARE EQUAL

If you are unable to find lactose-free cow's milk, then you could use calcium-fortified non-dairy milk products, which have had calcium added. These include rice milk, oat milk, almond milk, soy milk, coconut milk, and quinoa milk. However, not all of these are considered good alternatives, particularly in regards to their calcium and protein content. This is something to bear in mind if you are someone who makes your own non-dairy milk at home, such as almond milk.

When selecting a milk alternative, look for a product with a minimum of 100 mg of calcium per ½ cup. This detail can be found on the nutrition information panel on the product label. As different brands add different amounts of calcium, it is important to always check the nutrition information panel before purchase.

In Australia, some health organisations consider calcium-fortified soy milk as the best alternative to cow's milk as it contains the most protein. Some other good alternatives include calcium-fortified rice and oat milks. As rice and oats are both grains, they tend to be higher in carbohydrates and lower in protein than soy milk.

Generally speaking, almond and quinoa milks are not great alternatives, as some manufacturers do not add enough calcium or any at all, particularly if they are labelled organic. Coconut milk is also much higher in saturated fat than all milk alternatives, and often does not contain enough calcium.

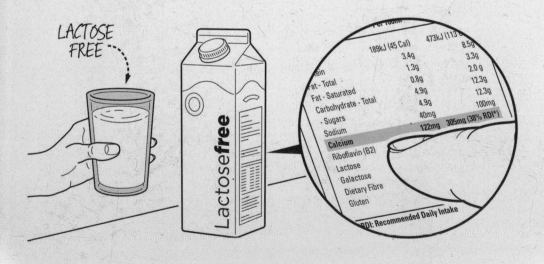

LACTOSE FREE

Per 100ml		
	189kJ (45 Cal)	473kJ (113
	3.4g	8.5g
...ein	1.3g	3.3g
Fat - Total	0.8g	2.0 g
Fat - Saturated	4.9g	12.3g
Carbohydrate - Total	4.9g	12.3g
- Sugars	40mg	100mg
Sodium	122mg	305mg (38% RDI*)
Calcium		
Riboflavin (B2)		
Lactose		
Galactose		
Dietary Fibre		
Gluten		

RDI: Recommended Daily Intake

2 CHEESE & YOGHURT

You might be surprised to know that cheese, especially hard cheese, doesn't actually contain much lactose, which means that people with an intolerance may be able to eat small amounts with little to no side effects. While fresh yoghurt has a much higher lactose content than cheese, this lactose content decreases day by day because of the natural bacteria that it contains. This means that people with lactose intolerance may also be able to eat yoghurt with little to no side effects, particularly if it is closer to its use-by date. In saying this, I do not recommend that you eat yoghurt that has passed its use-by date, for health and safety reasons.

It is possible to find cheeses and yoghurts that are lactose-free or ones that are made from soy. As these products are not very common, they may be more expensive. Just remember that if you choose non-dairy products, check the label to make sure they are fortified with calcium. If you want to avoid soy products altogether, then I advise getting the recommended serves of dairy from non-dairy milk products that have been fortified with good amounts of calcium.

Should I be taking a calcium supplement if I am lactose-intolerant?

The biggest problem with limiting or removing dairy products from your diet is that these are some of our best sources of calcium. By replacing these foods with suitable alternatives, it is possible to still meet your calcium needs without having to take a supplement. If you are lactose intolerant and unable to follow the guidelines that I have provided, then I recommend speaking with a health professional to determine whether you need to take a calcium supplement.

FAQ

Q CAN I STILL HAVE PROTEIN POWDER IF I AM LACTOSE-INTOLERANT?

A Some people who are lactose-intolerant are concerned about consuming whey protein because it comes from cow's milk. Generally speaking, whey protein isolates (WPI) are very low in lactose and can still be used by some as part of a low lactose diet. However, if you are aiming to follow a completely lactose-free diet, then you can replace whey protein powders with non-dairy protein powders such as soy, rice, or pea proteins.

NOTE: Whey and soy proteins are known as complete proteins, because they contain all of the nine amino acids that the body cannot produce itself. Rice and pea proteins, on the other hand, are incomplete proteins, as they do not contain all of these nine amino acids. Much like protein intake for vegetarians and vegans, if you make a conscious effort to include food from all food groups in recommended amounts throughout the day, then you should be able to get enough of these essential amino acids.

GLUTEN INTOLERANCE & CELIAC DISEASE

What is gluten?

Gluten is a protein found in grains such as wheat, barley, and rye.

What is gluten intolerance?

An intolerance or sensitivity to gluten is a negative reaction to foods containing gluten. Symptoms may include bloating and altered bowel motions after eating foods containing gluten. While these symptoms can be severe in some cases, they do not cause damage to the small intestine.

What is celiac disease?

Celiac disease is a condition where the immune system reacts negatively to gluten, which can cause damage to the small intestine. It may prevent you from absorbing nutrients properly, which can potentially result in nutritional deficiencies or, in some cases, malnourishment. The only way to successfully treat celiac disease is through a strict gluten-free diet.

NOTE: Celiac disease and gluten intolerance are very different conditions. If you think you are reacting to foods containing gluten, it is important that you see a health professional to investigate further.

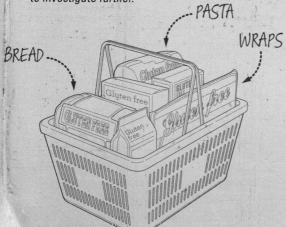

If I'm avoiding gluten, how does this affect me following the meal plans?

If you are gluten-intolerant or have been diagnosed with celiac disease, then you will need to avoid all gluten-containing products. The most common sources of gluten are breads, wraps, pasta, and oats, and you will need to replace these with gluten-free alternatives, of which there are plenty. Fortunately, a number of the grain foods that I have included in my meal plans, such as brown rice and quinoa, are naturally gluten-free, so you will not need to replace these foods.

BREAD, WRAPS & PASTA Many supermarkets now stock gluten-free versions of these foods. Before purchasing one of these products, check that the label clearly states it is gluten-free.

OATS While oats do not contain gluten, they do contain a protein called avenin that has similar properties. There is much debate as to whether oats are safe to eat for people with celiac disease, and different countries have different recommendations. In Australia, it is recommended that people with celiac disease completely avoid oats, whereas in the UK they are allowed in small amounts.

The main issue is that it is quite common for oats to become contaminated with wheat at various stages of their production. For example, they might be grown next to each other, be transported or stored together, or processed using the same equipment. If you have celiac disease, please refer to your local celiac organisation for further guidance on oats. Some people with gluten intolerance can tolerate small amounts of uncontaminated oats without any negative side effects. If you need to avoid oats, they can easily be replaced with gluten-free alternatives, such as rice flakes or quinoa flakes.

PEANUT & TREE NUT ALLERGIES

What are they?

Peanut and tree nut allergies are a negative reaction to proteins found in these foods that involves the immune system. Symptoms can vary from stomach discomfort and altered bowel motions to skin reactions and swelling around the mouth and throat. These symptoms can occur within 30 minutes of eating the allergen. In some cases, the reaction can be severe and even life-threatening (anaphylaxis, for example) and may occur within a few minutes of eating.

Peanuts aren't actually nuts at all—they are a type of legume and are quite different to tree nuts (such as almonds, walnuts, cashews, hazelnuts, brazil nuts, and pecans). This means that if you are allergic to peanuts, it is possible that you may not be allergic to tree nuts, and vice versa. However, as with oats, it is quite common for manufacturers to use the same equipment during processing. So unless you are growing your own nuts at home, it is generally recommended that you avoid both types in case of cross-contamination.

WHAT IF I HAVE OTHER SPECIAL DIETARY NEEDS?

If you have any other special dietary needs or intolerances that affect your ability to follow my meal plans, I recommend that you see an accredited practising dietitian, who will help tailor a nutrition plan specifically to your needs.

How do nut allergies affect the meal plans?

When adjusting your diet to suit a peanut or tree nut allergy, it is important to understand that these foods provide our bodies with healthy fats, including essential ones that the body is unable to produce on its own. Rather than eliminating these foods altogether, I recommend replacing any nuts or nut butters with nut-free alternatives, such as pumpkin or sunflower-seed spreads. You could also use a vegetable-based oil instead of a nut-based one, or use wholemeal flour in place of almond meal in your cooking. If you are unable to find a substitute for a particular meal, you can always add additional healthy fat servings to another meal on that day, such as eating extra avocado with your eggs at breakfast, or using a touch more olive oil in your salad dressing. These minor adjustments can help you achieve the recommended servings of healthy fats and ensure that you are not missing out on the nutrients that these foods provide.

It can be hard to avoid tree nuts and peanuts in everyday life, especially when it comes to packaged foods. Fortunately, most government regulations require that any food product that contains peanuts or tree nuts, or may have come into contact with them during production, must clearly state this on the label.

This highlights the importance of reading labels before purchasing food and also making enquiries at restaurants to ensure that the food you eat does not trigger an allergic reaction.

MY MEAL PLANS

Eating healthy doesn't have to be complicated. My meal plans are flexible and use a wide variety of foods from all six food groups (see the AGHE information on page 22).

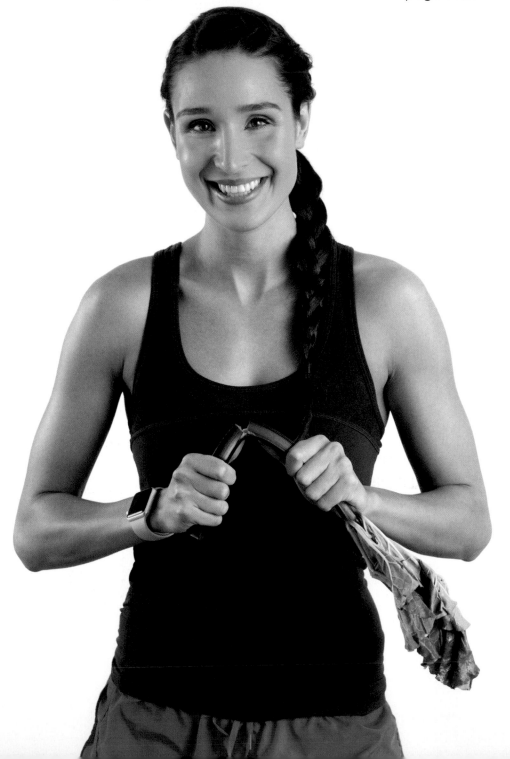

THESE SIX FOOD GROUPS REPRESENT THE BUILDING BLOCKS OF GOOD NUTRITIONAL HEALTH.

GRAINS

6 RECOMMENDED DAILY SERVINGS

Grain-based foods such as rice, quinoa, oats, muesli, breads, and cereals are our body's primary source of carbohydrates and preferred source of energy. These foods also provide other key nutrients, including protein, fibre, B group vitamins, and minerals such as iron, zinc, and magnesium.

HEALTHY FATS

2 RECOMMENDED DAILY SERVINGS

Foods such as avocados, nuts, and seeds provide us with essential fatty acids the body cannot produce on its own. These fatty acids supply the body with energy and contribute to the overall structure and function of our cells.

VEGETABLES & LEGUMES

5 RECOMMENDED DAILY SERVINGS

Vegetables are nutrient-dense and relatively low in energy. This means they contain lots of good stuff but don't provide many calories, which is great if you have a big appetite. They are of particular benefit as they contain an abundance of vitamins and minerals, fibre, and a range of phytochemicals (chemicals naturally found in plants that can help your body combat disease). Legumes, such as chickpeas and lentils, are a valuable source of protein.

FRUIT

2 RECOMMENDED DAILY SERVINGS

Fruit is a rich source of vitamins, including vitamin C and folate. It also provides us with potassium, fibre, and carbohydrates in the form of natural sugars. Fruit skins (the edible ones) are especially high in fibre.

DAIRY PRODUCTS & ALTERNATIVES

2½ RECOMMENDED DAILY SERVINGS

Milk, cheese, and yoghurt are particularly rich in calcium, a mineral that is important for bone and muscle health. These foods also provide our bodies with protein, iodine, vitamin A, vitamin D, riboflavin (vitamin B2), vitamin B12, and zinc.

LEAN MEAT, SEAFOOD, EGGS & MEAT ALTERNATIVES

2½ RECOMMENDED DAILY SERVINGS

This food group typically includes red meat (beef, lamb, kangaroo), poultry (chicken and turkey), seafood, eggs, and also legumes. These foods are our body's best source of protein. They also provide us with a long list of minerals (including iodine, iron, and zinc), vitamins, and healthy fats. For vegetarians or vegans, this group primarily consists of eggs, legumes, tofu, and tempeh.

FOOD GROUPS	COMMON FOODS AND SAMPLE SERVINGS
GRAINS	1 slice whole wheat bread or raisin bread ½ medium whole wheat roll or whole wheat wrap 1 oz muesli, rolled oats or quinoa flakes 3½ oz cooked quinoa or rice 3 oz cooked whole wheat pasta 3½ oz cooked rice vermicelli noodles 2 whole wheat crispbreads
VEGETABLES & LEGUMES	NON-STARCHY VEGETABLES 1 large handful lettuce leaves, baby spinach, arugula, or kale 1 medium carrot, cucumber, tomato, zucchini, small onion, or beetroot ½ medium bell pepper or eggplant 2 celery stalks 5 oz tinned crushed tomatoes STARCHY VEGETABLES ½ medium potato or sweet potato ½ ear of corn or ⅓ cup tinned or frozen corn kernels 2¾ oz cooked or tinned legumes (kidney beans, chickpeas, lentils)
FRUIT	1 medium apple, banana, orange, or mango, or small pear 6 oz mixed berries or 5¾ oz blueberries or raspberries 9 oz watermelon or strawberries 1 large handful grapes (~ 25), cherries (~ 20) 1 oz dried sultanas, or 1 oz dried goji berries or cranberries ½ cup freshly squeezed fruit juice
DAIRY PRODUCTS & ALTERNATIVES	1 cup low-fat milk or calcium-fortified milk 7 oz low-fat plain yoghurt or soy yoghurt 1½ oz reduced-fat (hard) cheese 2 oz low-fat salt-reduced feta or 3½ oz low-fat ricotta 4½ oz low-fat cottage cheese
LEAN MEAT, SEAFOOD, EGGS & MEAT ALTERNATIVES	2⅓ oz cooked lean red meat (beef, lamb, kangaroo) 3 oz cooked chicken or 3 oz cooked turkey 3½ oz cooked white fish fillet or tinned tuna 2½ oz cooked salmon fillet, or smoked or tinned salmon 2 large eggs 5¼ oz cooked or tinned legumes (kidney beans, chickpeas, lentils) 6 oz tofu or 3 oz tempeh
HEALTHY FATS	1½ teaspoons monounsaturated or polyunsaturated oil ⅓ oz nuts or 2 teaspoons nut paste 1 oz avocado (~ ⅛ avocado)

I HAVE USED THESE FOOD GROUPS TO ESTABLISH A COMPREHENSIVE 28-DAY MEAL PLAN THAT PROVIDES FOR ALL YOUR NUTRITIONAL NEEDS.

As you can see, each of these six food groups provides our bodies with a unique set of nutrients. This emphasises how important it is to consume foods from all of these food groups and in balanced amounts.

Just as we need nutrients in different amounts, we also need to consume a different number of servings from each of these groups. I have provided examples of sample servings for each of these food groups (see opposite for the more common foods, and pages 370–371 for a comprehensive list).

It is important not to confuse "serving size" with "portion size." For example, six servings of grains is *not* six meals worth of grains, but the total amount of grains that you should be eating every day.

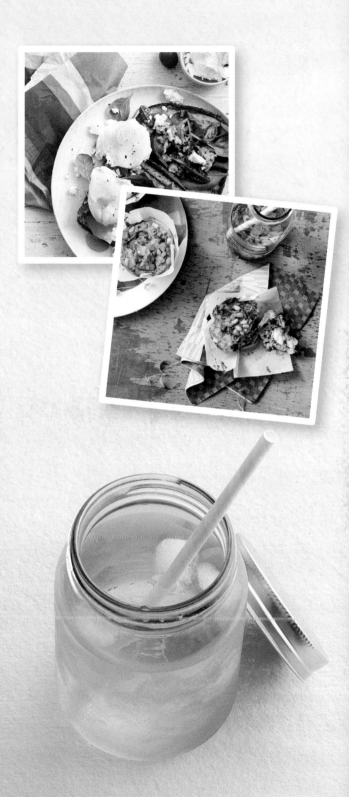

FAQ

Q DO I NEED TO TAKE SUPPLEMENTS?

A In my opinion, there is no substitute for a healthy lifestyle consisting of both a well-balanced diet and regular exercise or activity. As their name suggests, supplements are designed to *supplement* a healthy diet or lifestyle. Just like exercise cannot outweigh a poor diet, neither can supplements. It is important that you consume foods from all of the food groups and in balanced amounts, so that you can obtain all of the nutrients that you need consistently.

In the instance where you cannot eat foods from a particular food group because you have an allergy or intolerance, then a multivitamin supplement may be needed to help you fill any nutritional gaps. However, I recommend that you seek advice from a health professional before taking any vitamin supplement.

IT'S AS EASY AS A, B, C, D !

Each recipe in this book is coded
with one of the following icons:

If you come across a meal within the
28-day meal plan that does not suit your
taste preferences, you can replace it with
another recipe labelled with the same icon.

For example, if you don't feel like
Oat Porridge with Poached Pear, an "A"
option for breakfast, you can replace it
with Passionfruit Parfait, or Macerated
Strawberries, or any other breakfast
meal in the book with the same icon.

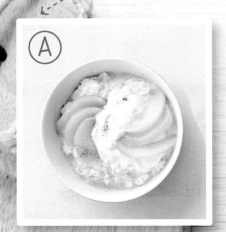 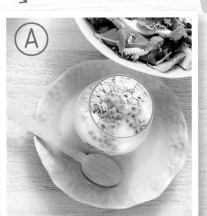 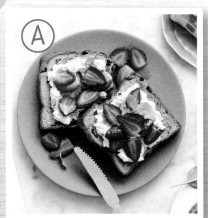

WHILE IT IS IMPORTANT
FOR YOU TO MEET ALL
OF THE RECOMMENDED
FOOD GROUP SERVINGS
THROUGHOUT THE DAY,
WHICHEVER WAY YOU
DO THAT IS UP TO YOU!

FLEXIBLE OPTIONS

Everyone's food preferences are diverse. The beauty of my method is that the meal plans can be adapted **to give you plenty of variety** and to suit *your* preferences.

To help you do this, I have provided four flexible meal variations—A, B, C, and D. While each variation contains the same number of meals and the required number of servings from all of the main food groups, they differ in the way these food groups are distributed throughout the day. This means you can have different types of foods at different times of the day during the week **to suit your individual lifestyle and preferences**.

For example, each meal in Option D contains a small serving of grains, whereas Option C contains more grain servings earlier in the day, but none at dinner. To keep it convenient and simple, the plan has varying days with varying layouts to suit all meal types.

	OPTION **A**	OPTION **B**	OPTION **C**	OPTION **D**
Breakfast	2 servings grains 1 serving fruit 1 serving dairy products & alternatives	1 serving grains ½ serving vegetables & legumes 1½ servings fruit 1½ servings dairy products & alternatives 1 serving healthy fats	2 servings grains ½ serving fruit ¾ serving dairy products & alternatives ½ serving healthy fats	2 servings grains 1 serving vegetables & legumes ½ serving dairy products & alternatives 1 serving lean meat, seafood, eggs & meat alternatives 1 serving healthy fats
A.M. Snack	1 serving grains 1 serving vegetables & legumes ½ serving lean meat, seafood, eggs & meat alternatives	½ serving fruit 1 serving healthy fats	1 serving grains 1½ servings fruit 1 serving dairy products & alternatives	1 serving grains 1 serving fruit ½ serving dairy products & alternatives
Lunch	1 serving grain 2 servings vegetables & legumes 1 serving lean meat, seafood, eggs & meat alternatives	2 servings grains 1½ servings vegetables & legumes ½ serving dairy products & alternatives 1 serving lean meat, seafood, eggs & meat alternatives	2 servings grains 1½ servings vegetables & legumes 1 serving lean meat, seafood, eggs & meat alternatives	1 serving grains 1½ servings vegetables & legumes ½ serving dairy products & alternatives ½ serving lean meat, seafood, eggs & meat alternatives
P.M. Snack	1 serving fruit 1½ servings dairy products & alternatives	1 serving grains 1 serving vegetables & legumes ½ serving lean meat, seafood, eggs & meat alternatives	1 serving grains ¼ serving dairy products & alternatives	1 serving grains ½ serving vegetables & legumes ½ serving dairy products & alternatives
Dinner	2 servings grains 2 servings vegetables & legumes 1 serving lean meat, seafood, eggs & meat alternatives 2 servings healthy fats	2 servings grains 2 servings vegetables & legumes ½ serving dairy products & alternatives 1 serving lean meat, seafood, eggs & meat alternatives	3½ servings vegetables (1 starchy) ½ serving dairy products & alternatives 1½ servings lean meat, seafood, eggs & meat alternatives ½ serving healthy fats	1 serving grains 2 servings vegetables & legumes 1 serving fruit ½ serving dairy products & alternatives 1 serving lean meat, seafood, eggs & meat alternatives 1 serving healthy fats

MEAL PLANS

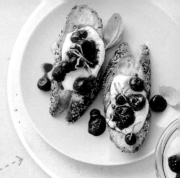

As you can see from these weekly meal plans, there is so much more to healthy eating than just chicken and broccoli!

WEEK ONE

	DAY 1 A	DAY 2 B	DAY 3 C	DAY 4 D	DAY 5 A	DAY 6 B	DAY 7 C
Breakfast	Quinoa Porridge with Fresh Figs (page 96)	Green Smoothie Bowl (page 100)	Whipped Peanut Butter & Banana (page 104)	Salmon & Dill Toast Topper (page 108)	Berry & Yoghurt Breakfast Bruschetta (page 112)	Berry-Nana Smoothie Bowl (page 116)	Homemade Granola (page 120)
Snack A.M.	Rice Crackers with Beetroot Dip (page 96)	Apple with Nut Butter (page 100)	Berry Mousse Parfait (page 104)	Crispbreads with Blueberries & Ricotta (page 108)	Tuna Rice Cakes (page 112)	Almonds & Grapes (page 116)	Honey Bear Smoothie (page 120)
Lunch	Moroccan Chicken Pita (page 96)	Chicken Yiros with Homemade Tzatziki (page 100)	San Choy Bow (page 104)	Caprese Salad (page 108)	Pasta Salad with Baked Tomatoes & Greens (page 112)	Black Bean, Tomato & Corn Quesadilla (page 116)	Black Rice Salad with Tuna (page 120)
Snack P.M.	Berry Swirl (page 97)	Crispbreads with Hummus & Tomato (page 101)	Rice Crackers with Minted Yoghurt (page 105)	Crispbreads with Tomato, Feta, and Basil (page 109)	Cherry Ripe Smoothie (page 113)	Crispbreads with White Bean Dip & Bell Pepper (page 117)	Pita Triangles with Tzatziki (page 121)
Dinner	Coconut Chilli Shrimp with Greens (page 97)	Peri Peri Chicken with Rice Salad (page 101)	Greek-style Baked Fish (page 105)	Grilled Chicken with Asian Slaw & Noodles (page 109)	Nasi Goreng with Egg (page 113)	Pulled Pork & Slaw Slider (page 117)	Stuffed Sweet Potato (page 121)

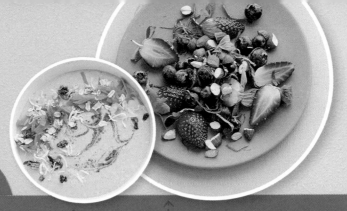

	DAY 1	DAY 2	DAY 3	DAY 4	DAY 5	DAY 6	DAY 7
	D	A	B	C	D	A	B
Breakfast	Super Green Baked Eggs (page 124)	Medjool Date Parfait (page 128)	Carrot Cake Smoothie Bowl (page 132)	Overnight Oats with Raspberries (page 136)	Chia Seed Omelette (page 140)	Banana & Ricotta Breakfast Wrap (page 144)	Green Smoothie Bowl with Mango (page 148)
Snack A.M.	Berry Yoghurt & Muesli (page 124)	Baked Chips with Carrot Hummus (page 128)	Berry Salad with Nuts (page 132)	Peachy Keen Smoothie (page 136)	Maple Banana Yoghurt & Muesli (page 140)	Pita Triangles with Lentil & Semi-dried Tomato Pate (page 144)	Strawberries with Chocolate Sauce (page 148)
Lunch	Quinoa & Roast Vegetable Salad (page 124)	Savoury Crepe (page 128)	Falafel Pita Sandwich (page 132)	Moroccan Chicken Salad (page 136)	Caesar Salad (page 140)	Mexican Salad (page 144)	Zucchini Fritter Pita (page 148)
Snack P.M.	Tomato & Cheese Toastie (page 125)	Stewed Apple with Honeyed Yoghurt (page 129)	Rice Cakes with Hummus, Tomato & Spinach (page 133)	Ricotta on Rye (page 137)	Rice Cakes with Semi-dried Tomato & Ricotta (page 141)	Passionfruit & Mango Mousse (page 145)	Egg & Cucumber Crispbreads (page 149)
Dinner	Stuffed Squid (page 125)	Chicken Paella (page 129)	Fish Tacos (page 133)	Zucchini Pasta Bolognese (page 137)	Lamb Tagine with Couscous (page 141)	Pumpkin & White Bean Risotto (page 145)	Shrimp Saganaki with Spinach Rice (page 149)

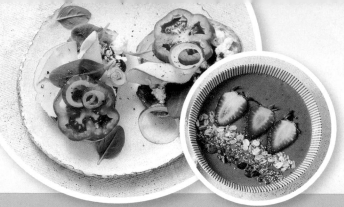

	DAY 1	DAY 2	DAY 3	DAY 4	DAY 5	DAY 6	DAY 7
	C	D	A	B	C	D	A
Breakfast	Strawberries, Ricotta and "Nutella Drizzle" on Toast (page 152)	Breakfast Burrito (page 156)	Oat Porridge with Poached Pear (page 160)	Red Velvet Smoothie Bowl (page 164)	Chia Berry Yoghurt & Muesli (page 168)	Breakfast Salad (page 172)	Passionfruit Parfait (page 176)
Snack A.M.	Mango Tango Smoothie (page 152)	Crispbreads with Blueberries & Ricotta (page 156)	Crispbreads with Smoked Salmon & Cucumber (page 160)	Banana & Peanut Butter Stack (page 164)	Peachy Keen Smoothie (page 168)	Apricot & Plum Parfait (page 172)	Rice Crackers with Carrot Hummus (page 176)
Lunch	Asian Noodle Salad (page 152)	Greek Pasta Salad (page 156)	Sushi Salad (page 160)	Turkey & Cranberry Toast Topper (page 164)	Vegetarian Salad Wrap (page 168)	Carrot & Chickpea Open Sandwich (page 172)	Chicken, Pumpkin & Quinoa Salad (page 176)
Snack P.M.	Rice Crackers with Cilantro & Garlic Yoghurt (page 153)	Pita Triangles with Beetroot Yoghurt Dip (page 157)	Sticky Date Smoothie (page 161)	Crispbreads with Hummus & Tomato (page 165)	Rice Crackers with Minted Yoghurt (page 169)	Rice Cakes with Semi-dried Tomato & Ricotta (page 173)	Peach Protein Smoothie (page 177)
Dinner	Moussaka (page 153)	"Fish and Chips" (page 157)	Pad Thai with Chicken (page 161)	Chicken, Sweet Potato, Caramelised Onion & Arugula Pizza (page 165)	Niçoise Salad (page 169)	Brown Rice, Chicken & Orange Salad (page 173)	Beef Stir-fry (page 177)

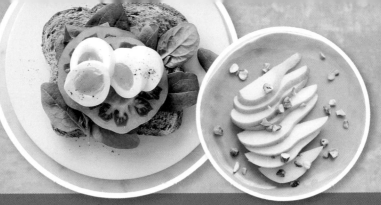

	DAY 1	DAY 2	DAY 3	DAY 4	DAY 5	DAY 6	DAY 7
	B	C	D	A	B	C	D
Breakfast	Tropical Smoothie Bowl (page 180)	Healthy Bircher (page 184)	Mushroom Bruschetta (page 188)	Macerated Strawberries (page 192)	Pumpkin Pie Smoothie Bowl (page 196)	Breakfast Berry Crumble (page 200)	Breakfast Stack with Dukkah (page 204)
Snack A.M.	Fruit Salad with Chia Seed Dressing (page 180)	Choc Raspberry Smoothie (page 184)	Crispbreads with Blueberries & Ricotta (page 188)	Egg on Toast with Spinach (page 192)	Pear & Pistachios (page 196)	Honey Bear Smoothie (page 200)	Apple & Rhubarb Compote with Muesli (page 204)
Lunch	Taco Salad (page 180)	Italian Pasta Salad (page 184)	Tuna & Brown Rice Salad (page 188)	Vietnamese Chicken Rolls (page 192)	Turkey & Rainbow Salad Sandwich (page 196)	Zesty Tuna Wrap (page 200)	Open Sandwich with Salmon (page 204)
Snack P.M.	Crispbreads with White Bean Dip & Bell Pepper (page 181)	Ricotta on Rye (page 185)	Tomato & Cheese Toastie (page 189)	Toffee Apple Smoothie (page 193)	Rice Cakes with Hummus, Tomato & Spinach (page 197)	Rice Crackers with Homemade Tzatziki (page 201)	Pita Triangles with Beetroot Yoghurt Dip (page 205)
Dinner	Beetroot Risotto with Salmon (page 181)	Greek-style Chicken Kebabs (page 184)	Chicken Enchiladas (page 189)	Massaman Beef Curry (page 193)	Spaghetti Marinara (page 197)	Falafel & Roast Pumpkin Salad (page 201)	Jerk Chicken with Rice & Beans (page 205)

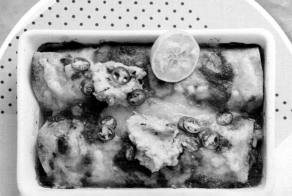

HEALTHY EATING & LIFESTYLE

In my experience, people who consider their health from
a holistic point of view are far more successful at achieving their goals.
To do this means being aware of all aspects of your health and
maintaining a consistent balance. Here are some ways to incorporate
balance into your diet and lifestyle.

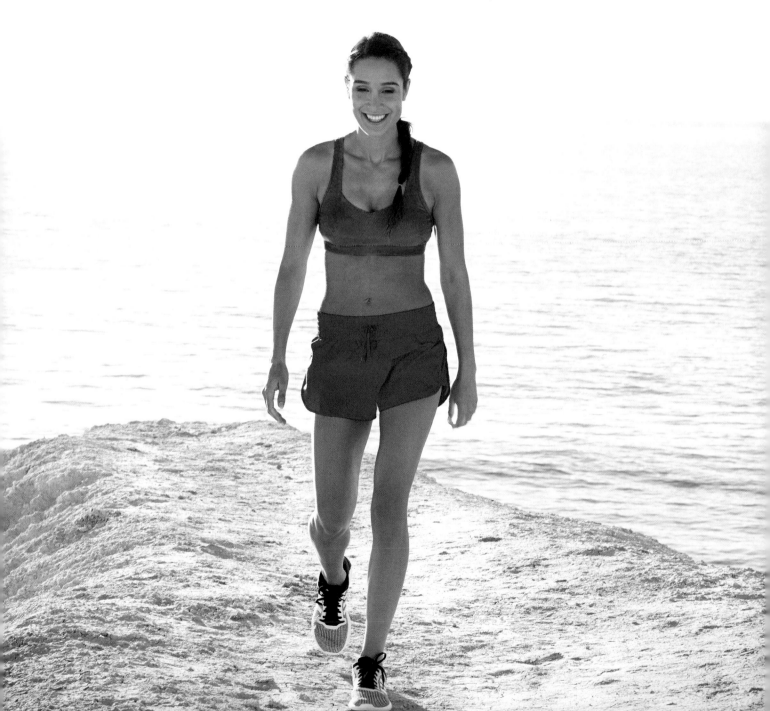

CHEAT MEALS

What is a "cheat meal"?

A cheat meal is an indulgence in food or drink enjoyed once a week. My understanding is that the concept of cheat meals originated in bodybuilding, where they were used to cause a deliberate spike in hormone activity and help promote sustained fat loss.

Many people are under the impression that they have a dramatic impact on your health goal, but my experience has shown me that cheat meals are not necessary for continued progress.

However, when embarking on a new healthy lifestyle, many people tend to struggle with cravings for their favourite foods and beverages. As you adopt a new diet and exercise routine, it is quite common to feel unsatisfied from meals or develop strong cravings. Having a cheat meal once a week has allowed many of my clients to continue to maintain their progress without overindulging multiple times throughout the week. Rather than providing any nutritionally scientific validity, in my experience cheat meals have proved an effective way of relieving psychological stress, which has allowed my clients to continue with training and healthy lifestyle management in the longer term.

"CHEAT MEAL" SUGGESTIONS

Tips to use when having a cheat meal:

1. It's called a cheat meal, not a cheat day. Try not to go on a binge for hours. 45–60 minutes is a typical meal time when dining, so try and stick to that.

2. Don't force yourself to overeat, or go out of your way to eat more than usual. There is no point in forcing yourself to have a big cheat meal.

3. Try not to regret it. There's nothing wrong with indulging, so don't punish yourself for it.

Many of my clients have found that when they overeat, they can hold a little extra water weight for the 24–48 hours following a cheat meal. Whether this is actually physical or psychological is hard to determine. Regardless, there is no need to be concerned as it's common for your body to bloat a little after large meals.

FOLLOWING A HEALTHY LIFESTYLE PLAN DOESN'T MEAN GOING WITHOUT —IT'S FINE TO TREAT YOURSELF ONCE IN A WHILE IF YOU'RE FOLLOWING A BALANCED DIET. THIS IS WHY I'VE INCLUDED NAUGHTY MADE NICE OPTIONS (SEE PAGE 335). AS HEALTHIER VERSIONS OF YOUR FAVOURITE SWEET TREATS, THESE RECIPES ARE PERFECT FOR SATISFYING A SUGAR CRAVING.

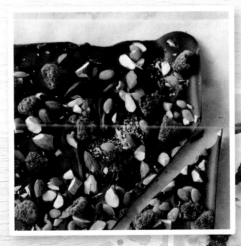

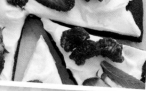

ALCOHOL

Let's be honest, alcohol is not a nutrient your body needs to survive! But in some countries, it's a big part of the culture and there can be a lot of pressure to join in when friends are having a drink. However, I must emphasise that I do not promote or condone the consumption of any alcoholic or recreational drug substance.

Alcohol is classified as a macronutrient as it provides seven calories per gram—almost TWICE as many calories as protein and carbohydrates. This means that drinking alcohol (even in small amounts) can seriously increase the number of calories you consume on a particular day, especially if the alcohol is mixed with drinks that are high in refined sugar.

The metabolism (or breakdown) of alcohol also interferes with the metabolism of other nutrients. This means it essentially pushes to the front of the queue to be metabolised first, leaving carbohydrates, proteins, and fats waiting in line. This is because alcohol cannot be stored for later use by the body in the same way as other macronutrients, so your body works furiously to get it out of your system first.

The by-products of alcohol metabolism can also be severely detrimental to your body, especially your liver, which is where the majority of alcohol metabolism occurs. Alcohol is essentially a poison that, if consumed regularly, does just that—poisons your body. For this reason, it is not something I recommend to my clients.

DINING OUT

At times during your healthy lifestyle journey, it is likely you'll find yourself in situations where you can't have a homemade meal. And if you are someone who enjoys dining out regularly, then the foods you choose can have a significant impact on your health and fitness goals. If you have just started a healthy lifestyle, sometimes you may need to adjust your food choices when dining out to suit your new goals. Here are five tips to help you maintain your healthy lifestyle habits when eating out.

1 DINING OUT DOESN'T HAVE TO BE A CHEAT MEAL

Just because you're eating out doesn't mean you have to make bad choices—there are plenty of ways to dine out regularly while maintaining a healthy diet. I suggest choosing a dish that matches what you would typically eat at that time of the day had you made it yourself. For example, if you tend to dine out at breakfast time, then an egg dish or the housemade granola could work perfectly. If you dine out more at lunch or dinner, this might mean sticking to things such as lean proteins, light condiments, vegetables, and salads.

On the other hand, if you don't dine out often and see it as a special occasion to get out of the house and enjoy yourself, you may want to indulge in foods you hardly ever get a chance to eat. This is totally okay as well! I believe that life is all about balance, and should include the occasional treat. As we all know, when someone else cooks it and cleans up, it always tastes better anyway!

2 CHOOSE YOUR RESTAURANT CAREFULLY

If you are planning to go out for a meal (that isn't a cheat meal), be smart about your choice of cuisine or restaurant. The menu at your local pub is likely to include lots of meals that are crumbed, fried, and covered in salt, leaving you with few healthy options to choose from. However, an Asian or Mediterranean-style restaurant will have more options as these cuisines tend to use more fresh ingredients.

I know that sometimes choosing the restaurant will be completely out of your control. Rather than raising your white flag and going for the greasiest thing on the menu, try to make the most of a bad situation! For example, if you want to order the fried chicken, you could ask for the chicken to be grilled instead. Similarly, if a group of your friends decide to order pizza, you could ask for a thinner base and choose a topping of fresh vegetables and lean proteins, rather than processed ones. A simple change in ingredient can have a big impact.

3 CHOOSE THE RIGHT SAUCE

Keep sauces to a minimum and try to select a healthier option where possible. For example, choose a red sauce over a white one—white sauces tend to be much higher in oil and fat. While we do need some fats in our diet, some restaurants can be very heavy-handed and we could be consuming far more than we intended without even knowing it. Another great tip is to ask for the sauce to be served on the side. This means that you (and you alone!) can determine how much you have.

4 FILL UP ON THE GOOD STUFF

Rather than going for white bread smothered in butter or a bowl of wedges, try and go for something a little lighter. Some good examples include a soup or a side of salad or steamed veggies. These types of foods contain beneficial nutrients and very few calories. They are also jam-packed with fibre, which can help us to recognise when we are full and stop us from going overboard!

5 PRACTISE PORTION CONTROL

Be mindful of your portions and understand when you should stop. Just having a massive plate full of food in front of you doesn't mean you have to eat every last crumb, especially if you know you are going to make yourself sick. Be aware that most restaurant portions are bigger than they need to be, and it is up to you to listen to your body and know when to stop. It can take a little longer for your stomach to recognise when it is full, so it is important that you eat slowly. If you are really enjoying your meal and don't want it to go to waste, then ask the waiter to put what's left in a doggy bag! It also means you will have one less meal you need to prepare for tomorrow, which is an added bonus!

FOOD CRAVINGS

We all experience food cravings. Whether you have a sweet tooth or enjoy a salty snack, I am sure cravings have hit you at one point or another. Sometimes when we succumb to these cravings they can leave us feeling guilty for having strayed from our healthy lifestyle habits.

WHAT A LOT OF PEOPLE DON'T KNOW IS THAT MOST OF THE TIME FOOD CRAVINGS ARE NOT NECESSARILY A RESULT OF HUNGER, BUT A COMBINATION OF PSYCHOLOGICAL AND BIOLOGICAL FACTORS.

In other words, your body behaves differently when it comes to hunger and cravings.

When you are hungry, your body signals to your brain that it is time to eat. This is a natural response that helps us stay alive and function properly from day to day. When your blood sugar levels begin to drop, your body releases a hormone called ghrelin that tells your brain you need food. Another hormone called leptin lets us know to stop eating once we begin to feel full. When it comes to cravings, it is a little more complicated than just providing your body with something that it needs (such as food, water, or sleep) ...

So, why do we experience food cravings?

1 PLEASURE & REWARD

The mind is complex, and when you are craving something it is not necessarily because you need it to survive. The insula, hippocampus, and caudate are the parts of the brain that are believed to be responsible for food cravings. These parts of the brain are in charge of short- and long-term memory creation, your social emotions, and the dopamine reward system (dopamine is a feel-good hormone that is linked to the feeling of pleasure, and sometimes to addictions).

If you have had nothing but pleasurable experiences when eating chocolate cake, then it is perfectly understandable for your brain to tell you that it will make you feel better!

2 EMOTIONAL EATING

Your emotions, particularly stress, can play a huge role in food cravings. As I mentioned previously, when you eat foods that contain refined carbohydrates, salt, and sugar, your body may produce feel-good hormones, such as dopamine, which can cause you to crave these foods again and again. These hormones can also help us feel relaxed, which is why you're more likely to reach for the chocolate instead of the carrots when you are feeling stressed or anxious. This is important to understand, so that you aren't too hard on yourself.

However, it is also important to know what causes your cravings, as this can help you curb them. If you are a highly stressed person, eating junk food and takeaway every day may not be the best solution for you. Instead, you can equip yourself with this knowledge and try to find different outlets for your stress. Taking a long relaxing walk, practising yoga, or reading a book are just a few strategies that you can use to help you handle your emotions and occupy your mind.

3 NUTRITIONAL DEFICIENCIES

In order for our body to function at its best, we need to fill it with the right type and amount of nutrients. If you are lacking in certain nutrients, your body may develop cravings for foods that contain these. This is why when so many people go on extreme or "fad" diets, they may find themselves experiencing intense cravings. This can be your body's way of communicating that it is lacking certain nutrients—especially if you have been cutting out one or more food groups.

How do I fight food cravings?

If you experience cravings when you are feeling particularly down, stressed, anxious, or it's that time of the month, learn to recognise these behaviours and come up with strategies to cope. Understand that you are craving that food for a reason, and take the time to delve a little deeper into why you may be feeling a certain way at that particular time.

When it comes to nutritional deficiencies, the best thing you can do is eat a wholesome, balanced diet that includes foods from all food groups. Try to get all of your important nutrients from foods rather than supplements, and always pick foods that have been processed as little as possible.

If you are someone who struggles with cravings A LOT, remove the foods that you crave from your pantry. By stocking up on junk food and chocolate, you are making it easy for yourself to access these when cravings hit. Instead, fill your fridge and pantry with healthy snacks and other foods you can eat that will fill you up and not leave you wanting more!

I WANT YOU TO REMEMBER
IT IS OKAY TO INDULGE
A LITTLE ONCE IN A WHILE.
NEVER DEPRIVE YOURSELF
AND NEVER FEEL LIKE YOU
CAN'T EAT SOMETHING.
BE AWARE OF WHAT IT IS
THAT YOU ARE PUTTING
INTO YOUR BODY, AND HOW
IT WILL MAKE YOU FEEL.

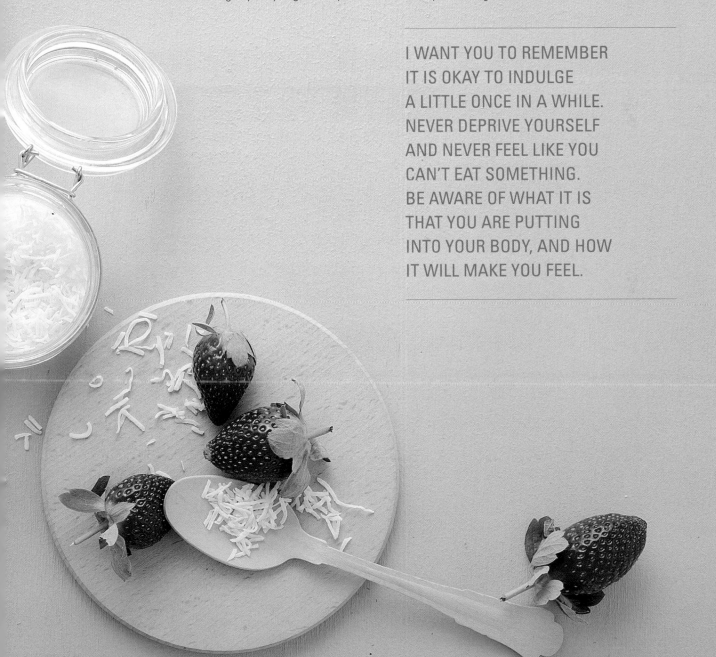

HYDRATION

As part of a holistic approach to your health, it is important to make a conscious effort to stay hydrated throughout the day.

Why is water important?

It is a well-known fact that we can survive weeks without food, but only a few days without water. While water does not provide us with energy, it is considered an essential nutrient that we need in large amounts every single day.

When we don't drink enough water, we will often become thirsty. This in a built-in mechanism that allows our body to recognise that we need more water. However, when the body loses large amounts of water and this is not replaced, we can become dehydrated. This may result in confusion, headaches, loss of strength and fatigue, which can dramatically impair your ability to exercise. For example, if you lose more than 5 per cent of your body weight in water, your ability to move and work can be decreased by as much as 30 per cent.

It is important that we consume enough water every single day to avoid becoming dehydrated and help our body function at its best.

How much do we need to drink?

As a general rule, it is recommended that we drink around eight glasses of water per day (around 2 litres). In saying that, many factors will influence how much water you need to drink. For example, if you are doing a workout, then you will need to drink more water than if you were having a rest day. Also, if it is really hot and humid outside, then you will need to drink more water than if it was a cold, wintry day. This is because physical activity, heat, and humidity can cause the body to lose more water.

AS A GENERAL RULE, I RECOMMEND DRINKING AN EXTRA ONE TO TWO GLASSES OF WATER FOR EVERY 30 MINUTES SPENT EXERCISING.

I *always* carry a drink bottle with me to ensure I stay hydrated throughout the day. It is also really important that each time you work out, you have a drink bottle on hand so you can regularly sip water before, during, and after your workout. This often means my car is full of empty bottles—haha!

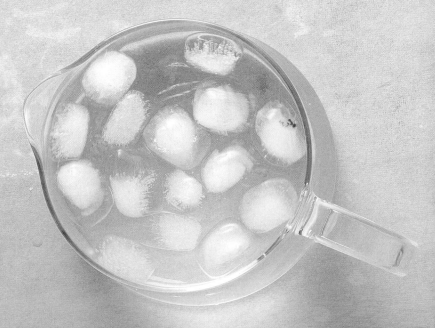

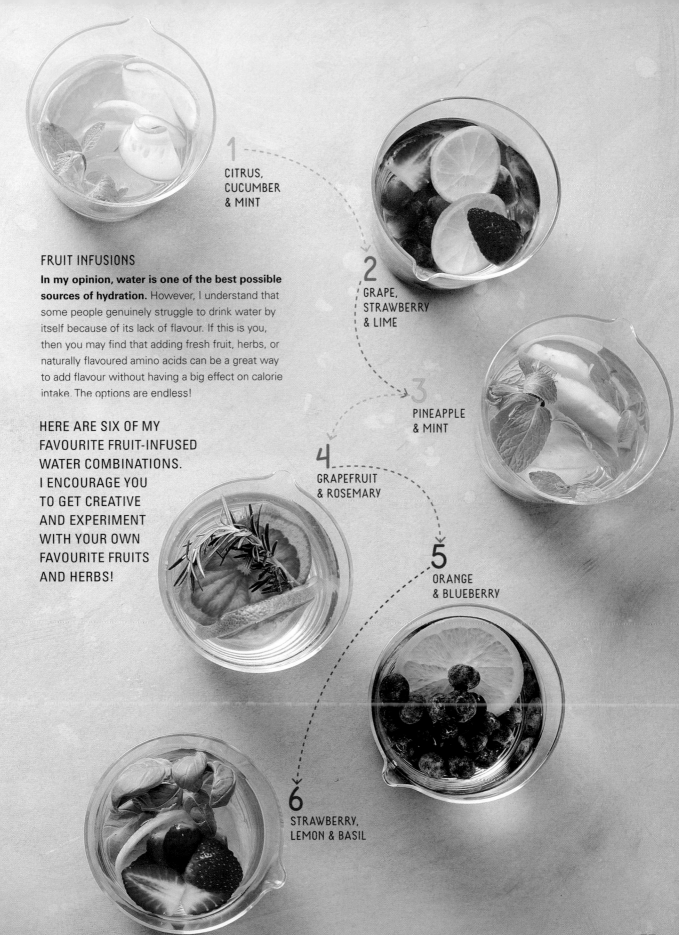

1
CITRUS,
CUCUMBER
& MINT

FRUIT INFUSIONS

In my opinion, water is one of the best possible sources of hydration. However, I understand that some people genuinely struggle to drink water by itself because of its lack of flavour. If this is you, then you may find that adding fresh fruit, herbs, or naturally flavoured amino acids can be a great way to add flavour without having a big effect on calorie intake. The options are endless!

HERE ARE SIX OF MY
FAVOURITE FRUIT-INFUSED
WATER COMBINATIONS.
I ENCOURAGE YOU
TO GET CREATIVE
AND EXPERIMENT
WITH YOUR OWN
FAVOURITE FRUITS
AND HERBS!

2
GRAPE,
STRAWBERRY
& LIME

3
PINEAPPLE
& MINT

4
GRAPEFRUIT
& ROSEMARY

5
ORANGE
& BLUEBERRY

6
STRAWBERRY,
LEMON & BASIL

What else can I drink?

Some other alternatives that can be used to replace water on occasion include mineral or sparkling water, herbal teas, fruit-based teas, black tea, or coffee.

When selecting water alternatives, it is important to consider whether the replacement contains additives or chemicals. For example, caffeine is a natural chemical found in both black tea and coffee beans. As well as giving us a little pick-me-up, caffeine can also act as a diuretic, which increases water loss by the body. Soft drinks and even fruit juices may contain lots of sugar and artificial ingredients, which do not always have much to offer nutritionally. This does not mean that you cannot drink coffee or soft drinks, but instead that you should not rely on these to meet your water requirements on a regular basis.

HERBAL TEAS

PEPPERMINT

This tea can be used to help settle your stomach when you are feeling full, bloated, or a bit gassy! I love having peppermint tea at night time, as it helps my body digest the food I have eaten and helps me feel rejuvenated.

LEMONGRASS

This lemony flavoured tea is jam-packed full of healing properties. It can help settle your stomach after a meal, calm your nervous system, and reduce anxiety, and improve circulation throughout the body.

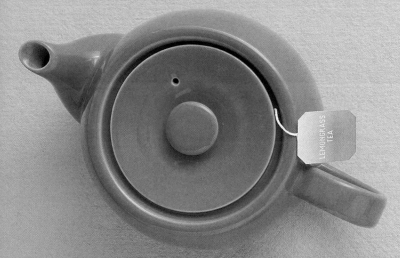

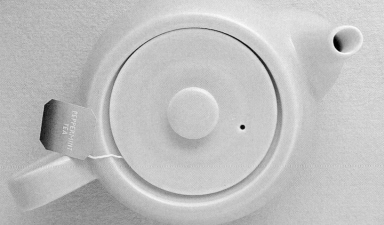

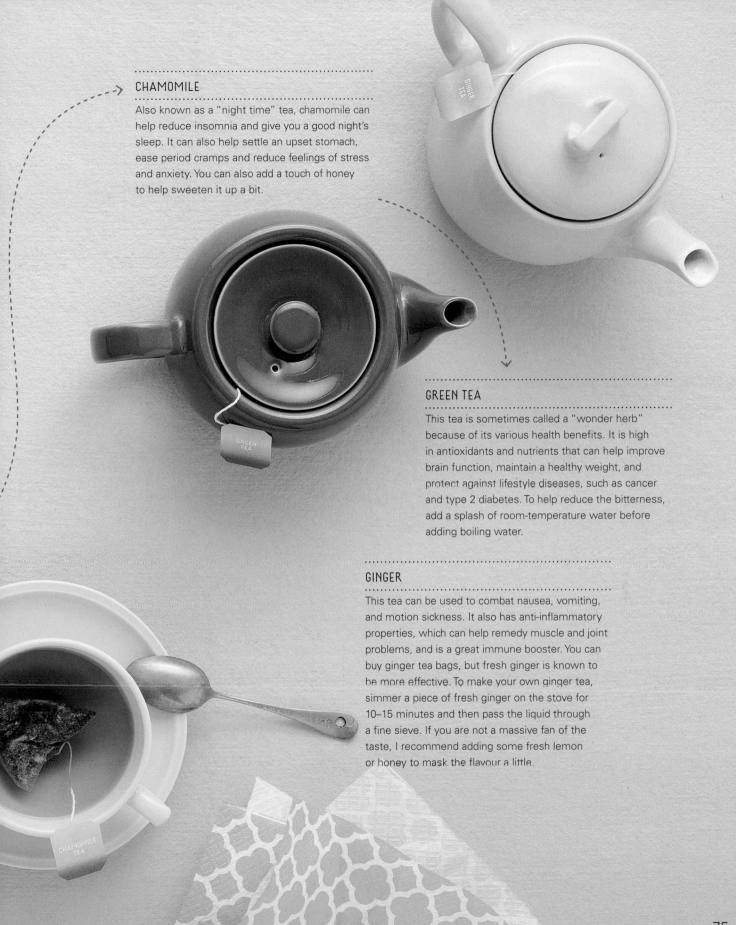

CHAMOMILE

Also known as a "night time" tea, chamomile can help reduce insomnia and give you a good night's sleep. It can also help settle an upset stomach, ease period cramps and reduce feelings of stress and anxiety. You can also add a touch of honey to help sweeten it up a bit.

GREEN TEA

This tea is sometimes called a "wonder herb" because of its various health benefits. It is high in antioxidants and nutrients that can help improve brain function, maintain a healthy weight, and protect against lifestyle diseases, such as cancer and type 2 diabetes. To help reduce the bitterness, add a splash of room-temperature water before adding boiling water.

GINGER

This tea can be used to combat nausea, vomiting, and motion sickness. It also has anti-inflammatory properties, which can help remedy muscle and joint problems, and is a great immune booster. You can buy ginger tea bags, but fresh ginger is known to be more effective. To make your own ginger tea, simmer a piece of fresh ginger on the stove for 10–15 minutes and then pass the liquid through a fine sieve. If you are not a massive fan of the taste, I recommend adding some fresh lemon or honey to mask the flavour a little.

COOKING TIPS & TRICKS

A little bit of organisation can go a long way to making your healthy lifestyle a lot more simple. Remember, simplicity is a key aspect in maintaining health. So here are some simple tips for preparing food, organising your fridge and freezer, and stocking up on the essentials!

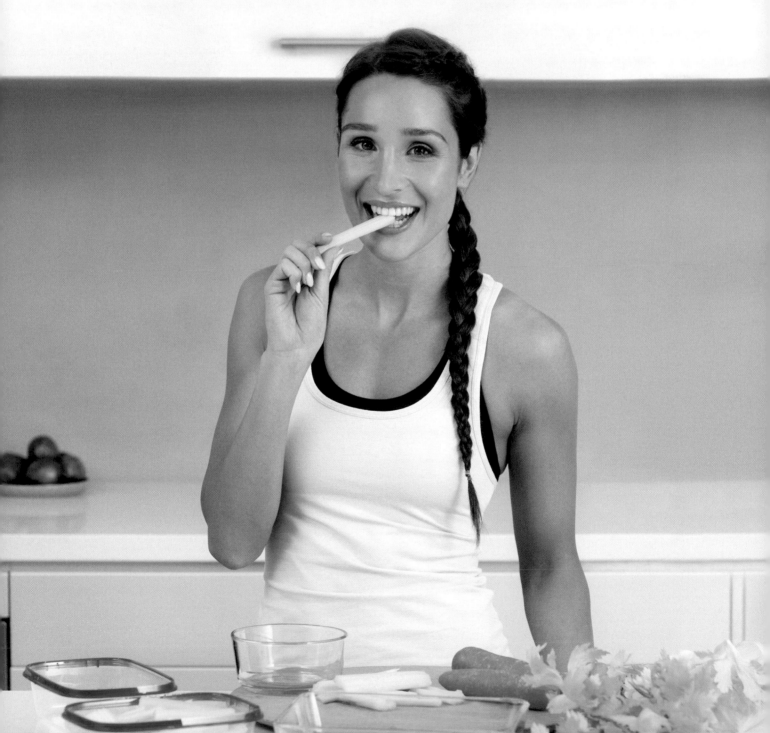

DID YOU KNOW THAT COOKING FOOD CAN CHANGE ITS WEIGHT?

When it comes to adjusting recipes to suit your taste preferences or swapping foods to tailor a meal plan to your needs, it is important to understand the effect that cooking has on an ingredient's weight. This is particularly important to remember for grains and protein foods (such as meat or beans) **as the servings sizes for these foods are based on their cooked value**.

When rice is cooked, it absorbs the water or liquid that it is cooked in, which causes its weight to increase. Meats like chicken will lose some water during the cooking process, causing their weight to decrease.

As a general rule:

- **The weight of grain foods will double or triple when cooked.**

- **The weight of meat foods will decrease by 20–30% when cooked.**

For example, 1 serving of grains is equivalent to 3 ounces of cooked brown rice or quinoa. So if you're wanting 1 serving of rice for lunch, make sure you're not adding 3 ounces of uncooked rice to the pot, as this will be too much!

Throughout this book, I have used raw or uncooked weights for the majority of grain and protein foods. If you are tailoring any of my recipes or creating your own using serving recommendations, it is important that you consider the change in weight of those ingredients for that particular meal. To help you with this, I have provided conversion charts on pages 372–373.

INGREDIENT SWAPS MADE EASY

If you don't like a particular food, you can replace it with another from the same food group. For example, if you don't like apples, when you make the Apple with Nut Butter on page 100, you can use 1 medium banana instead of 1 medium apple, and call it Banana with Nut Butter! See pages 370–371 for sample servings for each of the main food groups.

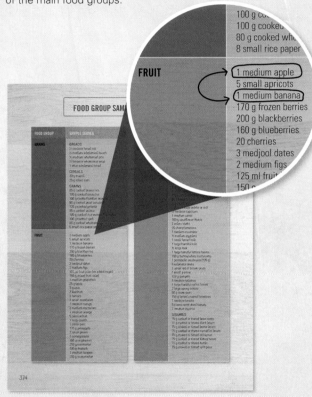

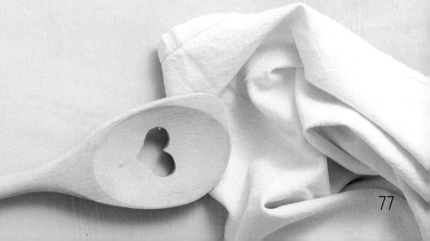

77

MEAL PREPARATION

Remember this saying from the front of the book: "Failing to plan is planning to fail"? This may sound a bit harsh, but it can certainly be true when it comes to healthy eating. Most of us are pretty busy in our day-to-day lives. Whether you are a mum, a student, working full time, or all three, it can be hard to cook all your meals at home each and every day. This is where meal preparation (or "meal prep") can quickly become your best friend! When you've had a busy day and are really hungry, and the last thing on your mind is preparing a meal from scratch, meal prep can help you avoid reaching for junk or convenience foods.

So, what is meal prep?

Meal prep is any sort of food preparation that can be done in advance to help you save time. It can vary from simply grouping ingredients together in a container in the fridge to slicing and chopping ahead of time or cooking entire meals. How much meal prep you do will depend on your lifestyle as well as the type of meals you are cooking.

If this is a relatively new concept for you, then you may need to use a little bit of trial and error until you find a routine that works. Just remember that there is no right or wrong way—how much or how little you do is completely up to you!

For example, if you grab a takeaway croissant for breakfast but you have no trouble cooking other meals, you might only need to prep breakfast meals. Likewise, if you struggle to make your dinner because you work late, you might only need to focus on preparing dinners. For some people, meal prep might involve preparing all their meals. It all depends on you and your lifestyle.

How do I do meal prep?

1 INVEST IN SOME GOOD-QUALITY CONTAINERS

The first step to successful meal prep is to invest in some good-quality airtight containers to store your food. These can be either glass or plastic (ideally BPA-free and microwave-safe if you are going to reheat food in them). If your plan is to prepare several days' worth of food at once, it is also a good idea to buy containers that are the same size so they stack easily in your fridge or your cupboard. No one likes having to play an unexpected game of Tetris when they're in a hurry!

REMEMBER, THERE ARE NO RULES FOR MEAL PREP! IF YOU CAN ONLY MANAGE A FEW DAYS' WORTH OF FOOD AT A TIME, THEN THAT IS FINE ... IT IS ALL ABOUT FINDING A ROUTINE AND A SYSTEM THAT WORKS FOR *YOU* AND *YOUR LIFESTYLE*.

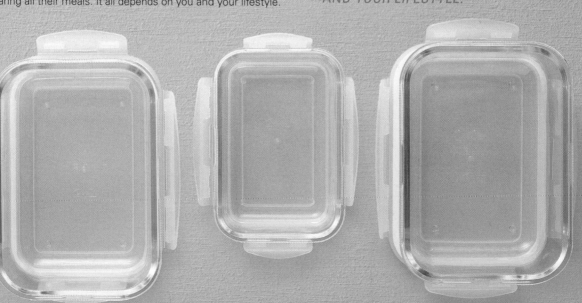

② WRITE A LIST

Now that you have your containers sorted, the next thing you need to do is to write a shopping list. There is no use going to the grocery store, throwing random things into your cart and hoping for the best ... every mission requires a well-thought-out plan! I recommend writing down the name of each breakfast, lunch, dinner, and/or snack meal that you will be preparing, and then breaking these down into a list of ingredients and amounts. Once you have done this for each of your meals, you can then write one comprehensive shopping list.

Once again, if you are new to meal prep, organising a whole week's worth of meals can be intimidating, so try to stick to a few days at a time if this seems more manageable. I also recommend sticking to tried and tested recipes, especially if you plan on cooking in bulk. There is nothing worse than spending money and time on a bunch of food that you don't really like the taste of!

SHOPPING LIST

GREEN SMOOTHIE BOWL

1 small handful baby spinach leaves

1 frozen medium banana, chopped

2⅓ oz strawberries

7 oz low-fat plain yoghurt

½ cup low-fat milk

¼ tsp matcha powder (optional)

1 oz natural muesli

1½ tsps goji berries

2 tsps chia seeds

③ GET PREPARING!

Once you have all your ingredients, it's time to start preparing. Sometimes the type of meal you are making will determine how much prep you should do. For example, salads and veggie sticks are best eaten fresh, so rather than chopping these up three days before, I just group them together in a container in the fridge and chop them up on the morning I need them. For more complex dishes, such as curries or stir-fries, I chop up all of the vegetables I need and pop them in a container in the fridge so they're ready to go when it's time to cook (except for ingredients that tend to go brown when chopped, such as potatoes or sweet potatoes, which I would leave until the last minute).

It's also really important that you consider food safety during your meal prep. Some foods, such as rice and meat, should not be kept in the fridge for more than a couple of days once cooked. While I sometimes cook these things in bulk, I will generally only prepare a few days' worth of ingredients at a time to avoid food-borne illnesses.

See pages 82–83 for all you need to know about how to prep veggies ...

④ STORE YOUR PREPARED FOOD CORRECTLY

Once you've finished preparing your meals, it is important that you store them correctly to prevent any risk of food poisoning. All fresh fruits, vegetables and cooked meals should be kept in the fridge, and then eaten as soon as possible once you remove them from the fridge. If you have made foods such as pasta sauces or soups in bulk, allow them to cool and then freeze what you won't eat within a couple of days.

⑤ ENJOY THE FRUITS OF YOUR LABOUR!

TURN THE PAGE TO SEE HOW I PREP FOR A TYPICAL DAY OF MY MEAL PLAN ...

Here's how I would prep a typical day's worth of meals from my meal plan

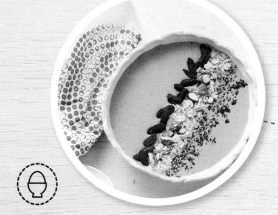

BREAKFAST

GREEN SMOOTHIE BOWL

If I was at home and in no particular rush, I would make my smoothie bowl fresh. To make things a little easier, I would put all of the ingredients together in a container beforehand so they're ready to put in the blender (but I would peel the banana at the last minute so that it doesn't go brown). I would measure out each of the toppings so I can sprinkle them on as soon as I'm done blending. If I was really short of time, I would blend the ingredients for the smoothie bowl together the night before and place them in a container in the fridge.* I would measure the toppings out and combine them in a single container, to sprinkle straight on to the smoothie bowl the next morning.

Just be wary that some smoothie bowl ingredients, such as spinach or berries, can lose their vibrant colour over time, so it's possible that your bowl might be a slightly different colour in the morning. This certainly doesn't mean it is no longer edible, it just might not look as pretty!

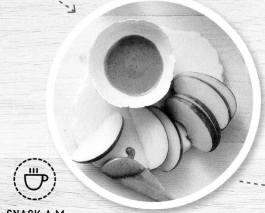

SNACK A.M.

APPLE with NUT BUTTER

I would thoroughly wash my apple and dry with paper towel. Apples tend to go brown once chopped, so if I had plenty of time I would slice it at the last minute. If not I would slice my apple before I left home and store it in a container with a squeeze of fresh lemon juice to slow down that natural browning process. I would weigh out my nut butter in advance and place it in a container in the fridge.

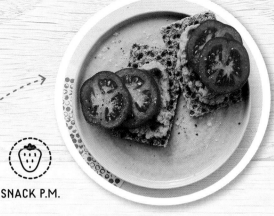

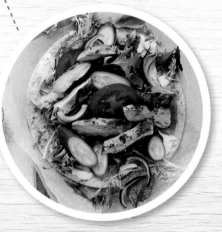

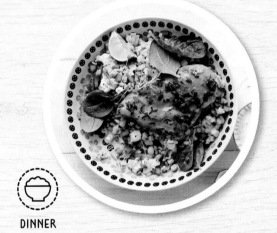

SNACK P.M.

CRISPBREADS with HUMMUS and TOMATO

Like the tzatziki, if I needed hummus for a few different meals, I would make a big batch and then weigh it out into smaller containers. I would wash and dry the tomato and keep it in the fridge in the same container as my crispbreads, and slice it just before serving.

DINNER

PERI PERI CHICKEN with RICE SALAD

Brown rice is a staple for me, so I cook it in batches and store it in the refrigerator. **Remember though: cooked rice should not be kept any longer than a few days. I wouldn't suggest cooking a week's worth all in one go.** I would pre-marinate the chicken and keep it in the freezer to defrost when I need it. To help make the rice salad a little easier to prepare, I would place the bell pepper, onion, and cucumber together in a container in the fridge, but only chop them up at the last minute before adding the corn and spinach. The yoghurt dressing could also be made the night before, or fresh on the day depending on how much time you have.

LUNCH

CHICKEN GYROS

Tzatziki is a staple I use all the time—to dip freshly cut vegetables in, or as a sauce for a gyro, in a wrap or with my favourite cooked protein. As it can last a few days in the fridge, I make a large batch and then weigh it out into smaller containers for each of the meals I plan to use it. For the chicken, I would pre-slice and marinate it in advance, then I would cook the chicken and store it in a container in the fridge overnight, ready to reheat it in the microwave just before serving. However, if I was not eating it for a couple of days, I would freeze the sliced, marinated chicken and defrost it ready to cook the night before I needed it. I would place the vegetables in a container and slice them fresh the morning of or just before serving. This meal is an excellent example of how meal prep can be flexible. Remember that it is not always possible to prep all of your meals in advance, so it is important to adapt to suit the meal or how busy you are.

As you can see, setting some time aside to prepare your meals can make healthy eating easy!

VEGETABLE PREPARATION TECHNIQUES

SLICING is usually the first cutting technique we learn. It involves cutting food crossways or lengthways to a desired thickness. It is also the start of other cutting techniques such as julienne and diced. Sliced vegetables can be used in sandwiches or salads, for example.

JULIENNE means to cut into thin, long matchstick-like strips. This cut works best for harder vegetables such as carrots, beetroot, and bell pepper.

SHREDDING can be achieved with a grater or a knife depending on your skill level or the vegetable you are using. Vegetables such as carrots, cucumbers, and zucchini are best shredded using a grater. For vegetables such as Chinese cabbage, lettuce, and other leafy greens, it is easier to shred them with a knife.

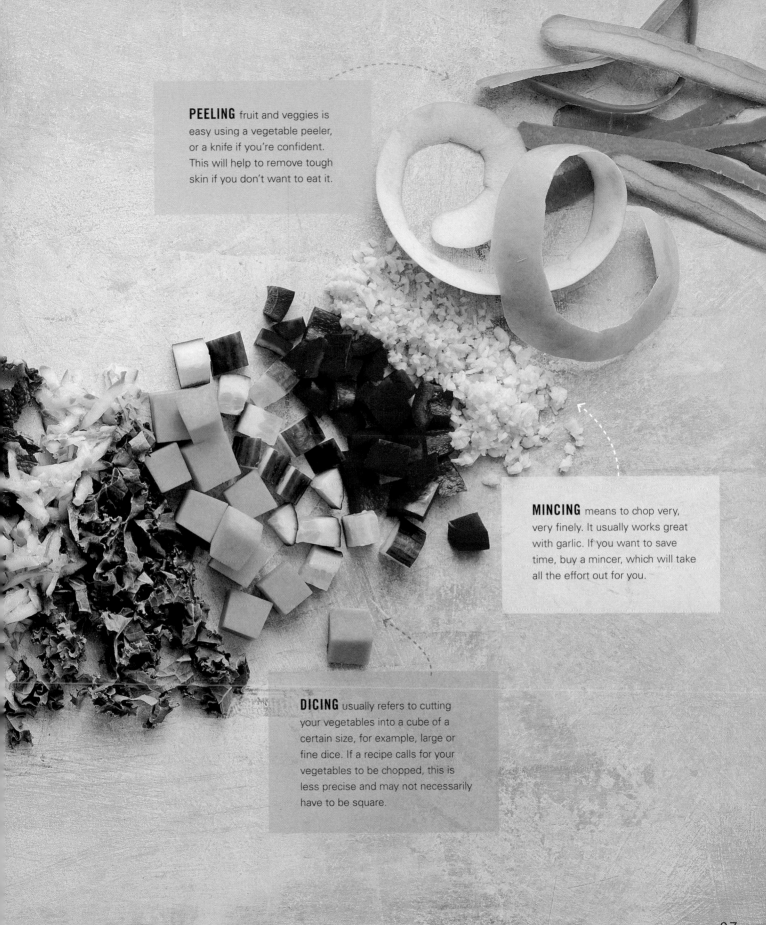

PEELING fruit and veggies is easy using a vegetable peeler, or a knife if you're confident. This will help to remove tough skin if you don't want to eat it.

MINCING means to chop very, very finely. It usually works great with garlic. If you want to save time, buy a mincer, which will take all the effort out for you.

DICING usually refers to cutting your vegetables into a cube of a certain size, for example, large or fine dice. If a recipe calls for your vegetables to be chopped, this is less precise and may not necessarily have to be square.

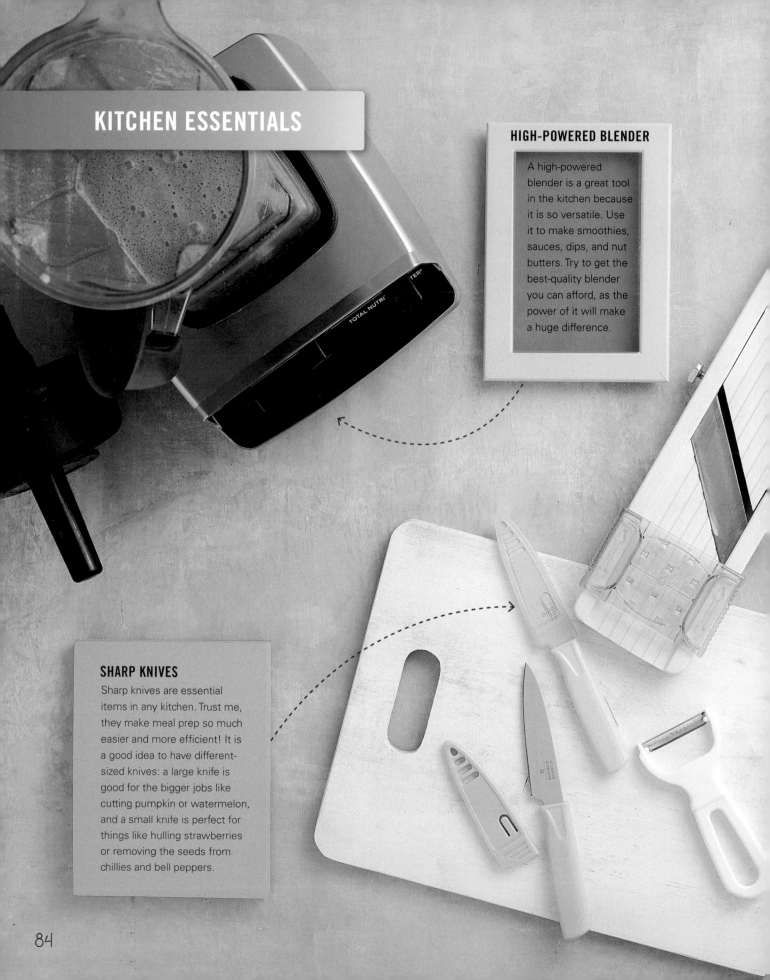

KITCHEN ESSENTIALS

HIGH-POWERED BLENDER

A high-powered blender is a great tool in the kitchen because it is so versatile. Use it to make smoothies, sauces, dips, and nut butters. Try to get the best-quality blender you can afford, as the power of it will make a huge difference.

SHARP KNIVES

Sharp knives are essential items in any kitchen. Trust me, they make meal prep so much easier and more efficient! It is a good idea to have different-sized knives: a large knife is good for the bigger jobs like cutting pumpkin or watermelon, and a small knife is perfect for things like hulling strawberries or removing the seeds from chillies and bell peppers.

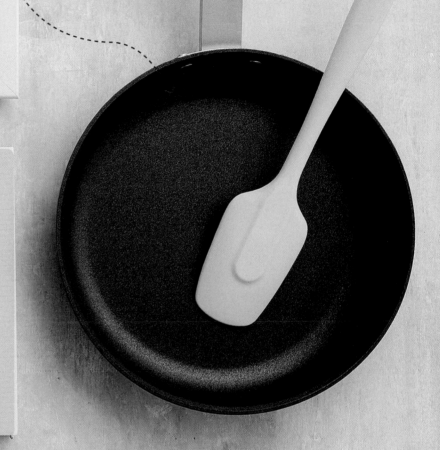

NON-STICK FRY PAN

A good-quality non-stick fry pan is absolutely essential in my kitchen. By choosing a non-stick one you should be able to reduce or even eliminate the need to use oils and fats to cook your food. Good-quality fry pans cook your food evenly and are generally easier to clean.

MANDOLINE & JULIENNE PEELER

This is a handy kitchen gadget that can save you a lot of time! A mandoline will slice your fruit and vegetables super-fine, super-quick. Most mandolines come with a separate julienne attachment that you can use to quickly whip up a salad using veggies such as cucumbers, carrots, and beetroot.

CHOPPING BOARDS

Chopping boards are an essential item in any kitchen. I recommend having separate boards for meats and fresh fruits and vegetables, to prevent contamination. Wooden boards are great, as they have natural antibacterial properties and can last a really long time if you look after them properly. They are also gentle on your knives. Plastic boards are cheap, so it's easy to have a few different-coloured ones to help avoid cross-contamination (and being cheap, when they look a bit overused they are easy to replace). Glass or marble boards look good but can blunt your knives and have very little grip when you are chopping food.

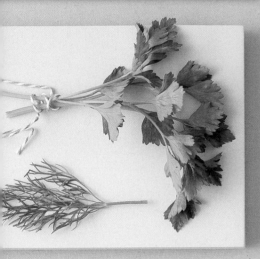

CONDIMENTS

HERBS & SPICES

One of the best ways to add flavour and zest to your meals is with herbs (dried or fresh) and spices. Here are some of my favourites.

BASIL is great for adding flavour to a pasta sauce, or try adding a few fresh basil leaves to your wraps.

CHILLI POWDER will add a kick to any dish. Just remember to start with small amounts and then increase to your liking.

CINNAMON complements both sweet and savoury dishes. Simply use it to top your toast or low-fat yoghurt, or stir it into your porridge with some toasted nuts. Use it in cooked fruit dishes. It can also be added to stews and chillis in combination with other spices.

CUMIN, together with **CHILLI POWDER** and **GARLIC**, can season vegetables or Mexican-style dishes.

DILL is great with fresh vegetables and salmon. It also pairs especially well with cucumbers, making it a great addition to homemade tzatziki.

DRIED OR FRESH THYME is especially tasty when used to season beans or egg dishes. You can sprinkle it with a small amount of olive oil over vegetables, such as potatoes, before roasting them. It also goes well with lemon.

MINT can be used to make iced or hot tea. Add it to a grain salad with dried fruit and nuts, or toss it with fresh berries for a refreshing and healthy dessert.

OREGANO is especially good in tomato-based dishes, and is very common in Italian and Greek cooking. Use it in soups or sprinkle it over vegetables before cooking. Also try sprinkling it over homemade pizzas.

PARSLEY can be a main ingredient in salads, such as tabouli, or can be used as a garnish for a bit of extra flavour. Toss some fresh parsley through brown or wild rice with a squeeze of lemon juice. Or add it to soups, pasta dishes, eggs, or salads.

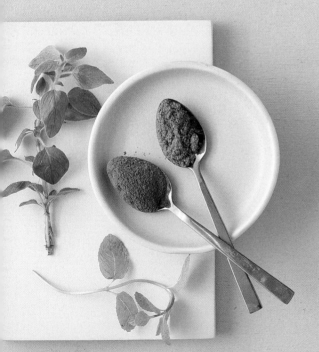

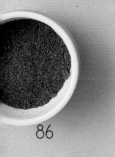

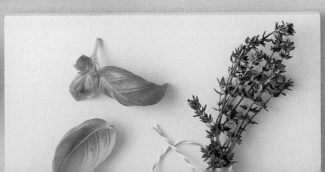

COOKING OILS

There are many different types of oils out there, and often people don't realise that some are better suited to certain cooking methods than others. Some oils are suited to cooking with at high heat, while others are best kept away from heat altogether and just used for their flavour in a dressing. I always try to select the oil that is best suited to the cooking method and flavour of the dish. Regardless of your choice of oil, it is important to remember that oils are quite calorie-dense and therefore should be used in moderation.

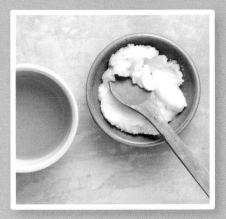

These oils are suitable for cooking at high heat.

AVOCADO OIL This oil is full of healthy fats and very versatile when it comes to cooking—it's suitable for sautéing, frying, stir-frying, and baking. Its lovely flavour makes it a great addition to dressings.

PEANUT OIL Peanut oil has a distinctive nutty flavour and is perfect for stir-fries and Asian dishes. It contains heart-healthy plant sterols (an essential plant fat), which are known to lower cholesterol.

RICE BRAN OIL Rice bran oil is extracted from the germ of rice grains. It has a mild flavour and is suitable for any type of cooking. It is rich in antioxidants, vitamin E, and plant sterols.

These oils break down more easily when exposed to light, heat, and air, which means they are not the best option to choose when cooking.

CHIA SEED OIL This oil is high in omega-3 fatty acids, which are essential for overall health and to help combat inflammation in the body. It has a neutral flavour that works well in salad dressings and smoothies. It is best kept in the fridge.

FLAXSEED OIL This oil is also an excellent source of omega-3 fatty acids. It can work well in salad dressings or drizzled over steamed vegetables. It is best kept in the fridge.

Some oils have amazing health benefits because of their nutritional content but may not be suitable to cook with over high heat as they can break down (oxidise) and potentially create unhealthy trans fats during this process. The following oils are suitable for cooking at low- medium heat.

OLIVE OIL Olive oil is considered a heart healthy oil as it helps to raise good (HDL) cholesterol and lower bad (LDL) cholesterol. It is suitable for cooking, like sautéing over low heat, but really shines in salad dressings, cold dishes, or drizzled over steamed vegetables. You may have noticed there are a few different types of olive oil. Extra virgin olive oil generally has more antioxidants and a bolder flavour than the others.

COCONUT OIL Coconut oil is suitable for baking or sautéing. It can have a distinctive taste, so can alter the flavour of the dish you use it in. This "coconutty" flavour can work well in soups, stews, curries, and baking, as well as in raw desserts. Coconut oil can be stored in the cupboard for months without going "off."

SESAME OIL There are two types of sesame oil: light (made from untoasted sesame seeds) and dark (made from toasted sesame seeds). Sesame oil may be linked to lowering blood pressure and reducing the risk of heart disease. While sesame oil has quite a distinctive taste it can work really well in salad dressings and Asian sauces.

ORGANISING YOUR FRIDGE FOR MAXIMUM FRESHNESS

Anybody who lives a healthy lifestyle knows the struggle is real when it comes to consuming your fruits and veggies before they go bad. Most people don't have time to go food shopping every two or three days, so they buy their produce in bulk once a week, hoping to get through it all. Sometimes life happens and we don't manage to eat everything, so inevitably we end up throwing some out. Knowing how to store food in your fridge correctly can minimise this problem, and help your produce stay fresher for MUCH longer!

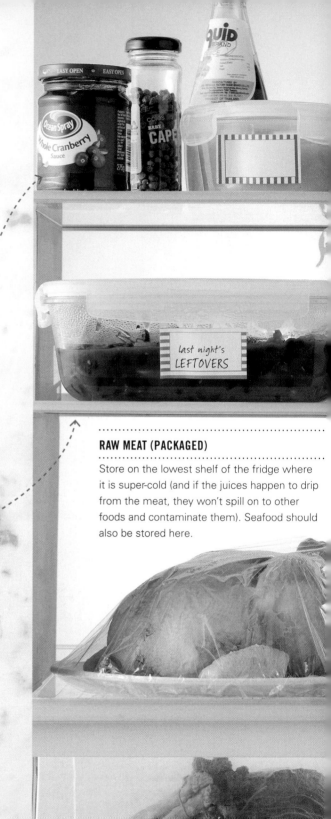

CONDIMENTS

Condiments, such as sauces and dressings, should go in the fridge doors because they are the least prone to spoiling and the doors are the warmest part of the fridge. You can also store drinks there too, just not dairy-based ones.

LEFTOVERS & READY-TO-EAT FOODS

Store foods such as leftovers, hummus, and other ready-to-eat foods on the top shelf. You can also store drinks here. Fresh herbs can be stored on the upper shelves in a jar filled with water.

FRUITS & VEGETABLES

Whole fruits and veggies belong in the crisper drawer, which may have separate compartments, so you can have your veggies on one side where there is low humidity, and your fruit on the other. Keep them in their original packaging or in a plastic bag if possible. If you have a crisper that isn't separated into two compartments, try to keep fruits and veggies away from each other—many fruits contain a chemical called ethylene that causes them to ripen faster and this may affect your veggies.

RAW MEAT (PACKAGED)

Store on the lowest shelf of the fridge where it is super-cold (and if the juices happen to drip from the meat, they won't spill on to other foods and contaminate them). Seafood should also be stored here.

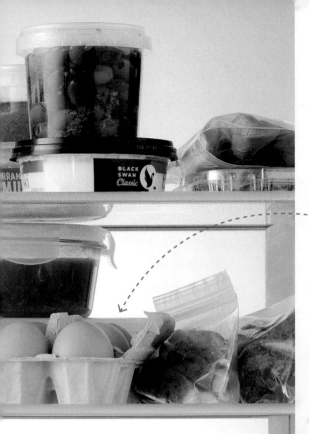

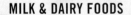

EGGS

These are best stored where the temperature is most consistent, which is not—contrary to what you may have been told—in the fridge doors! Store them on the middle shelf and keep them in their cartons instead of transferring them to egg holders.

MILK & DAIRY FOODS

Milk should be on the bottom shelf where it is coldest, all the way at the back. This also applies to yoghurts, cottage cheese, and the like.

THINGS NOT TO REFRIGERATE

Some things just shouldn't be refrigerated even though they may fall into one of the above categories. Potatoes, onions, and pumpkins should be stored in a cool, dark area with low moisture, such as a cupboard or pantry. Tomatoes also don't like to be refrigerated so keep those at room temperature.

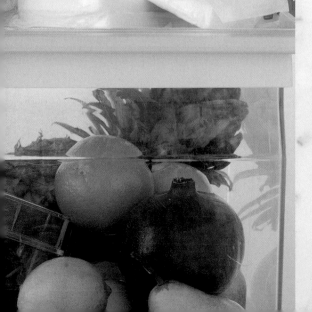

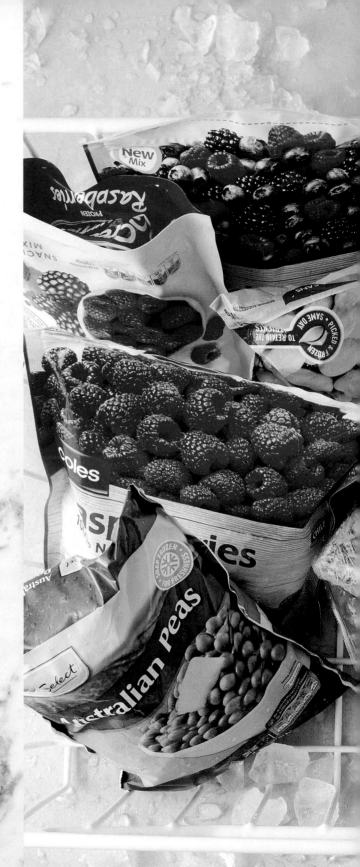

ORGANISING YOUR FREEZER

To avoid being stuck with a week's worth of the same meal, I recommend dividing food into smaller, meal-size portions before freezing, so you only take out the amount you need. Unfortunately, nothing lasts forever, so it is important that you follow recommended freezing times for foods.

RED MEAT (FRESH)	4–12 MONTHS, DEPENDING ON TYPE
RED MEAT (COOKED)	2–3 MONTHS
POULTRY (FRESH)	9–12 MONTHS
POULTRY (COOKED)	4–6 MONTHS
FISH AND SHELLFISH	2–6 MONTHS, DEPENDING ON TYPE
LEFTOVER MEALS (SOUPS, STEWS, AND CASSEROLES)	2–3 MONTHS

THAWING

When thawing frozen meat such as chicken or beef, place it in a container and store it in the bottom of your fridge. Make sure that the meat is thawed all the way through before using. This may take one to two days from the time you take it out of the freezer.

When defrosting leftover meals, allow these to thaw in your fridge as above. It is important to never re-freeze food that has already been frozen and then thawed. This is to avoid the potential risk of food poisoning from harmful bacteria.

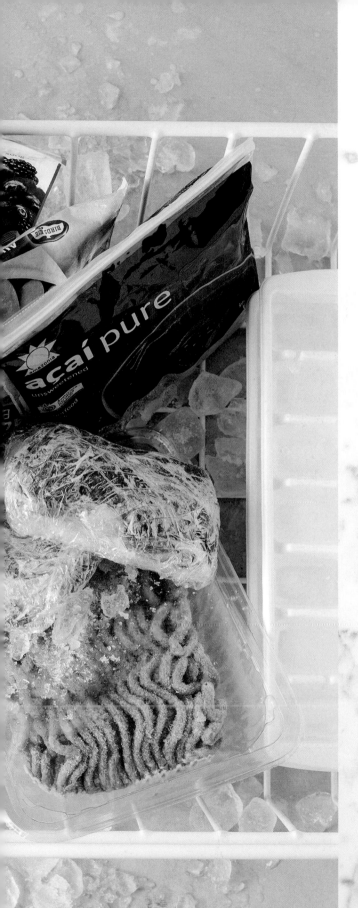

NOURISH YOUR BODY WITH WHOLESOME FOODS AND EXERCISE REGULARLY.

You deserve to feel amazing!

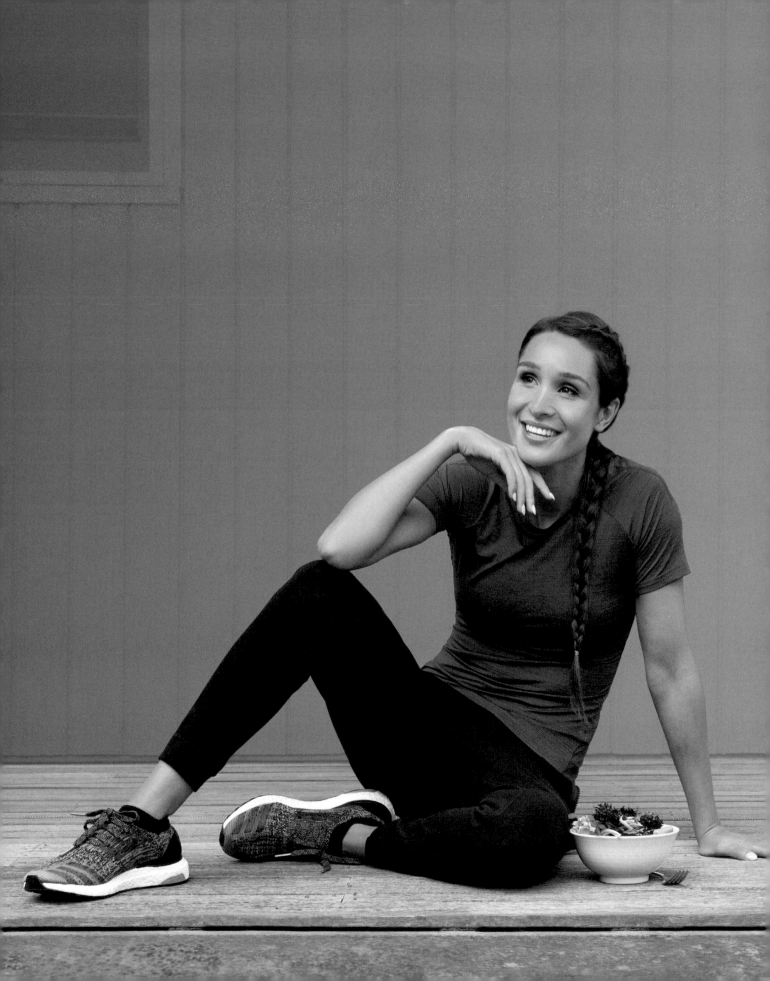

2

RECIPES
FOR THE
28-DAY
MEAL PLAN

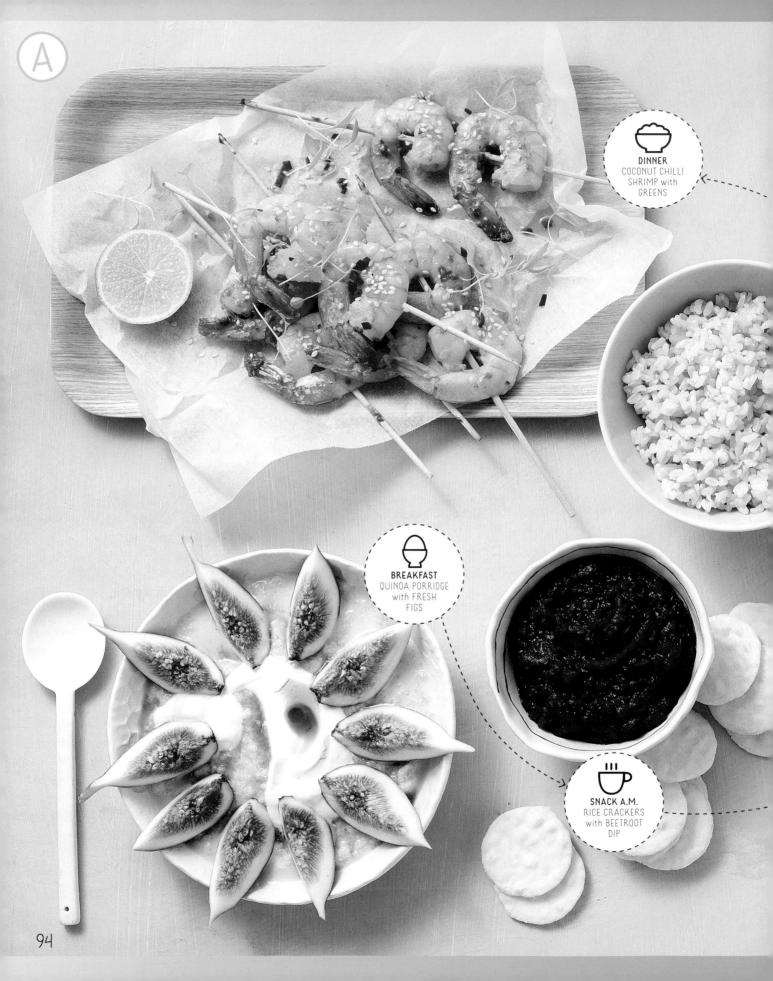

A

DINNER
COCONUT CHILLI
SHRIMP with
GREENS

BREAKFAST
QUINOA PORRIDGE
with FRESH
FIGS

SNACK A.M.
RICE CRACKERS
with BEETROOT
DIP

94

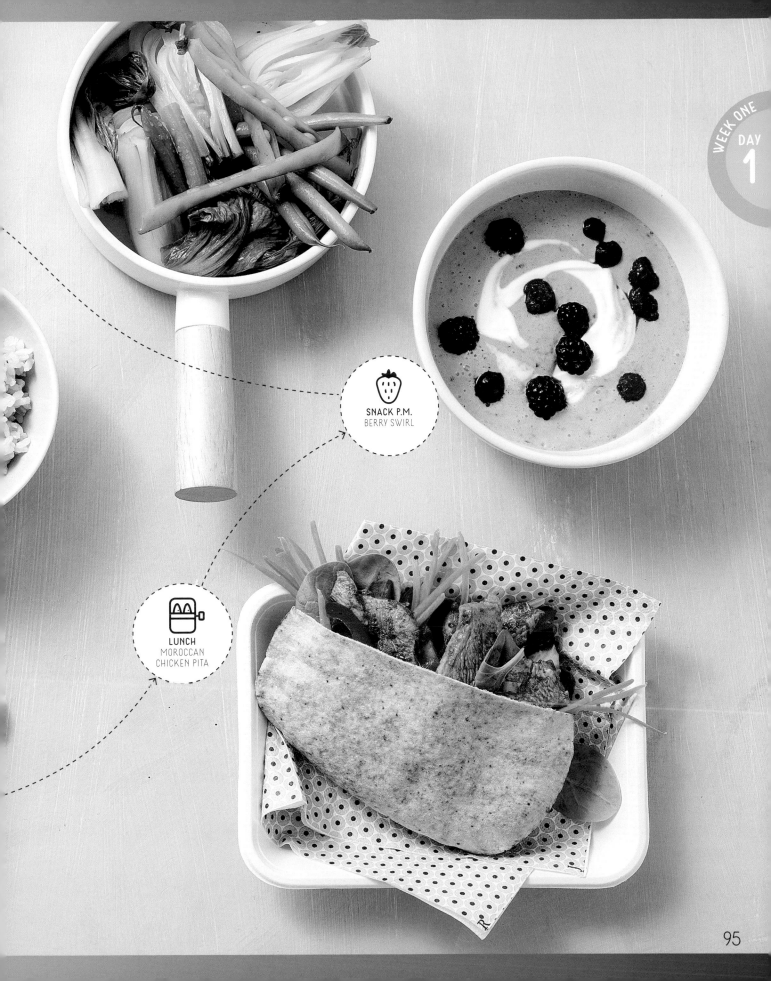

SNACK P.M.
BERRY SWIRL

LUNCH
MOROCCAN
CHICKEN PITA

QUINOA PORRIDGE with FRESH FIGS

BREAKFAST | **SERVES** 1 | **PREP TIME** 5 MINUTES | **COOKING TIME** 5 MINUTES | **DIFFICULTY** EASY

½ teaspoon pure vanilla extract

½ cup low-fat milk

3 oz quinoa flakes

3½ oz low-fat plain yoghurt

2 teaspoons pure maple syrup

2 medium figs, sliced

In a small saucepan, bring ½ cup of water, vanilla, and half of the milk to the boil over high heat. Add the quinoa and reduce the heat to low. Simmer for 5 minutes or until thickened, stirring occasionally.

Meanwhile, place the yoghurt and maple syrup in a small bowl and mix until well combined.

To serve, pour the quinoa porridge into a bowl. Top with the remaining milk, sliced figs, and maple yoghurt.

RICE CRACKERS with BEETROOT DIP

SNACK A.M. | **SERVES** 1 | **PREP TIME** 5 MINUTES | **DIFFICULTY** EASY

1 small beetroot, scrubbed and grated

2¾ oz tinned cannellini beans, drained and rinsed

¼ garlic clove, crushed

pinch of ground coriander

pinch of ground cumin

pinch of sweet paprika

lemon juice, to taste

sea salt and ground black pepper, to taste

12 plain rice crackers

Place the beetroot, cannellini beans, garlic, coriander, cumin, paprika, and 2 teaspoons of water in a food processor and process until smooth. Season with lemon juice, salt, and pepper, if desired.

Place the beetroot dip in a small bowl and serve with the rice crackers.

MOROCCAN CHICKEN PITA

LUNCH | **SERVES** 1 | **PREP TIME** 10 MINUTES + 30 MINUTES MARINATING TIME | **COOKING TIME** 8 MINUTES | **DIFFICULTY** EASY

¼ teaspoon cayenne pepper

¼ teaspoon ground cinnamon

½ teaspoon ground cumin

½ teaspoon ground coriander

½ teaspoon smoked paprika

1 teaspoon sea salt

½ garlic clove, crushed

juice of ½ lemon

3½ oz boneless skinless chicken breast, cut into thin strips

oil spray

1 small handful baby spinach leaves

¼ medium red bell pepper, seeds removed and thinly sliced

½ medium carrot, grated

½ medium tomato, chopped

½ whole wheat pita bread

Place the cayenne, cinnamon, cumin, coriander, paprika, salt, garlic, and lemon juice in a small bowl and stir until well combined. Place the chicken in the bowl and rub with the spice mix. Ensure that all the chicken is coated. Cover with plastic wrap and refrigerate for 30 minutes to marinate.

Heat a non-stick fry pan over medium heat and spray lightly with oil spray. Add the chicken strips and cook for 3–4 minutes on each side or until lightly browned and cooked through. Remove from the heat and set aside.

To serve, layer the chicken, spinach, bell pepper, carrot, and tomato within the pita half.

BERRY SWIRL

SNACK P.M. | **SERVES** 1 | **PREP TIME** 5 MINUTES | **DIFFICULTY** EASY

6 oz frozen mixed berries, thawed

10¾ oz low-fat plain yoghurt

Place half of the berries and half of the yoghurt in a high-powered blender and blend until smooth.

To serve, place the remaining yoghurt in a serving bowl. Add the berry yoghurt and swirl through with a spoon. Top with the remaining berries.

COCONUT CHILLI SHRIMP with GREENS

DINNER | **SERVES** 2 | **PREP TIME** 15 MINUTES + 1–2 HOURS MARINATING TIME | **COOKING TIME** 35 MINUTES | **DIFFICULTY** EASY

½ cup light coconut milk

finely grated zest and juice of 1 lime

1 garlic clove, crushed

1 fresh long red chilli, finely chopped

2 teaspoons fish sauce

2 teaspoons salt-reduced tamari or soy sauce

20 medium raw shrimp, peeled and deveined, tails intact

4¼ oz brown rice

½ lb bok choy, chopped

15 green beans, trimmed and halved

3 oz snow peas, trimmed

1 tablespoon chopped fresh cilantro

⅔ oz sesame seeds

lime wedges, to serve

Whisk the coconut milk, lime zest and juice, garlic, chilli, fish sauce, and tamari or soy sauce together in a large bowl. Add the shrimp and toss well to combine. Cover with plastic wrap and refrigerate for 1–2 hours to marinate, if possible.

Soak 10 wooden skewers in cold water for 30 minutes. This will help stop them from burning when cooking the shrimp.

Place the rice and 1¼ cups of water in a small saucepan over high heat and bring to the boil, stirring occasionally. Cover and reduce the heat to medium–low. Simmer for 20–25 minutes or until the liquid is absorbed and the rice is tender. Remove from the heat and leave to stand, covered, for 5 minutes.

Preheat the barbecue or chargrill over medium–high heat. Thread the shrimp onto the skewers. Grill for about 3 minutes on each side or until cooked to your liking. Once cooked, brush over again with the marinade.

Fill a saucepan with water until 2 in deep and insert a steamer basket. Cover with a lid and bring the water to the boil over high heat, then reduce the heat to medium. Add the bok choy and green beans and steam for 3 minutes, covered. Add the snow peas and steam for a further 2–3 minutes or until the vegetables are tender-crisp.

To serve, place the rice, shrimp skewers, and steamed greens on two serving plates. Sprinkle over the sesame seeds and cilantro. Serve with lime wedges on the side.

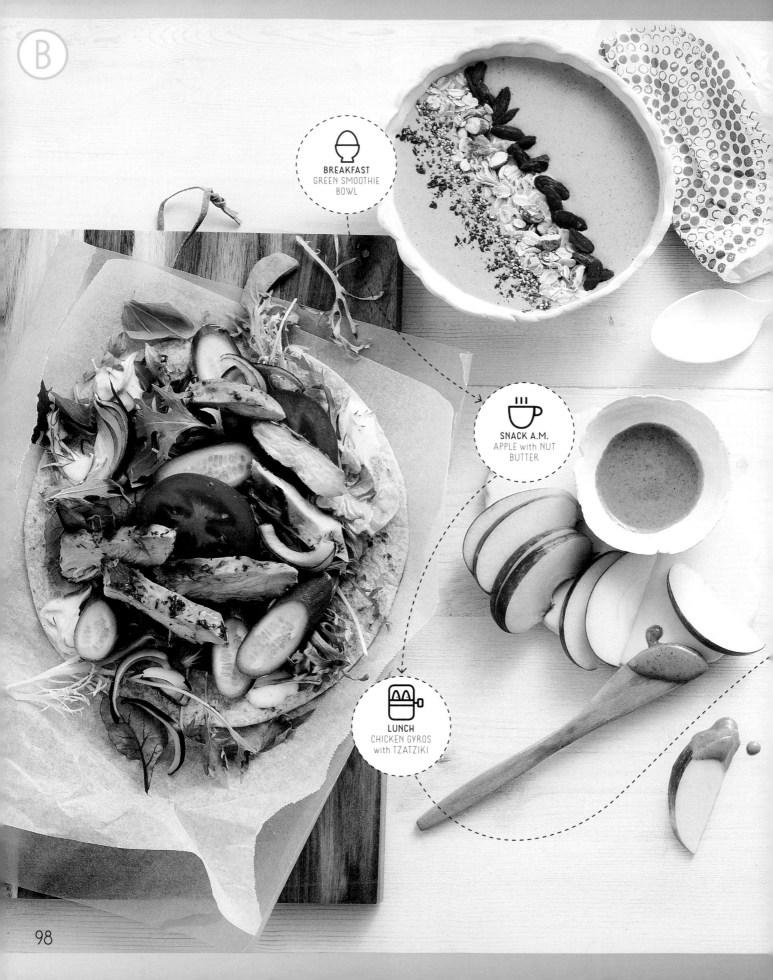

B

BREAKFAST
GREEN SMOOTHIE
BOWL

SNACK A.M.
APPLE with NUT
BUTTER

LUNCH
CHICKEN GYROS
with TZATZIKI

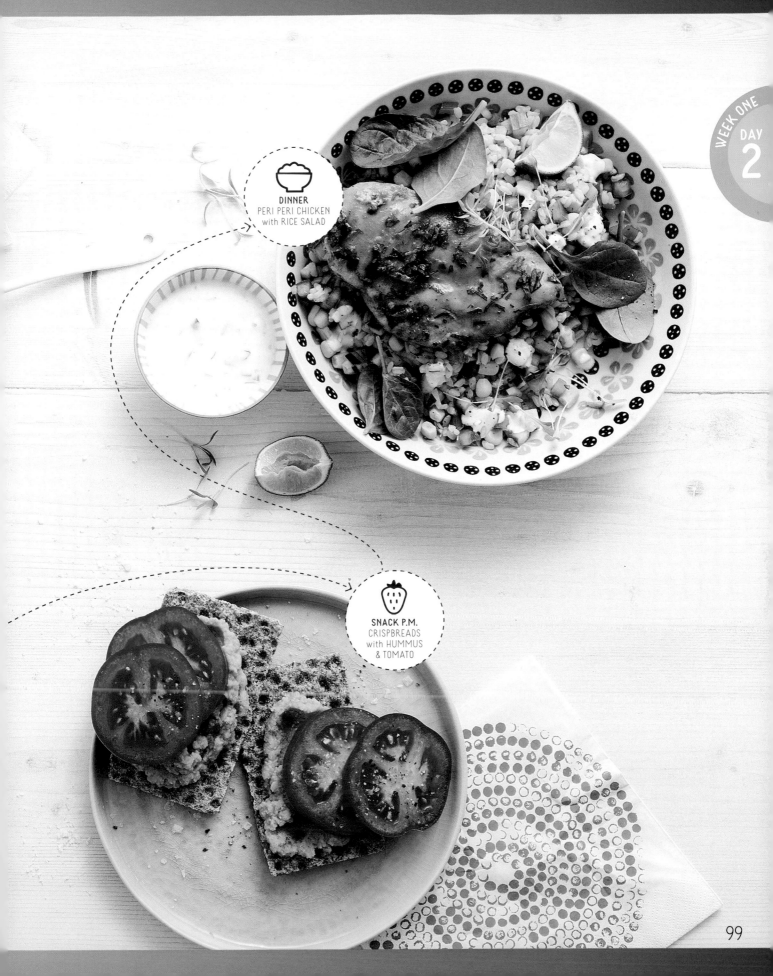

DINNER
PERI PERI CHICKEN
with RICE SALAD

SNACK P.M.
CRISPBREADS
with HUMMUS
& TOMATO

GREEN SMOOTHIE BOWL

1 small handful baby
spinach leaves

1 frozen medium banana,
chopped

2⅓ oz strawberries

7 oz low-fat plain yoghurt

½ cup low-fat milk

¼ teaspoon matcha (green
tea) powder (optional)

TOPPINGS

1 oz natural muesli

1½ teaspoons goji berries

2 teaspoons chia seeds

Place the spinach, banana, strawberries, yoghurt, milk,
and matcha (if using) in a high-powered blender and
blend until smooth.

To serve, pour the smoothie mixture into a serving bowl
and top with the muesli, goji berries, and chia seeds.

APPLE with NUT BUTTER

SNACK A.M. | **SERVES** 1 | **PREP TIME** 2 MINUTES | **DIFFICULTY** EASY

2 teaspoons 100% natural
nut butter of your choice

½ medium apple, cored
and sliced

To serve, spread the nut butter over the apple slices.

CHICKEN GYROS with TZATZIKI

LUNCH | **SERVES** 1 | **PREP TIME** 15 MINUTES + 30 MINUTES MARINATING TIME | **COOKING TIME** 15 MINUTES | **DIFFICULTY** EASY

3½ oz boneless skinless
chicken breast, cut into
bite-sized pieces

1 whole wheat wrap

3½ oz tzatziki (see page 254)

½ medium tomato, sliced

¼ Lebanese cucumber, sliced

¼ small red onion, thinly
sliced

1 small handful lettuce leaves

MARINADE

½ garlic clove, crushed

1 teaspoon lemon juice

½ teaspoon finely chopped
fresh rosemary

½ teaspoon finely chopped
fresh oregano

To make the marinade, whisk the garlic, lemon juice,
rosemary, and oregano together in a medium bowl.

Place the chicken in the bowl containing the marinade and
stir to combine. Cover with plastic wrap and refrigerate for
30 minutes to marinate.

Heat a non-stick fry pan over medium–high heat and
spray lightly with oil spray. Add the chicken and cook for
8–12 minutes or until the chicken is cooked through, stirring
occasionally. Transfer to a heatproof bowl and set aside.
To save time, the chicken can be marinated and cooked
the night before and stored in an airtight container in
the refrigerator.

To serve, place the wrap on a serving plate. Spread half
of the tzatziki over the wrap and place the chicken,
tomato, cucumber, onion, and lettuce down the middle.
Fold over the end and roll up to enclose the filling.
Drizzle over the remaining tzatziki.

CRISPBREADS with HUMMUS & TOMATO

2¾ oz hummus (see page 254)

2 rye crispbreads

1 medium tomato, sliced

ground black pepper, to taste

To serve, spread the hummus over the crispbreads.
Top with the tomato and season with pepper, if desired.

PERI PERI CHICKEN with RICE SALAD

DINNER | SERVES 2 | PREP TIME 15 MINUTES + 1 HOUR MARINATING TIME | COOKING TIME 35 MINUTES | DIFFICULTY EASY

7 oz boneless skinless
chicken breast

oil spray

lime wedges, to serve

MARINADE

2 garlic cloves, crushed

¾ in fresh ginger, peeled
and grated

juice of 1 lemon

2 teaspoons honey

½ teaspoon dried chilli flakes

½ teaspoon sweet paprika

2 tablespoons chopped
fresh parsley

sea salt and ground black
pepper, to taste

RICE SALAD

4¼ oz brown rice

½ medium green bell pepper,
finely diced

½ small red onion,
finely diced

1 Lebanese cucumber,
finely diced

2 oz frozen corn kernels,
thawed

1 small handful baby spinach
leaves, shredded

DRESSING

7 oz low-fat plain yoghurt

lime juice, to taste

1 tablespoon chopped
fresh cilantro

To make the marinade, whisk the garlic, ginger, lemon juice, honey, chilli, paprika, parsley, salt, pepper, and 1 tablespoon of water together in a medium bowl.

Place the chicken in the bowl and rub with the marinade. Cover with plastic wrap and refrigerate for 1 hour to marinate.

To make the rice salad, place the rice and 1¼ cups (300 ml) of water in a small saucepan over high heat and bring to the boil, stirring occasionally. Cover and reduce the heat to medium–low. Simmer for 20–25 minutes or until the liquid is absorbed and the rice is tender. Remove from the heat and let stand, covered, for 5 minutes. Set aside to cool.

Place the rice, bell pepper, onion, cucumber, corn, and spinach in a bowl and toss gently to combine.

To make the dressing, whisk the yoghurt, lime juice, and cilantro together in a small bowl.

Heat a non-stick fry pan over medium heat and spray lightly with oil spray. Add the chicken and cook for 4–6 minutes on each side or until cooked through. Set aside to cool slightly.

To serve, place the rice salad on two serving plates and top with the peri peri chicken. Drizzle over the yoghurt dressing and serve with lime wedges on the side.

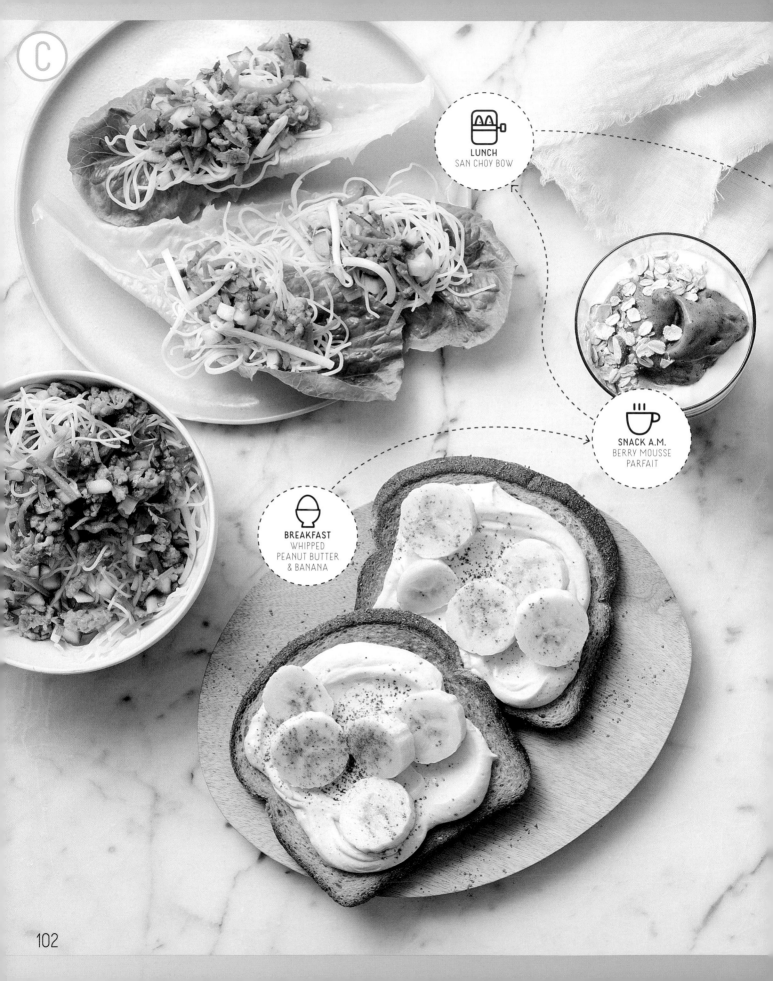

LUNCH
SAN CHOY BOW

SNACK A.M.
BERRY MOUSSE
PARFAIT

BREAKFAST
WHIPPED
PEANUT BUTTER
& BANANA

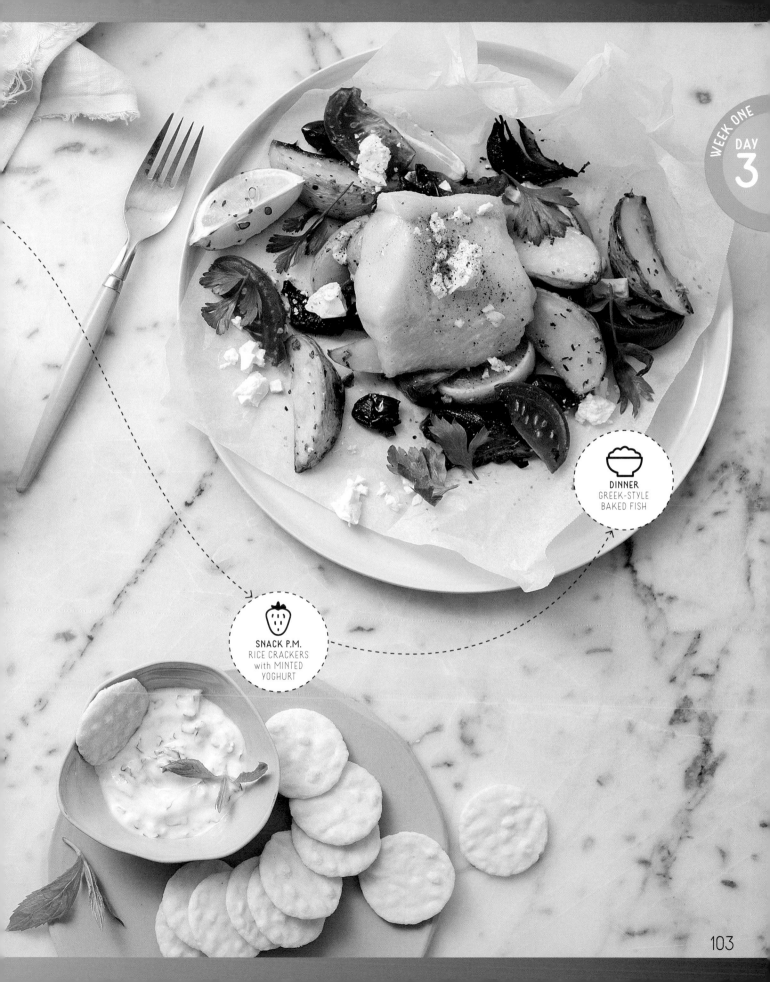

DINNER
GREEK-STYLE
BAKED FISH

SNACK P.M.
RICE CRACKERS
with MINTED
YOGHURT

103

WHIPPED PEANUT BUTTER & BANANA

BREAKFAST | SERVES 1 | **PREP TIME** 5 MINUTES | **COOKING TIME** 2 MINUTES | **DIFFICULTY** EASY

2 slices whole wheat bread

½ medium banana,
peeled and sliced

½ teaspoon raw cacao powder
(see page 49; optional)

WHIPPED PEANUT BUTTER

3 teaspoons 100% natural
peanut butter

5¼ oz low-fat plain yoghurt

Toast the bread to your liking.

To make the whipped peanut butter, place the peanut butter and yoghurt in a small bowl. Using a hand-held beater, whip the peanut butter and yoghurt until light and fluffy.

To serve, spread the whipped peanut butter over the toast and top with the banana. Lightly dust with cacao powder, if desired.

BERRY MOUSSE PARFAIT

SNACK A.M. | SERVES 1 | **PREP TIME** 5 MINUTES + 10 MINUTES CHILLING TIME | **DIFFICULTY** EASY

7 oz low-fat plain yoghurt

9 oz frozen mixed berries,
thawed

1 oz natural muesli

Place half of the yoghurt and half of the berries in a high-powered blender and blend until smooth.

Layer the berry yoghurt, plain yoghurt, muesli, and remaining berries in a glass.

Place in the refrigerator to chill for 10 minutes. Serve.

SAN CHOY BOW

LUNCH | SERVES 1 | **PREP TIME** 15 MINUTES + 10 MINUTES SOAKING TIME | **COOKING TIME** 10 MINUTES | **DIFFICULTY** EASY

3½ oz rice vermicelli
noodles

oil spray

½ garlic clove, crushed

½ in fresh ginger, peeled
and grated

3 oz lean ground pork

¼ Lebanese cucumber,
finely diced

1 small handful bean
sprouts

¼ medium carrot, grated

1 tablespoon chopped
fresh cilantro

½ teaspoon salt-reduced
tamari or soy sauce

½ teaspoon fish sauce

2 teaspoons lime juice

½ teaspoon honey

3 large romaine lettuce
leaves, left whole, base
trimmed

Place the noodles in a heatproof bowl and cover with boiling water. Leave for 10 minutes, then loosen the noodles with a fork. Drain and refresh under cool running water. Drain well and set aside to cool slightly. When cool enough to handle, cut into shorter lengths.

Heat a non-stick fry pan over medium–high heat and spray lightly with oil spray. Add the garlic, ginger, and ground pork and cook for 5–7 minutes or until the pork is browned, stirring frequently with a wooden spoon to break the meat up. Transfer to a heatproof bowl and set aside.

Add the noodles, cucumber, bean sprouts, carrot, and cilantro to the bowl containing the pork and stir gently to combine.

Whisk the tamari or soy sauce, fish sauce, lime juice, and honey together in a small bowl. Pour over the pork and noodle mixture and toss gently to combine.

To serve, place the lettuce leaves on a serving plate and fill with the san choy bow mixture.

RICE CRACKERS with MINTED YOGHURT

SNACK P.M. | **SERVES** 1 | **PREP TIME** 5 MINUTES | **DIFFICULTY** EASY

12 plain rice crackers

MINTED YOGHURT

1¾ oz low-fat plain yoghurt

2 tablespoons chopped
fresh mint

¼ garlic clove, crushed

lemon juice, to taste

sea salt and ground black
pepper, to taste

To make the minted yoghurt, whisk the yoghurt,
mint, garlic, lemon juice, salt, and pepper
together in a small bowl. To save time, the
minted yoghurt can be made the night before
and stored in an airtight container in
the refrigerator.

Serve the rice crackers with the minted yoghurt.

GREEK-STYLE BAKED FISH

DINNER | **SERVES** 2 | **PREP TIME** 15 MINUTES | **COOKING TIME** 50 MINUTES | **DIFFICULTY** EASY

1½ medium potatoes,
peeled and cut into wedges

1 small red onion,
halved and sliced

2 garlic cloves, crushed

1 teaspoon dried oregano

1½ teaspoons olive oil

sea salt and ground black
pepper, to taste

1 lemon, cut into wedges

2 medium tomatoes,
cut into wedges

8 kalamata olives

Two 6-oz white fish fillets

1 small handful fresh parsley,
chopped

2 oz salt-reduced low-fat
feta cheese, crumbled

Preheat the oven to 400°F (350°F convection) and line
a baking dish with parchment paper.

Place the potato, onion, garlic, oregano, oil, salt, and
pepper in a large bowl and toss gently to combine.
Ensure that all of the vegetables are lightly coated.

Place the vegetable mixture in the lined baking dish and
bake in the oven for 15 minutes. Turn the potato and
onion over and bake for a further 15 minutes. Add the
lemon, tomato, and olives and bake for 10 minutes.
Add the fish fillets and bake for a further 10 minutes
or until cooked through.

To serve, place the vegetables on two serving plates
and top with the baked fish. Sprinkle over the parsley
and feta.

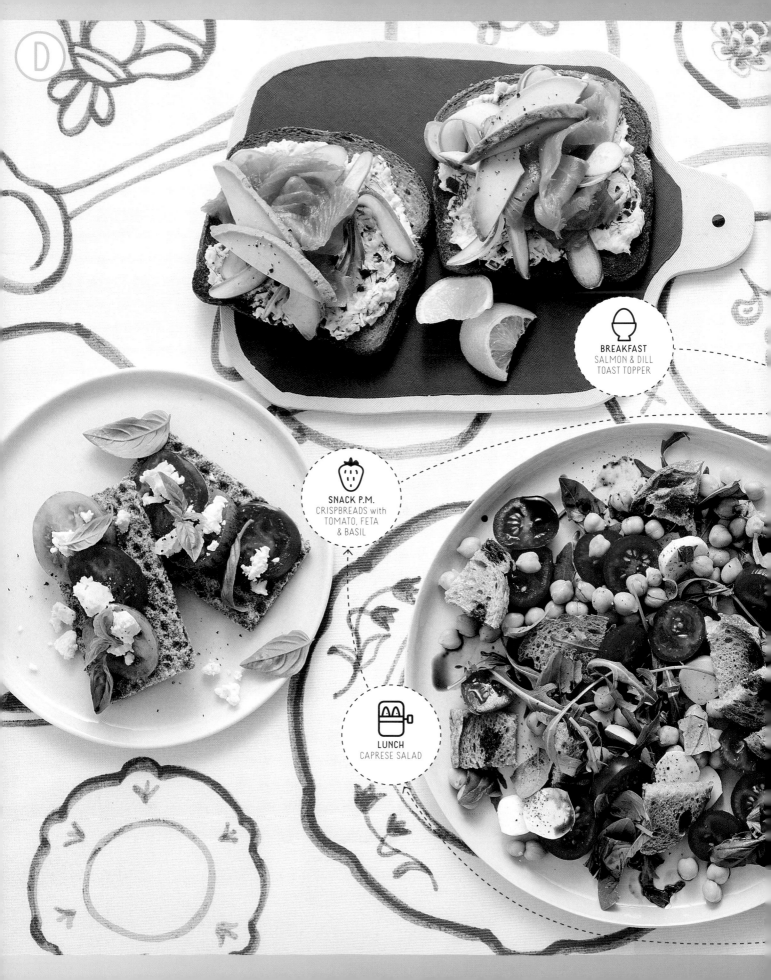

D

BREAKFAST
SALMON & DILL
TOAST TOPPER

SNACK P.M.
CRISPBREADS with
TOMATO, FETA
& BASIL

LUNCH
CAPRESE SALAD

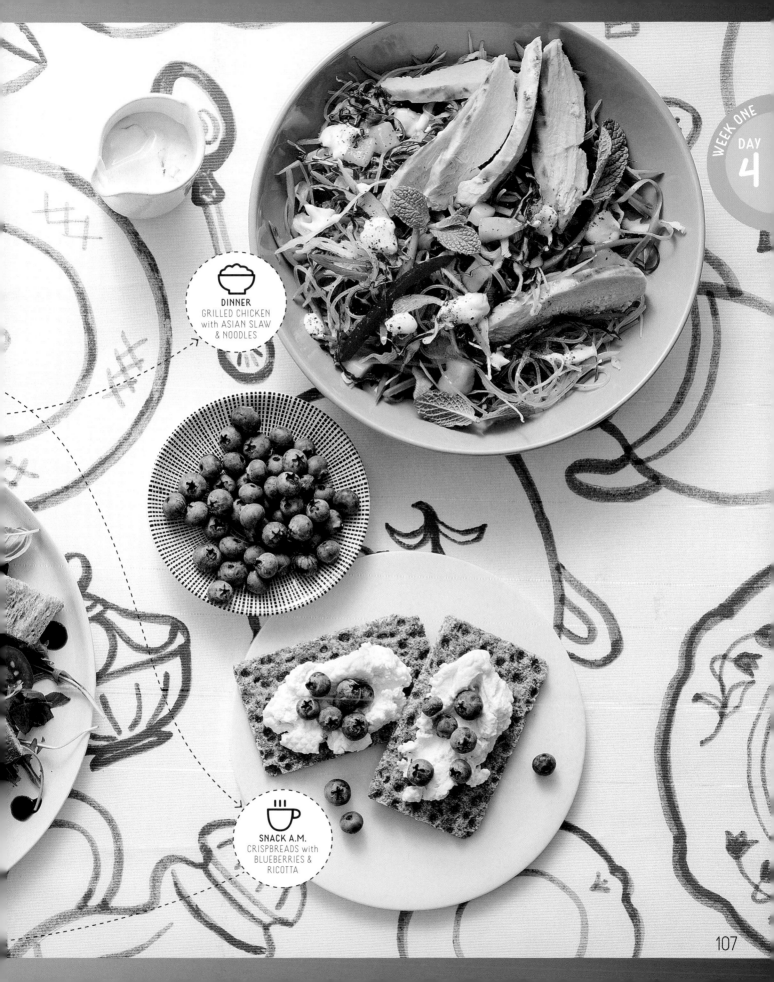

DINNER
GRILLED CHICKEN
with ASIAN SLAW
& NOODLES

SNACK A.M.
CRISPBREADS with
BLUEBERRIES &
RICOTTA

WEEK ONE

DAY
4

SALMON & DILL TOAST TOPPER

BREAKFAST | **SERVES** 1 | **PREP TIME** 10 MINUTES | **COOKING TIME** 2 MINUTES | **DIFFICULTY** EASY

2 slices whole wheat bread

1¾ oz low-fat ricotta cheese

¼ small red onion, finely diced

2 teaspoons finely chopped fresh dill

finely grated lemon zest and juice, to taste

¾ Lebanese cucumber, sliced

2½ oz smoked salmon

1 oz avocado, sliced

Toast the bread to your liking.

Place the ricotta, onion, dill, lemon zest, and juice in a small bowl and mix until well combined.

To serve, spread the ricotta mixture over the toast. Top with the cucumber, smoked salmon, and avocado.

CRISPBREADS with BLUEBERRIES & RICOTTA

SNACK A.M. | **SERVES** 1 | **PREP TIME** 2 MINUTES | **DIFFICULTY** EASY

1¾ oz low-fat ricotta cheese

2 rye crispbreads

5¾ oz blueberries

To serve, spread the ricotta over the crispbreads and top with the blueberries.

CAPRESE SALAD

LUNCH | **SERVES** 1 | **PREP TIME** 10 MINUTES | **COOKING TIME** 2 MINUTES | **DIFFICULTY** EASY

1 slice whole wheat bread

½ teaspoon balsamic vinegar

1 small handful arugula leaves

10 cherry tomatoes, halved

⅔ oz baby bocconcini (mozzarella) quartered

2½ oz tinned chickpeas, drained and rinsed

chopped fresh basil leaves, to taste

Toast the bread to your liking. Cut into small squares and set aside.

Whisk the vinegar and 1 teaspoon of water together in a small bowl.

To serve, place the arugula, tomato, bocconcini, chickpeas, and basil in a serving bowl. Drizzle over the dressing and toss gently to combine. Top with the croutons.

CRISPBREADS with TOMATO, FETA & BASIL

SNACK P.M. | SERVES 1 | PREP TIME 2 MINUTES | DIFFICULTY EASY

2 rye crispbreads

½ medium tomato, sliced

1 oz salt-reduced low-fat feta cheese, crumbled

fresh basil leaves, to serve

To serve, top the crispbreads with the tomato, feta, and basil leaves.

GRILLED CHICKEN with ASIAN SLAW & NOODLES

DINNER | SERVES 2 | PREP TIME 20 MINUTES + 10 MINUTES SOAKING TIME | COOKING TIME 10 MINUTES | DIFFICULTY EASY

3½ oz rice vermicelli noodles

oil spray

7 oz boneless skinless chicken breast, cut into thick strips

YOGHURT LIME DRESSING

7 oz low-fat plain yoghurt

2 tablespoons chopped fresh cilantro

2 teaspoons lime juice

3 teaspoons sesame oil

2 teaspoons salt-reduced tamari or soy sauce

2 teaspoons honey

pinch of ground ginger

ASIAN SLAW

1 medium carrot, grated

1¾ oz green cabbage, shredded

1¾ oz red cabbage, shredded

2 scallions, thinly sliced

½ medium red bell pepper, seeds removed and thinly sliced

1 medium mango, peeled and flesh sliced

2 tablespoons sultanas

2 tablespoons chopped fresh mint

Place the noodles in a heatproof bowl and cover with boiling water. Leave for 10 minutes, then loosen the noodles with a fork. Drain and refresh under cool running water. Drain well and set aside to cool.

Heat a large non-stick fry pan over medium heat and spray lightly with oil spray. Add the chicken strips and cook for 3–4 minutes on each side or until cooked through. Transfer to a plate and set aside to rest.

To make the yoghurt lime dressing, whisk the yoghurt, cilantro, lime juice, sesame oil, tamari or soy sauce, honey, and ginger in a small bowl.

To make the Asian slaw, place the carrot, green cabbage, red cabbage, scallions, bell pepper, mango, sultanas, and mint in a large bowl. Add the noodles. Drizzle over half of the dressing and toss gently to combine.

To serve, place the Asian slaw on two serving plates. Top with the chicken and drizzle over the remaining dressing.

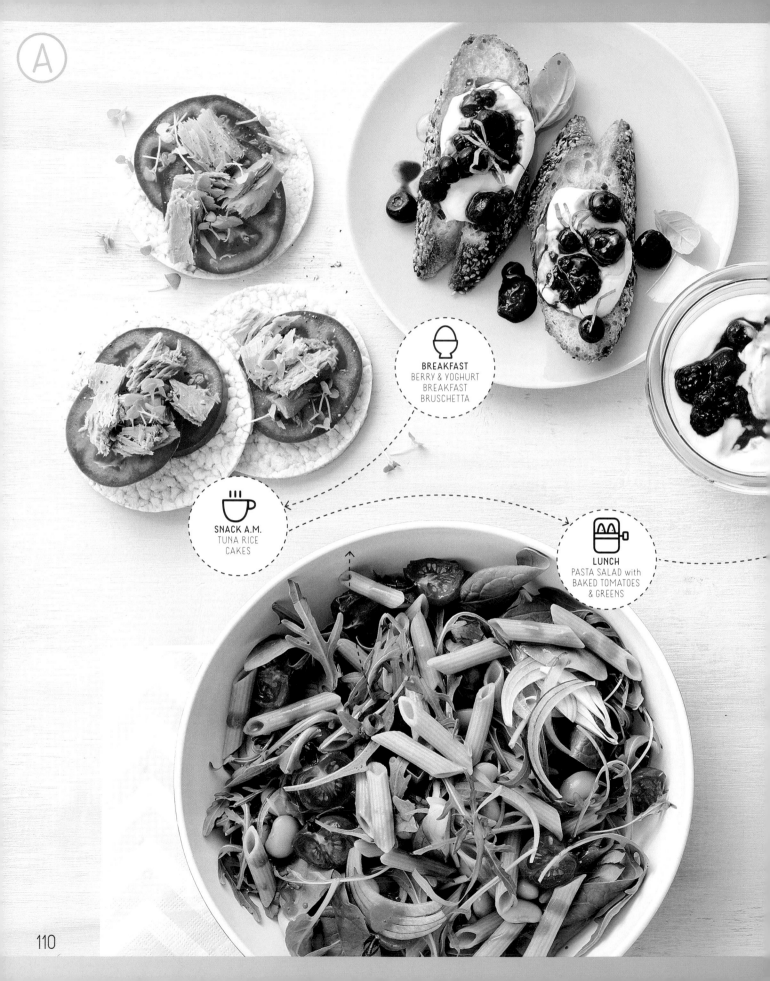

A

BREAKFAST
BERRY & YOGHURT
BREAKFAST
BRUSCHETTA

SNACK A.M.
TUNA RICE
CAKES

LUNCH
PASTA SALAD with
BAKED TOMATOES
& GREENS

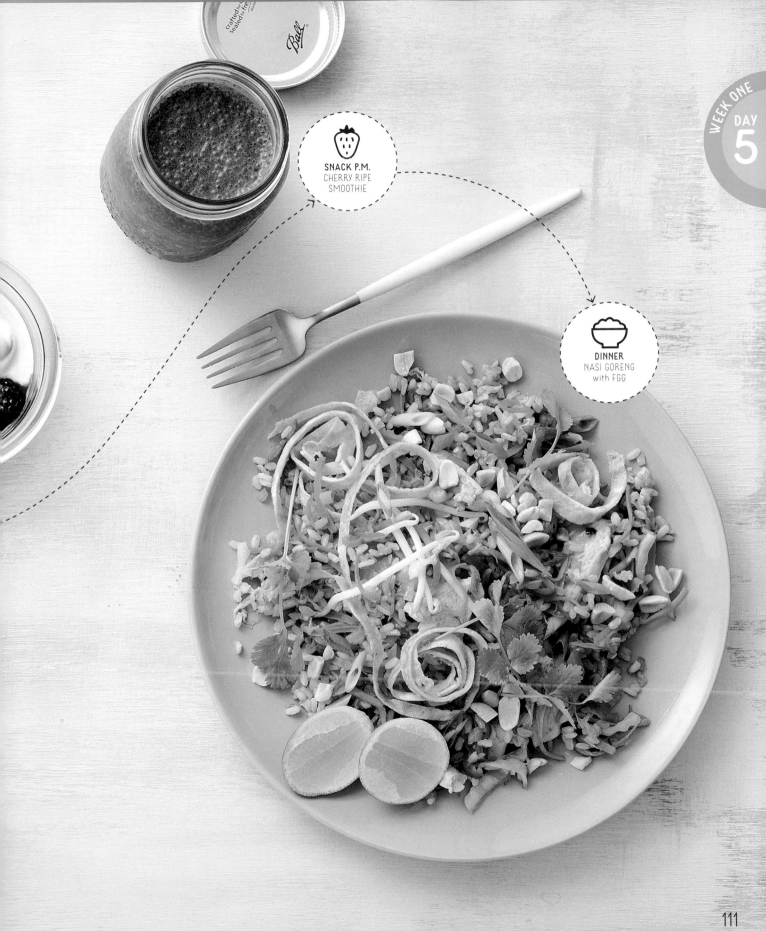

SNACK P.M.
CHERRY RIPE
SMOOTHIE

DINNER
NASI GORENG
with FGG

BERRY & YOGHURT BREAKFAST BRUSCHETTA

BREAKFAST | **SERVES** 1 | **PREP TIME** 5 MINUTES | **COOKING TIME** 2 MINUTES | **DIFFICULTY** EASY

7 oz low-fat plain yoghurt

2 teaspoons honey

¼ teaspoon pure vanilla extract

6 oz frozen mixed berries, thawed

2 teaspoons finely chopped fresh basil

2 slices whole wheat bread

Place the yoghurt, honey, and vanilla in a small bowl and mix until well combined.

Place the berries in a small bowl and lightly mash with a fork. Add the basil and stir to combine.

Toast the bread to your liking.

To serve, spread the yoghurt mixture over the toast and top with the berry mixture.

TUNA RICE CAKES

SNACK A.M. | **SERVES** 1 | **PREP TIME** 2 MINUTES | **DIFFICULTY** EASY

3 rice cakes

1 medium tomato, sliced

1¾ oz tinned tuna in springwater, drained

sea salt and ground black pepper, to taste

To serve, top the rice cakes with the tomato and tuna. Season with salt and pepper, if desired.

PASTA SALAD with BAKED TOMATOES & GREENS

LUNCH | **SERVES** 1 | **PREP TIME** 10 MINUTES | **COOKING TIME** 15 MINUTES | **DIFFICULTY** EASY

1½ oz whole wheat pasta

8 cherry tomatoes, halved

oil spray

pinch of dried oregano

pinch of dried thyme

sea salt and ground black pepper, to taste

1 small handful baby spinach leaves

1 small handful arugula leaves

¼ small red onion, thinly sliced

5¼ oz tinned butter beans, drained and rinsed

DRESSING

1 teaspoon balsamic vinegar

½ teaspoon Dijon mustard

Preheat the oven to 400°F (350°F/convection) and line a baking sheet with parchment paper.

Fill a large saucepan with water, add a pinch of salt and bring to a boil. Add the pasta and cook until al dente (see the pasta packet for the recommended cooking time). Drain and set aside to cool.

Meanwhile, place the tomatoes, cut-side up, on the lined baking sheet and spray lightly with oil spray. Sprinkle over the oregano and thyme and season with salt and pepper, if desired. Bake in the oven for 10–15 minutes or until soft and set aside to cool. To save time, you can cook the pasta and bake the tomatoes the night before and store in an airtight container in the refrigerator.

To make the dressing, whisk the vinegar, mustard, and 1 tablespoon of water together in a small bowl.

To serve, place the pasta, tomatoes, spinach, arugula, onion, and butter beans in a serving bowl. Drizzle over the dressing and toss gently to combine.

CHERRY RIPE SMOOTHIE

SNACK P.M. | **SERVES** 1 | **PREP TIME** 5 MINUTES | **DIFFICULTY** EASY

20 cherries, pitted

1 scoop (1 oz) protein powder, chocolate flavour (optional)

1 cup low-fat milk

3½ oz low-fat plain yoghurt

1 teaspoon raw cacao powder (see page 49)

Place the cherries, protein powder (if using), milk, yoghurt, and cacao powder in a high-powered blender and blend until smooth.

To serve, pour into a glass or shaker.

NASI GORENG with EGG

DINNER | **SERVES** 2 | **PREP TIME** 15 MINUTES | **COOKING TIME** 30 MINUTES | **DIFFICULTY** MEDIUM

4¼ oz brown rice

oil spray

2 large eggs, whisked

3 teaspoons sesame oil

½ small brown onion, finely diced

1 garlic clove, crushed

½ in fresh ginger, peeled and grated

¼ teaspoon ground turmeric

½ teaspoon ground cumin

3½ oz boneless skinless chicken breast, thinly sliced

1 fresh long red chilli, seeds removed and thinly sliced

1 tablespoon salt-reduced tamari or soy sauce

1 medium carrot, grated

1 large handful bean sprouts

3½ oz Chinese cabbage (wombok), shredded

1 tablespoon fresh cilantro

1 scallion, sliced

⅔ oz unsalted peanuts, chopped (about 2 tablespoons)

lime wedges, to serve

Place the rice and 1¼ cups of water in a small saucepan over high heat and bring to a boil, stirring occasionally. Cover and reduce the heat to medium–low. Simmer for 20–25 minutes or until the liquid is absorbed and the rice is tender. Remove from the heat and let stand, covered, for 5 minutes.

Meanwhile, heat a small non-stick fry pan over medium heat and spray lightly with oil spray. Pour in the egg and swirl to cover the base of the pan. Cook for 1–2 minutes or until the egg is set. Place the omelette on a plate and set aside to cool. When cool enough to handle, slice into thin strips.

Heat the oil in a large non-stick fry pan over medium heat. Add the onion and cook for 5 minutes or until soft and translucent. Add the garlic, ginger, turmeric, and cumin and cook for 1 minute or until fragrant.

Add the chicken and cook for 5 minutes until lightly browned on both sides.

Add the rice, chilli, and tamari or soy sauce and toss gently to combine.

Add the carrot, bean sprouts, and cabbage and cook for 3–4 minutes or until all the vegetables are tender.

To serve, place the nasi goreng on two serving plates and top with the egg, cilantro, scallion, and peanuts. Serve with lime wedges on the side.

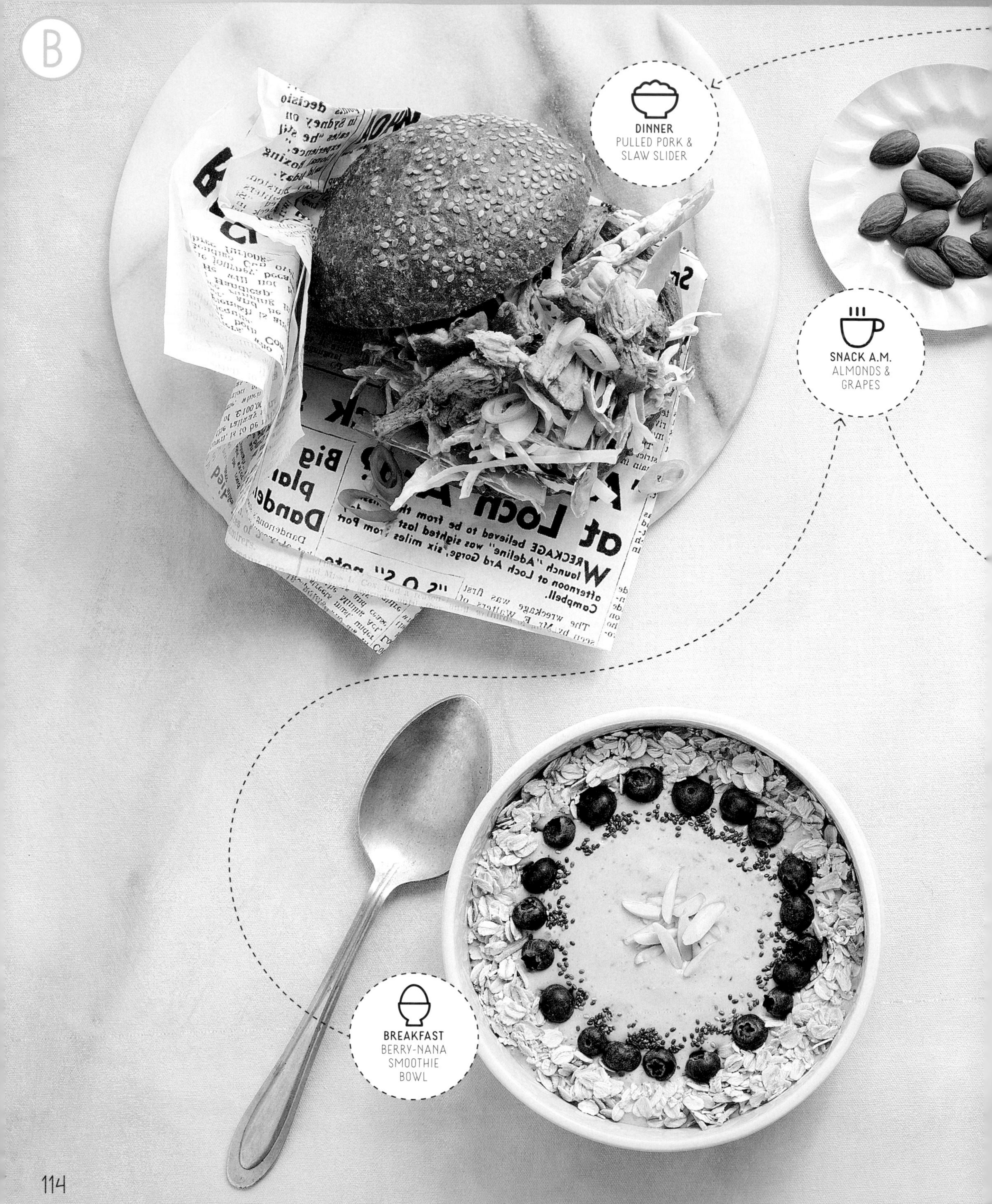

B

DINNER
PULLED PORK &
SLAW SLIDER

SNACK A.M.
ALMONDS &
GRAPES

BREAKFAST
BERRY-NANA
SMOOTHIE
BOWL

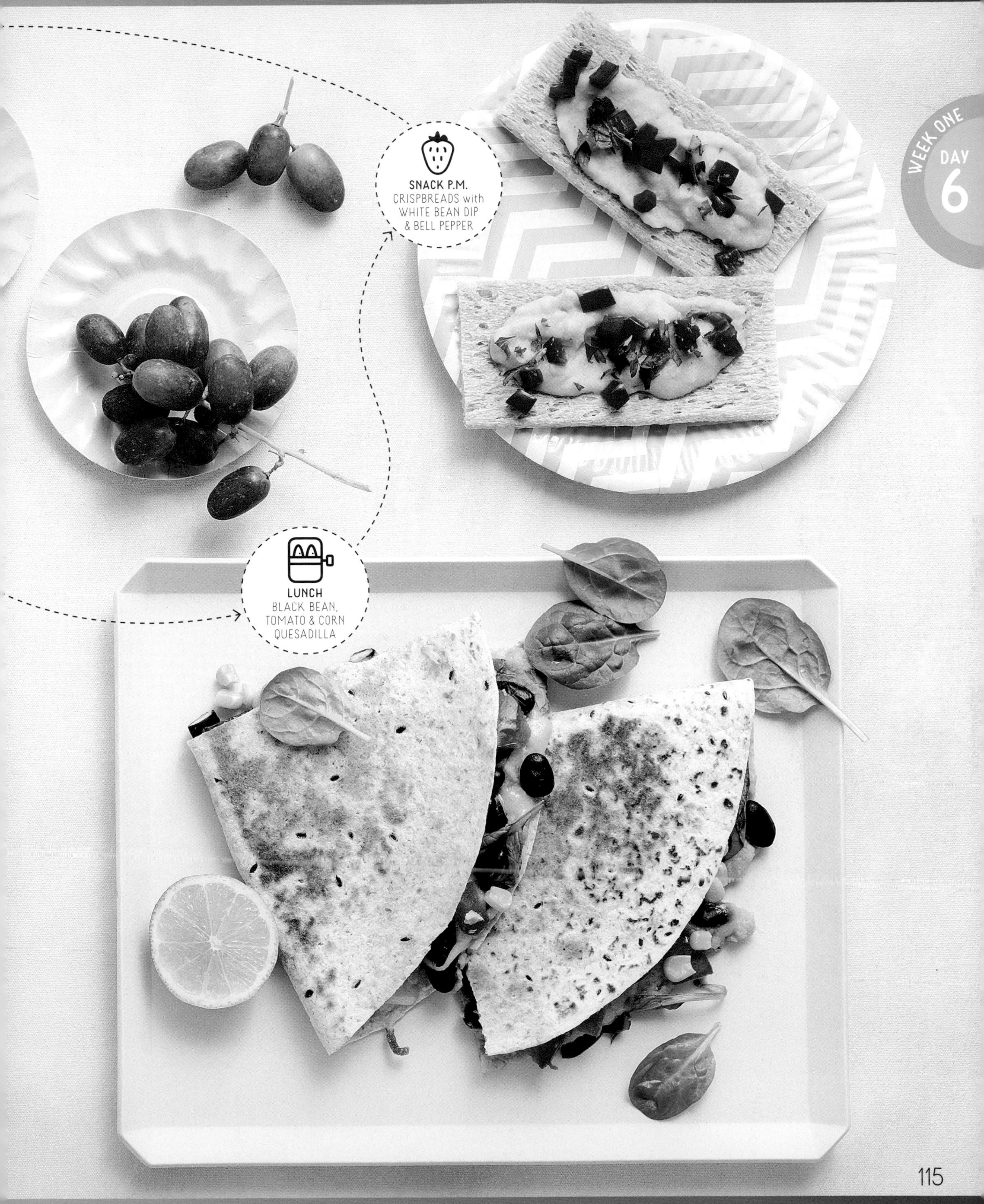

SNACK P.M.
CRISPBREADS with
WHITE BEAN DIP
& BELL PEPPER

LUNCH
BLACK BEAN,
TOMATO & CORN
QUESADILLA

BERRY-NANA SMOOTHIE BOWL

BREAKFAST | **SERVES** 1 | **PREP TIME** 5 MINUTES | **DIFFICULTY** EASY

2 oz blueberries

1 frozen medium banana, chopped

1 small handful baby spinach leaves

2 teaspoons acai berry blend powder (optional)

7 oz low-fat plain yoghurt

½ cup low-fat milk

TOPPINGS

1 oz natural muesli

1 tablespoon blueberries

1 teaspoon chia seeds

1 teaspoon slivered almonds

Place the blueberries, banana, spinach, acai berry powder (if using), yoghurt, and milk in a high-powered blender and blend until well combined.

To serve, pour the smoothie mixture into a bowl and top with muesli, blueberries, chia seeds and almonds.

ALMONDS & GRAPES

SNACK A.M. | **SERVES** 1 | **PREP TIME** 2 MINUTES | **DIFFICULTY** EASY

1 tablespoon whole almonds

12 grapes

To serve, place the almonds and grapes in a small bowl.

BLACK BEAN, TOMATO & CORN QUESADILLA

LUNCH | **SERVES** 1 | **PREP TIME** 10 MINUTES | **COOKING TIME** 5 MINUTES | **DIFFICULTY** EASY

2¾ oz tinned black beans, drained and rinsed

½ medium tomato, diced

2 tablespoons tinned corn kernels, drained and rinsed

2¾ oz hummus (see page 254)

1 whole wheat wrap

1 small handful baby spinach leaves

⅔ oz reduced-fat cheddar cheese, grated

Preheat a sandwich press.

Place the black beans, tomato, and corn in a small bowl and mix until well combined.

Spread the hummus over one half of the wrap and lay on the sandwich press. Top with the spinach, black bean mixture, and cheese. Fold in half to enclose the filling and gently press down the sandwich press lid.

Toast for 3–5 minutes or until the wrap is crisp and golden brown. Remove the quesadilla from the sandwich press and transfer to a serving plate. Serve.

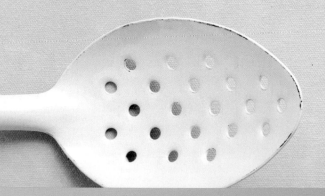

CRISPBREADS with WHITE BEAN DIP & BELL PEPPER

SNACK P.M. | **SERVES** 1 | **PREP TIME** 5 MINUTES | **DIFFICULTY** EASY

2 rye crispbreads

½ medium red bell pepper, seeds removed and sliced

chopped fresh parsley, to garnish (optional)

WHITE BEAN DIP

2¾ oz tinned cannellini beans, drained and rinsed

¼ garlic clove, crushed

lemon juice, to taste

2 teaspoons chopped fresh parsley

sea salt and ground black pepper, to taste

To make the white bean dip, place the cannellini beans, garlic, lemon juice, parsley, salt, black pepper, and 1 tablespoon of water in a food processor and pulse until smooth and creamy. To save time, you can make the white bean dip the night before and store in an airtight container in the refrigerator.

To serve, spread the dip over the crispbreads and top with the bell pepper and parsley (if using).

PULLED PORK & SLAW SLIDER

DINNER | **SERVES** 2 | **PREP TIME** 20 MINUTES | **COOKING TIME** 45 MINUTES | **DIFFICULTY** EASY

oil spray

6 oz blade pork steaks

½ teaspoon smoked paprika

½ teaspoon ground cumin

pinch of ground cinnamon

2 teaspoons pure maple syrup

sea salt and ground black pepper, to taste

½ cup salt-reduced vegetable stock

2 whole wheat bread rolls

SLAW

7 oz low-fat plain yoghurt

½ teaspoon Dijon mustard

1 tablespoon chopped fresh parsley

3½ oz green cabbage, finely shredded

1 medium carrot, grated

3 oz snow peas, trimmed and thinly sliced

2 scallions, thinly sliced

Preheat the oven to 300°F (266°F convection) and line an ovenproof dish with parchment paper.

Heat a large non-stick fry pan over medium–high heat and spray lightly with oil spray. Add the pork and cook for 3–4 minutes on each side or until browned. Remove from the heat.

Place the paprika, cumin, cinnamon, and maple syrup in a medium bowl and stir to combine. Place the pork steaks in the bowl and rub with the spice mix. Transfer to the prepared dish and season with salt and pepper, if desired. Pour in the stock and cover with a lid or foil. Braise in the oven for 20–35 minutes or until cooked through.

Meanwhile, to make the slaw, whisk the yoghurt, mustard, and parsley together in a small bowl. Place the cabbage, carrot, snow peas, and scallions in a bowl. Drizzle over the yoghurt dressing and toss gently to combine.

Transfer the pork to a clean chopping board and coarsely shred using two forks.

To serve, cut the bread rolls in half and toast lightly in a toaster or under a hot broiler. On one half of each roll, layer the pork and slaw. Top with the other half of the roll.

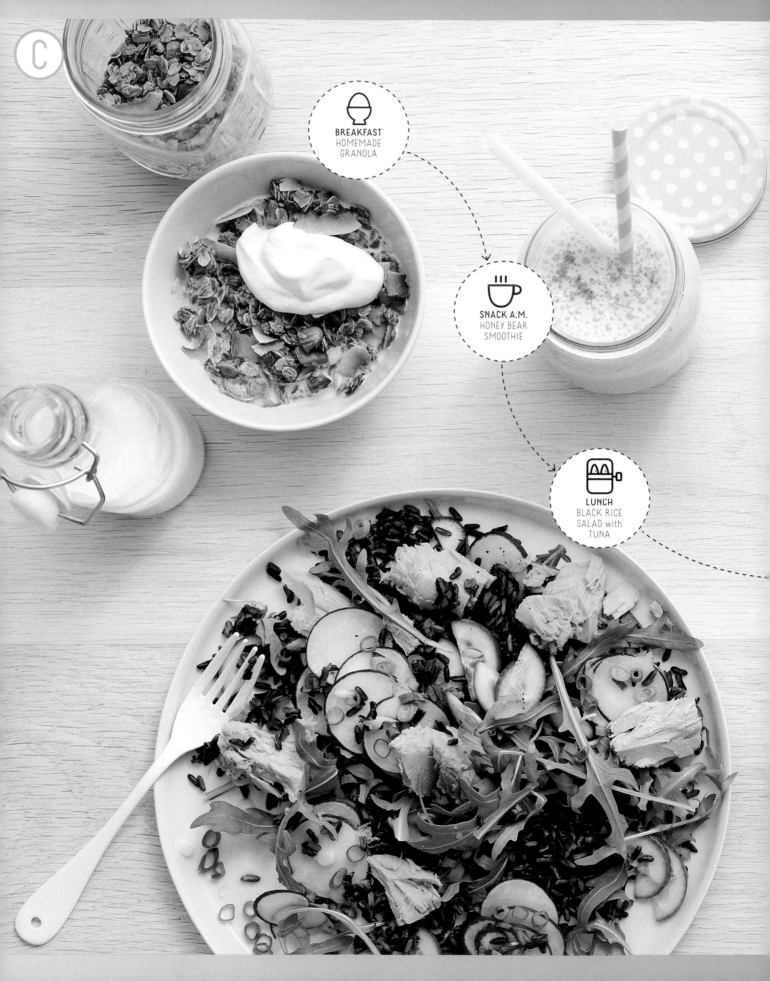

BREAKFAST
HOMEMADE
GRANOLA

SNACK A.M.
HONEY BEAR
SMOOTHIE

LUNCH
BLACK RICE
SALAD with
TUNA

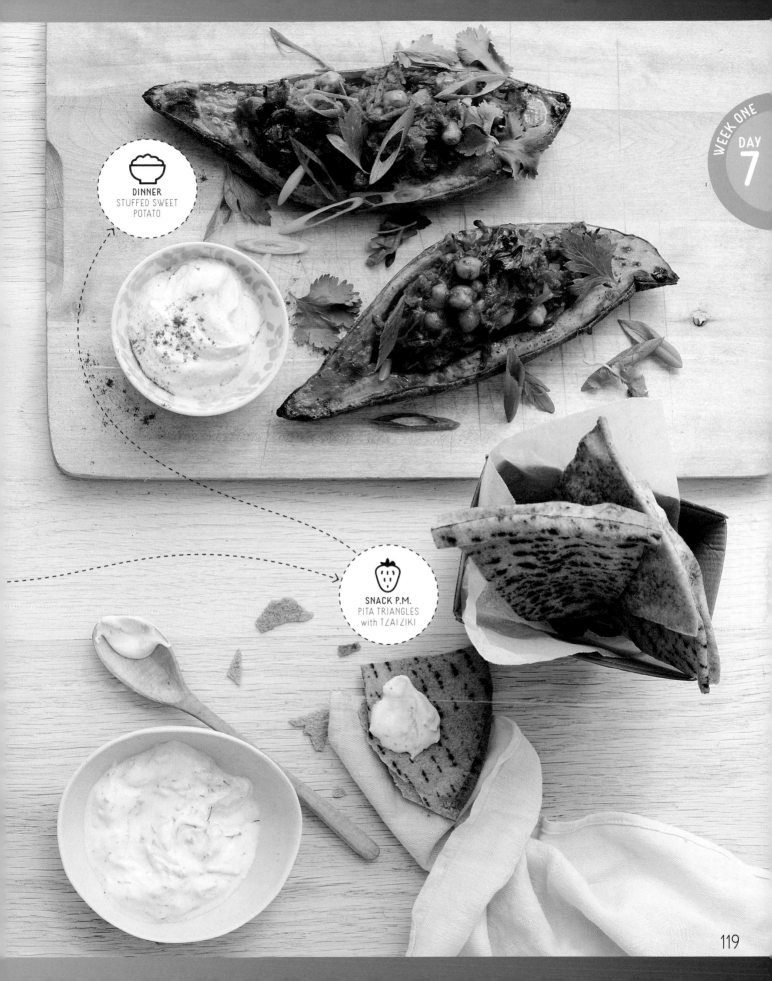

DINNER
STUFFED SWEET
POTATO

SNACK P.M.
PITA TRIANGLES
with TZATZIKI

119

HOMEMADE GRANOLA

2 tablespoons honey

½ cup pure maple syrup

1 teaspoon pure vanilla extract

10¾ oz rolled oats

1¼ oz almonds, chopped

1¼ oz pumpkin seeds (pepitas)

1 oz coconut flakes

1½ oz sultanas

1¾ oz dried cranberries

TO SERVE

½ cup low-fat milk

1¾ oz low-fat plain yoghurt

Preheat the oven to 300°F (266°F convection) and line two baking sheets with parchment paper.

Whisk the honey, maple syrup, and vanilla together in a large bowl. Add the oats, almonds, and pumpkin seeds and mix until well combined. Ensure that all ingredients are coated with the maple syrup mixture.

Evenly spread the granola over the two backing sheets and spread out thinly. Bake in the oven for 15 minutes, then stir in the coconut flakes. Ensure that the granola is spread out evenly and thinly again.

Bake for a further 10–15 minutes until golden and toasted, stirring every 3–4 minutes. Sprinkle the dried fruit over both sheets and stir. Set the sheets aside until the granola is completely cooled and crunchy.

Place 1 serving of the granola in the bowl and top with the milk and yoghurt. Store the remaining granola in an airtight container.

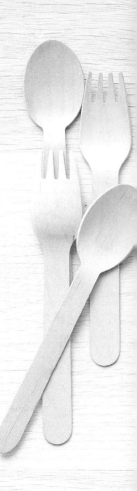

HONEY BEAR SMOOTHIE

1 oz rolled oats

1½ medium bananas, peeled and chopped

¾ cup low-fat milk

1¾ oz low-fat plain yoghurt

2 teaspoons honey

¼ teaspoon ground cinnamon

ice cubes

Place the oats, banana, milk, yoghurt, honey, cinnamon, and ice cubes in a high-powered blender and blend until smooth.

To serve, pour into a glass or shaker.

BLACK RICE SALAD with TUNA

2 oz black rice

3½ oz tinned tuna in springwater, drained

1 small handful arugula leaves

½ Lebanese cucumber, thinly sliced

½ scallion, thinly sliced

1 radish, halved and thinly sliced

DRESSING

¼ garlic clove, crushed

2 teaspoons white wine vinegar

¼ teaspoon Dijon mustard

sea salt and ground black pepper, to taste

Place the rice and 1 cup of water in a small saucepan over high heat and bring to a boil, stirring occasionally. Cover and reduce the heat to medium–low. Simmer for 35–40 minutes or until the liquid is absorbed and the rice is tender. Remove from the heat and leave to stand, covered, for 5 minutes. Set aside to cool.

To make the dressing, whisk the garlic, vinegar, mustard, salt, pepper, and 2 teaspoons of water together in a small bowl.

To serve, place the tuna, arugula, cucumber, scallion, radish, and black rice in a serving bowl. Drizzle over the dressing and toss gently to combine.

PITA TRIANGLES with TZATZIKI

SNACK P.M. | **SERVES** 1 | **PREP TIME** 5 MINUTES | **COOKING TIME** 12 MINUTES | **DIFFICULTY** EASY

½ whole wheat pita bread, cut into 4 wedges

oil spray

1¾ oz tzatziki (see page 254)

Preheat the oven to 400°F (350°F convection) and line a baking sheet with parchment paper.

Lay the pita wedges in a single layer on the lined baking sheet and spray lightly with oil spray. Bake in the oven for 5 minutes until they begin to colour. Turn the wedges over and bake for a further 5–8 minutes or until both sides are lightly coloured and set aside to cool.

Serve the pita triangles with the tzatziki.

STUFFED SWEET POTATO

DINNER | **SERVES** 2 | **PREP TIME** 15 MINUTES | **COOKING TIME** 50 MINUTES | **DIFFICULTY** EASY

1 medium sweet potato, washed, dried and halved lengthways

1½ teaspoons sunflower oil

sea salt and ground black pepper, to taste

oil spray

½ small brown onion, finely chopped

1 medium carrot, grated

2 garlic cloves, crushed

¼ teaspoon ground cumin

¼ teaspoon ground ginger

pinch of ground cinnamon

pinch of ground allspice

pinch of cayenne pepper

13½ oz tinned chickpeas, drained and rinsed

1 teaspoon pure maple syrup

5 oz tinned crushed tomatoes

2 large handfuls baby spinach leaves, shredded

2 tablespoons chopped fresh cilantro

1 large egg, lightly whisked

1 scallion, thinly sliced

SPICED YOGHURT DRESSING

7 oz low-fat plain yoghurt

pinch of sweet paprika

lemon juice, to taste

Preheat the oven to 400°F (350°F convection) and line a baking sheet with parchment paper.

Place the sweet potato, oil, salt, and pepper in a medium bowl and toss to combine. Ensure that the entire potato is lightly coated in the oil. Place the sweet potato on the baking sheet, cut-side up, and bake in the oven for 30–35 minutes or until tender. Set aside to cool slightly.

Meanwhile, heat a non-stick fry pan over medium heat and spray lightly with oil spray. Add the onion and carrot and cook for 3–4 minutes or until the onion starts to soften, stirring occasionally.

Add the garlic, cumin, ginger, cinnamon, allspice, and cayenne pepper and cook for 1 minute or until fragrant. Add the chickpeas, maple syrup, and tomatoes and cook for 5 minutes or until heated through, stirring frequently. Stir through the spinach and half of the cilantro. Set aside.

Leaving the sweet potato shell intact, scoop out the flesh and place in a bowl. Roughly mash the flesh with a fork. Add the egg and sweet potato mash to the chickpea and tomato mixture and mix until well combined.

Spoon the sweet potato and chickpea mixture into the sweet potato shells and return to the lined baking sheet. Spray the top lightly with oil spray and bake for 15 minutes, until heated through and light golden in colour.

To make the spiced yoghurt dressing, whisk the yoghurt, paprika, and lemon juice together in a small bowl.

To serve, place the stuffed sweet potato halves on two serving plates. Sprinkle over the sliced scallion and drizzle with the spiced yoghurt dressing.

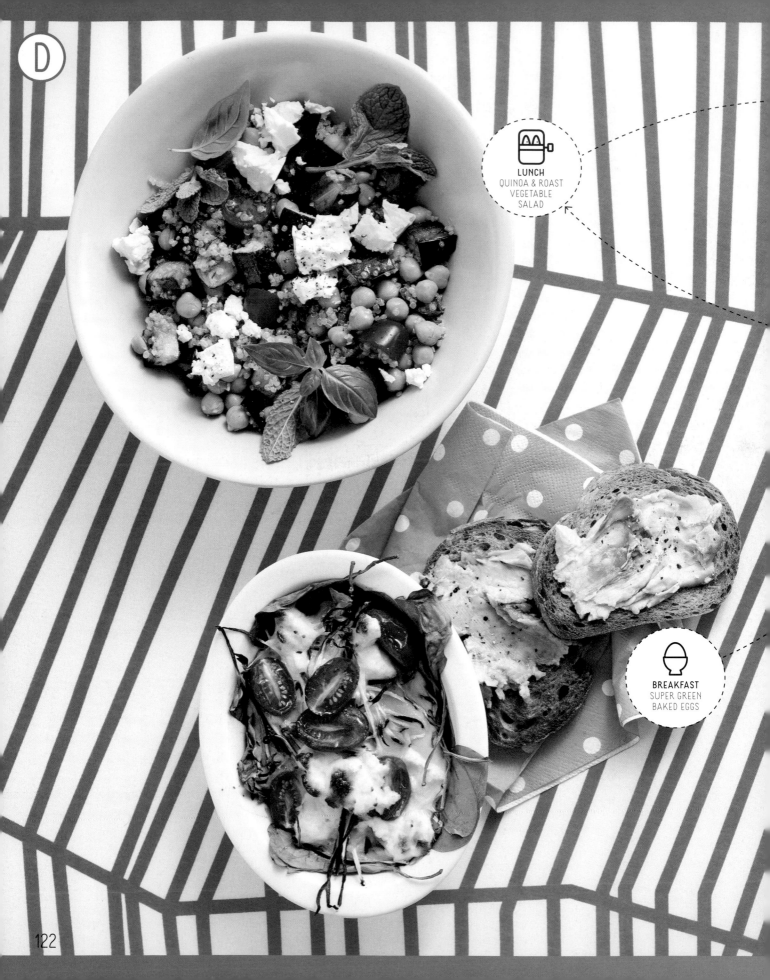

D

LUNCH
QUINOA & ROAST
VEGETABLE
SALAD

BREAKFAST
SUPER GREEN
BAKED EGGS

122

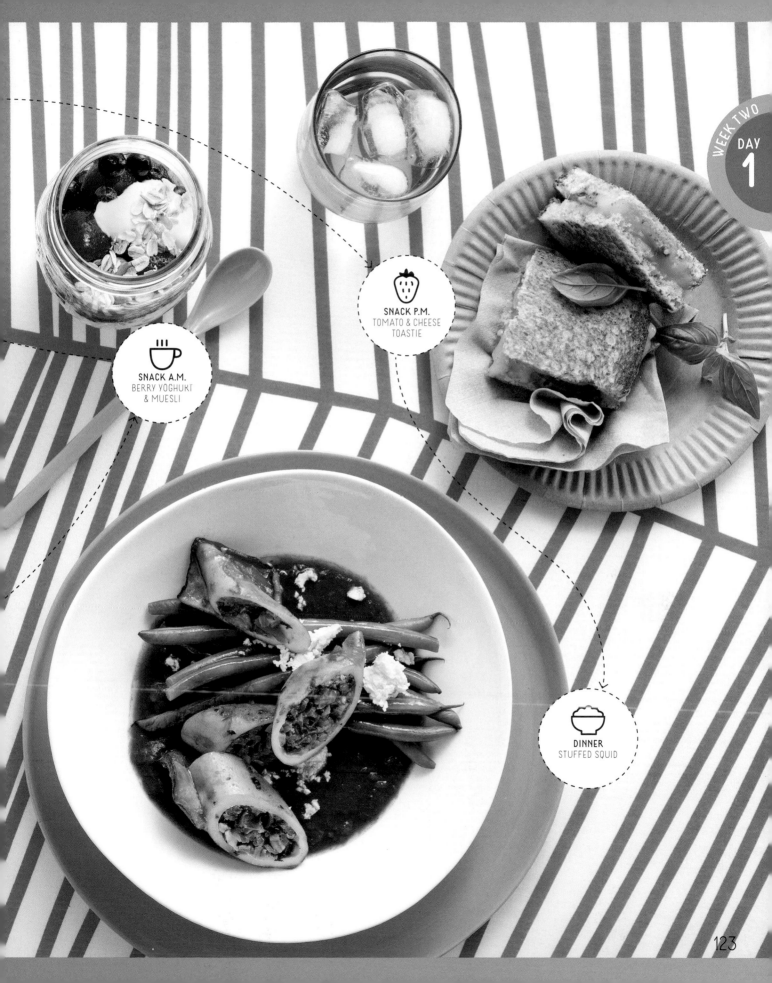

SNACK P.M.
TOMATO & CHEESE
TOASTIE

SNACK A.M.
BERRY YOGHURT
& MUESLI

DINNER
STUFFED SQUID

123

SUPER GREEN BAKED EGGS

BREAKFAST | SERVES 1 | PREP TIME 10 MINUTES | COOKING TIME 20 MINUTES | DIFFICULTY EASY

oil spray
¼ medium zucchini, grated
1 small handful baby spinach leaves
1¾ oz low-fat ricotta cheese
2 large eggs
sea salt and ground black pepper, to taste
3 cherry tomatoes, halved
2 slices whole wheat bread
1 oz avocado, mashed

Preheat the oven to 350°F (325°F convection) and lightly spray a 4 in diameter ramekin with oil spray.

Heat a non-stick fry pan over medium heat and spray lightly with oil spray. Add the zucchini and spinach and cook for 3–4 minutes or until the zucchini is soft and the spinach has wilted. Place in the prepared ramekin and top with the ricotta.

Whisk the eggs, salt, and pepper together in another small bowl. Pour into the ramekin and top with the cherry tomatoes. Bake in the oven for 10–15 minutes or until the egg has just set.

Meanwhile, toast the bread to your liking. Spread the avocado over the toast and serve with the baked eggs.

BERRY YOGHURT & MUESLI

SNACK A.M. | SERVES 1 | PREP TIME 2 MINUTES | DIFFICULTY EASY

3½ oz low-fat plain yoghurt
6 oz frozen mixed berries, thawed
1 oz natural muesli

To serve, place the yoghurt and berries in a small bowl or jar and top with the muesli.

QUINOA & ROAST VEGETABLE SALAD

LUNCH | SERVES 1 | PREP TIME 10 MINUTES | COOKING TIME 35 MINUTES | DIFFICULTY EASY

¼ medium eggplant, cut into ¾ in cubes
½ medium zucchini, cut into ¾ in cubes
oil spray
sea salt and ground black pepper, to taste
1 oz quinoa
2¾ oz tinned chickpeas, drained and rinsed
5 cherry tomatoes, halved

2 teaspoons chopped fresh basil
2 teaspoons chopped fresh mint
1 oz salt-reduced low-fat feta cheese, crumbled

DRESSING
1 tablespoon lemon juice
¼ garlic clove, crushed

Preheat the oven to 400°F (350°F convection) and line a baking sheet with parchment paper. Place the eggplant and zucchini on the lined baking sheet and spray lightly with oil spray. Season with salt and pepper, if desired. Roast in the oven for 10 minutes, then turn over and roast for a further 10 minutes until tender and lightly browned. Set aside to cool.

Place the quinoa and ½ cup of water in a saucepan over high heat and bring to the boil, stirring occasionally. Cover and reduce the heat to low. Simmer for 10–12 minutes or until the quinoa is tender. Drain off any excess liquid and set aside to cool. To save time, the vegetables and quinoa can be cooked the night before and stored in an airtight container in the refrigerator.

To make the dressing, whisk the lemon juice, garlic, and 1 tablespoon of water together in a small bowl.

To serve, place the roast vegetables, quinoa, chickpeas, tomato, basil, and mint in a serving bowl. Drizzle over the dressing and toss gently to combine. Top with the feta.

TOMATO & CHEESE TOASTIE

SNACK P.M. | **SERVES** 1 | **PREP TIME** 5 MINUTES | **COOKING TIME** 5 MINUTES | **DIFFICULTY** EASY

1 slice whole wheat bread, halved

½ medium tomato, sliced

⅔ oz reduced-fat cheddar cheese, sliced

sea salt and ground black pepper, to taste

fresh basil leaves, to serve

Preheat a sandwich press.

Place one half of the bread on a clean chopping board and top with the tomato and cheese. Season with salt and pepper, if desired. Top with the other half of the bread.

Place the sandwich on the sandwich press and gently press down the lid. Toast for 3–5 minutes or until the cheese is melted and the sandwich is golden. Garnish with basil and serve.

STUFFED SQUID

DINNER | **SERVES** 2 | **PREP TIME** 20 MINUTES | **COOKING TIME** 1 HOUR | **DIFFICULTY** MEDIUM

2½ oz plus 3 teaspoons olive oil

2 medium oranges, juiced

2½ oz couscous

½ small brown onion, finely diced

3 garlic cloves, crushed

½ medium carrot, grated

½ medium zucchini, grated

6⅔ oz tinned crushed tomatoes

sea salt and ground black pepper, to taste

½ teaspoon dried chilli flakes (optional)

chopped fresh parsley, to taste

⅔ lb squid (2 tubes), cleaned

1 tablespoon tomato paste

½ cup salt-reduced vegetable stock

12 green beans, trimmed

2 oz salt-reduced low-fat feta cheese, crumbled

In a small saucepan, bring ¼ teaspoon of the oil, the orange juice, and 2½ tablespoons of water to a boil. Add the couscous and remove from the heat. Let stand, covered, for 2–3 minutes before fluffing with a fork to help separate the grains.

Heat half of the remaining oil in a medium saucepan over medium heat. Add the onion and 2 cloves of the garlic and cook for 1–2 minutes or until fragrant, stirring constantly. Add the carrot and zucchini and cook for a further 3–4 minutes or until soft, stirring occasionally.

Add one-quarter of the crushed tomatoes, the salt, pepper, and chilli flakes (if using) and reduce the heat to medium–low. Cook for 7–10 minutes or until heated through, stirring occasionally. Remove from the heat and stir through the couscous and parsley.

Stuff the squid tubes with the tomato and couscous mixture and seal with a toothpick. Prick the squid tubes all over with the point of a sharp knife.

Heat the remaining oil in a medium saucepan over medium heat. Add the squid tubes and cook for 3 minutes on each side or until lightly browned.

Add the remaining garlic clove and crushed tomatoes, tomato paste, and stock and reduce the heat to medium–low. Simmer for 35–40 minutes until the squid tubes are tender and cooked through, turning occasionally.

Fill a saucepan with water until 2 in deep and insert a steamer basket. Cover with a lid and bring the water to a boil over high heat, then reduce the heat to medium. Add the beans and cook for 2–3 minutes, covered, or until tender-crisp. Refresh under cool running water.

To serve, place the tomato sauce in two serving bowls. Top with the green beans, followed by the stuffed squid and feta.

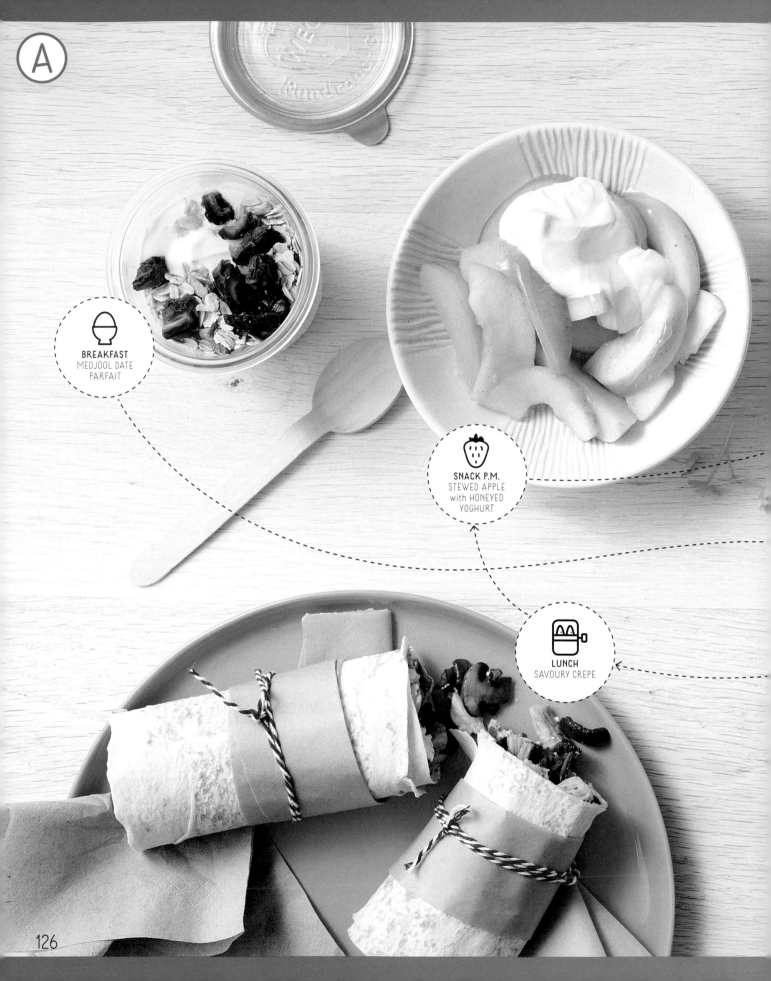

A

BREAKFAST
MEDJOOL DATE
PARFAIT

SNACK P.M.
STEWED APPLE
with HONEYED
YOGHURT

LUNCH
SAVOURY CREPE

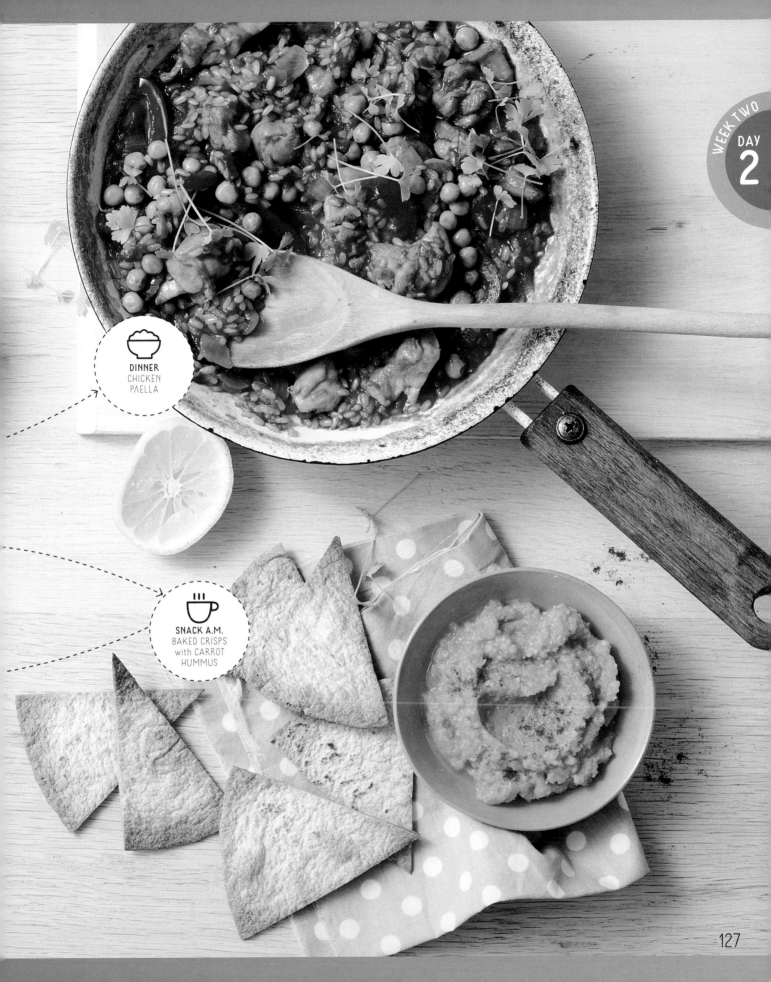

DINNER
CHICKEN
PAELLA

SNACK A.M.
BAKED CRISPS
with CARROT
HUMMUS

127

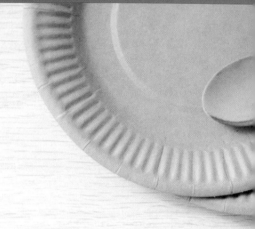

MEDJOOL DATE PARFAIT

BREAKFAST | **SERVES** 1 | **PREP TIME** 5 MINUTES + 10 MINUTES CHILLING TIME | **DIFFICULTY** EASY

7 oz low-fat plain yoghurt

2 oz natural muesli

3 medjool dates, pitted
and diced

Layer the yoghurt, muesli, and dates in a glass.

Place in the refrigerator to chill for 10 minutes. Serve.

BAKED CHIPS with CARROT HUMMUS

SNACK A.M. | **SERVES** 1 | **PREP TIME** 5 MINUTES | **COOKING TIME** 30 MINUTES | **DIFFICULTY** EASY

½ whole wheat wrap,
cut into 4–6 wedges

CARROT HUMMUS

1 medium carrot,
roughly chopped

2¾ oz tinned chickpeas,
drained and rinsed

¼ garlic clove, crushed

lemon juice, to taste

pinch of smoked paprika

sea salt, to taste

To make the carrot hummus, place the carrot in a small saucepan and fill with cold water until it just covers the carrot. Bring the water to a boil then reduce the heat to medium–low. Simmer for 15–20 minutes until tender. Drain and set aside to cool.

Place the carrot, chickpeas, garlic, lemon juice, paprika, and salt in a food processor and pulse until smooth and creamy. To save time, the carrot hummus can be made the night before and stored in an airtight container in the refrigerator.

Preheat the oven to 350°F (325°F convection) and line a baking sheet with parchment paper.

Lay the wrap wedges in a single layer on the lined baking sheet and bake in the oven for 3 minutes until they begin to colour. Turn the wedges over and bake for a further 3–5 minutes or until both sides are lightly coloured and set aside to cool.

Serve the baked chips with the carrot hummus.

SAVOURY CREPE

LUNCH | **SERVES** 1 | **PREP TIME** 5 MINUTES | **COOKING TIME** 10 MINUTES | **DIFFICULTY** EASY

oil spray

¼ small red onion, thinly sliced

4½ oz mushrooms, sliced

3 oz cooked boneless skinless
chicken breast, shredded

1 small handful baby
spinach leaves

sea salt and ground black
pepper, to taste

½ large whole wheat
lavash bread

Heat a non-stick fry pan over medium heat and spray lightly with oil spray. Add the onion, mushroom, and chicken and cook for 5 minutes or until the onion is soft and the chicken is warmed through, stirring occasionally.

Add the spinach and cook for 1–2 minutes or until wilted, stirring occasionally. Season with salt and pepper, if desired.

Warm the lavash in a dry pan over medium heat for 30 seconds. Remove from the heat and cut in half.

To serve, place the lavash halves on a serving plate and place the chicken and mushroom mixture down the middle of each. Fold over the ends and roll up to enclose the filling.

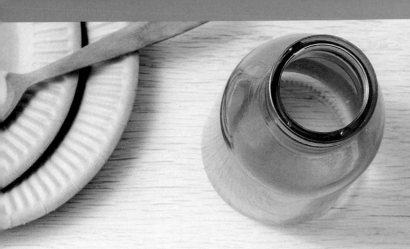

STEWED APPLE with HONEYED YOGHURT

SNACK P.M. | **SERVES** 1 | **PREP TIME** 5 MINUTES | **COOKING TIME** 5 MINUTES | **DIFFICULTY** EASY

1 medium apple, cored and sliced

ground cinnamon, to taste

10¾ oz low-fat plain yoghurt

1 teaspoon honey

Heat a small saucepan over medium heat. Add the apple, cinnamon, and 2 tablespoons of water and cook, covered, for 5 minutes or until the apple is soft, stirring occasionally.

Place the yoghurt and honey in a small bowl and mix until well combined.

To serve, top the stewed apple with the honey yoghurt.

CHICKEN PAELLA

DINNER | **SERVES** 2 | **PREP TIME** 10 MINUTES | **COOKING TIME** 50 MINUTES | **DIFFICULTY** EASY

¼ teaspoon saffron threads

3 teaspoons olive oil

7 oz boneless skinless chicken breast, cut into bite-sized pieces

sea salt and ground black pepper, to taste

½ small brown onion, diced

1 garlic clove, crushed

2 teaspoons sweet paprika

1¼ cups salt-reduced vegetable stock

4¼ oz brown rice

½ medium red bell pepper, seeds removed and sliced

5 oz tinned crushed tomatoes

1¾ oz frozen peas

2 teaspoons chopped fresh parsley

1 tablespoon pine nuts

lemon wedges, to serve

Place the saffron threads in a small bowl with 2 teaspoons of boiling water and set aside.

Heat half of the oil in a large non-stick fry pan over medium heat. Add the chicken and cook for 5–6 minutes or until browned. Transfer to a heatproof bowl and set aside to rest. Season with salt and pepper, if desired.

Heat the remaining oil in the pan over medium heat. Add the onion and cook for 3–4 minutes or until soft and translucent. Add the garlic and cook for 1 minute, stirring frequently. Add the paprika and cook for a further 2 minutes, stirring frequently.

Return the chicken to the pan. Add ½ cup of the stock and reduce the heat to medium–low. Simmer for 10 minutes or until almost all the liquid has evaporated, turning the chicken occasionally.

Add the rice, saffron mixture, bell pepper, crushed tomatoes, and ⅔ cup of stock to the pan. Simmer for 15 minutes or until almost all the liquid has been absorbed, stirring occasionally.

Add the peas and the remaining stock and simmer for a further 5–8 minutes until the stock has been absorbed and the rice is tender. If the stock is all used and the rice is not ready, just add ½ cup of hot water at a time until the rice is cooked. Stir through the parsley and pine nuts. Season with salt and black pepper, if desired.

To serve, place the chicken paella in two serving bowls. Serve with lemon wedges on the side.

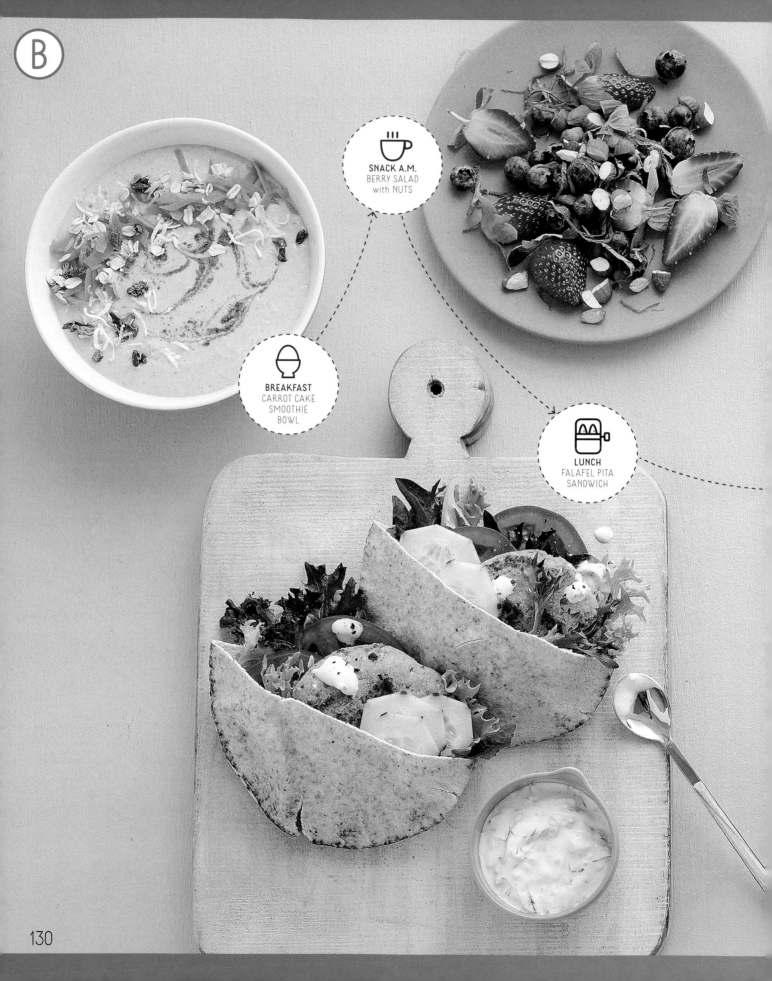

B

SNACK A.M.
BERRY SALAD
with NUTS

BREAKFAST
CARROT CAKE
SMOOTHIE
BOWL

LUNCH
FALAFEL PITA
SANDWICH

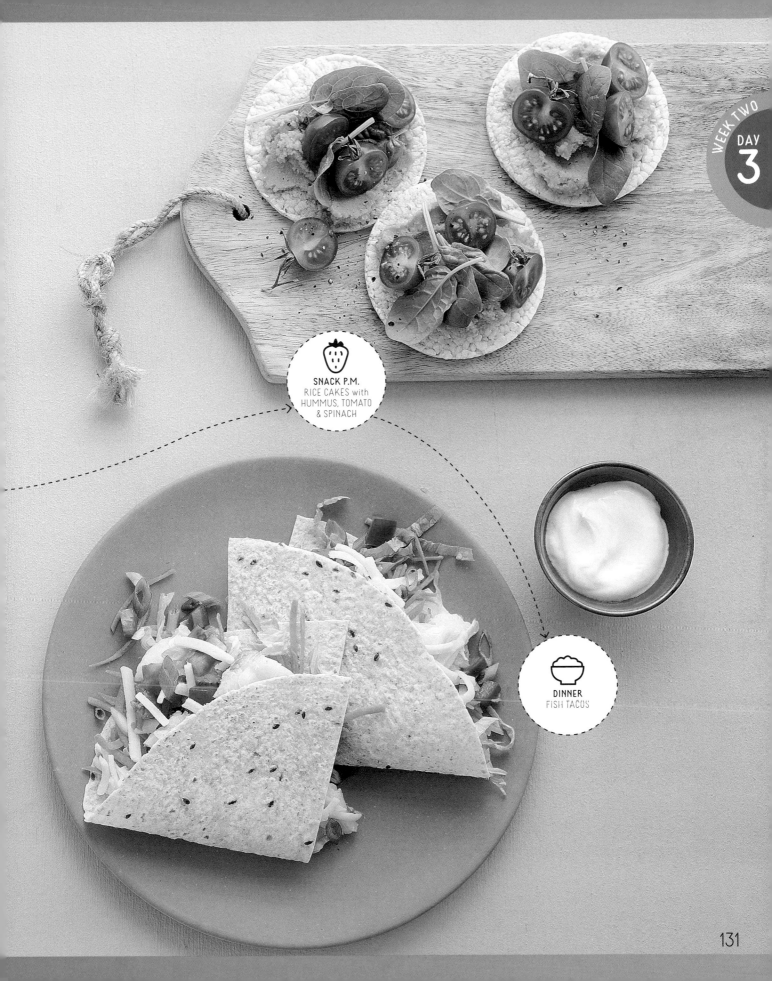

SNACK P.M.
RICE CAKES with
HUMMUS, TOMATO
& SPINACH

DINNER
FISH TACOS

CARROT CAKE SMOOTHIE BOWL

BREAKFAST **SERVES** 1 | **PREP TIME** 5 MINUTES + 30 MINUTES SOAKING TIME | **DIFFICULTY** EASY

1½ medjool dates, pitted

½ medium carrot, roughly chopped

1 medium banana, peeled and sliced

7 oz low-fat plain yoghurt

½ cup low-fat milk

½ teaspoon ground cinnamon

½ teaspoon ground ginger

1 teaspoon maca powder (see page 48; optional)

TOPPINGS

1 oz natural muesli

1 tablespoon shredded coconut

1 tablespoon raw cacao nibs

finely grated zest of ½ lemon

1 tablespoon finely grated carrot (optional)

In a heatproof bowl, cover the dates with boiling water and leave to soak for 30 minutes to soften. Drain.

Place the carrot, banana, yoghurt, milk, dates, cinnamon, ginger, and maca powder (if using) in a high-powered blender and blend until smooth.

To serve, pour the smoothie mixture into a bowl and top with the muesli, coconut, cacao nibs, lemon zest, and grated carrot (if using).

BERRY SALAD with NUTS

SNACK A.M. **SERVES** 1 | **PREP TIME** 5 MINUTES | **DIFFICULTY** EASY

2⅓ oz strawberries, halved or quartered

1½ oz blueberries

3–4 fresh mint leaves, chopped

1 tablespoon almonds, chopped

To serve, place the strawberries, blueberries, and mint in a small bowl and toss gently to combine. Sprinkle over the almonds.

FALAFEL PITA SANDWICH

LUNCH **SERVES** 1 | **PREP TIME** 15 MINUTES + 30 MINUTES CHILLING TIME | **COOKING TIME** 10 MINUTES | **DIFFICULTY** EASY

5¼ oz tinned chickpeas, drained and rinsed

¼ small brown onion, roughly chopped

½ garlic clove

¼ teaspoon ground cumin

¼ teaspoon ground coriander

1 tablespoon chopped fresh parsley

2 teaspoons whole wheat flour

sea salt and ground black pepper, to taste

oil spray

3½ oz tzatziki (see page 254)

1 whole wheat pita bread, halved

1 small handful lettuce leaves

½ medium tomato, sliced

½ Lebanese cucumber, sliced

Place the chickpeas, onion, garlic, cumin, coriander, parsley, flour, salt, and pepper into a food processor and blend until almost smooth. Shape the mixture into two even patties. Place on a plate, cover with plastic wrap, and refrigerate for 30 minutes.

Heat a non-stick fry pan over medium heat and spray lightly with oil spray. Add the falafels and cook for 4–5 minutes on each side until cooked through. To save time, the falafels can be made and cooked the night before and stored in an airtight container in the refrigerator.

To serve, spread half of the tzatziki over the inside of the pita bread. Fill with the lettuce, tomato, cucumber, and falafels. Drizzle over the remaining tzatziki.

RICE CAKES with HUMMUS, TOMATO & SPINACH

SNACK P.M. | **SERVES** 1 | **PREP TIME** 2 MINUTES | **DIFFICULTY** EASY

2¾ oz hummus (see page 254)

3 rice cakes

1 small handful baby spinach leaves

5 cherry tomatoes, halved

To serve, spread the hummus over the rice cakes. Top with the spinach and tomatoes.

FISH TACOS

DINNER | **SERVES** 2 | **PREP TIME** 10 MINUTES | **COOKING TIME** 10 MINUTES | **DIFFICULTY** EASY

oil spray

½ lb white fish fillet

sea salt and ground black pepper, to taste

2 whole wheat wraps

1 large handful romaine lettuce leaves, shredded

1 medium tomato, diced

1 medium carrot, grated

2 scallions, sliced

⅔ oz reduced-fat cheddar cheese, grated

DRESSING

3½ oz low-fat plain yoghurt

lemon juice, to taste

Heat a non-stick fry pan over medium–high heat and spray lightly with oil spray.

Season the fish fillet with salt and pepper, then place in the pan and cook for 2–3 minutes or until golden brown. Carefully flip the fish over and cook for a further 2–3 minutes or until the fish is opaque all the way through and flakes apart easily.

Transfer the fish to a plate and flake into large chunks using two forks.

To make the dressing, whisk the yoghurt and lemon juice together in a small bowl.

Meanwhile, warm the wraps in a large dry fry pan over medium–high heat for 30 seconds on each side. Remove from the heat and cut in half.

To serve, place the wrap halves on two serving plates. Top with the lettuce, tomato, carrot, scallions, cheese, and fish. Drizzle over the dressing and fold in half.

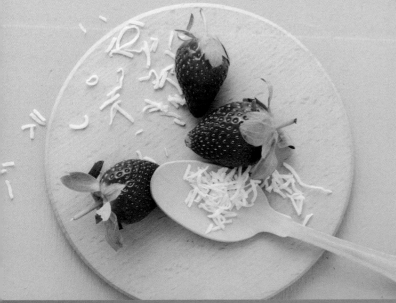

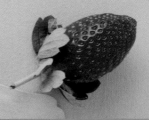

133

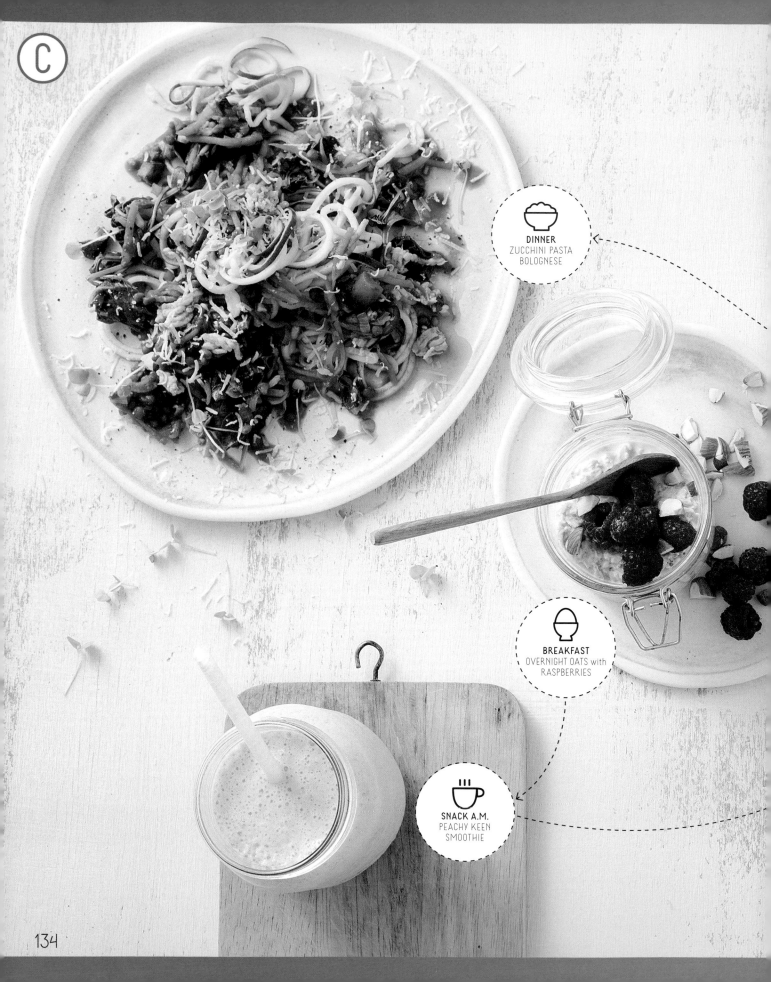

DINNER
ZUCCHINI PASTA
BOLOGNESE

BREAKFAST
OVERNIGHT OATS with
RASPBERRIES

SNACK A.M.
PEACHY KEEN
SMOOTHIE

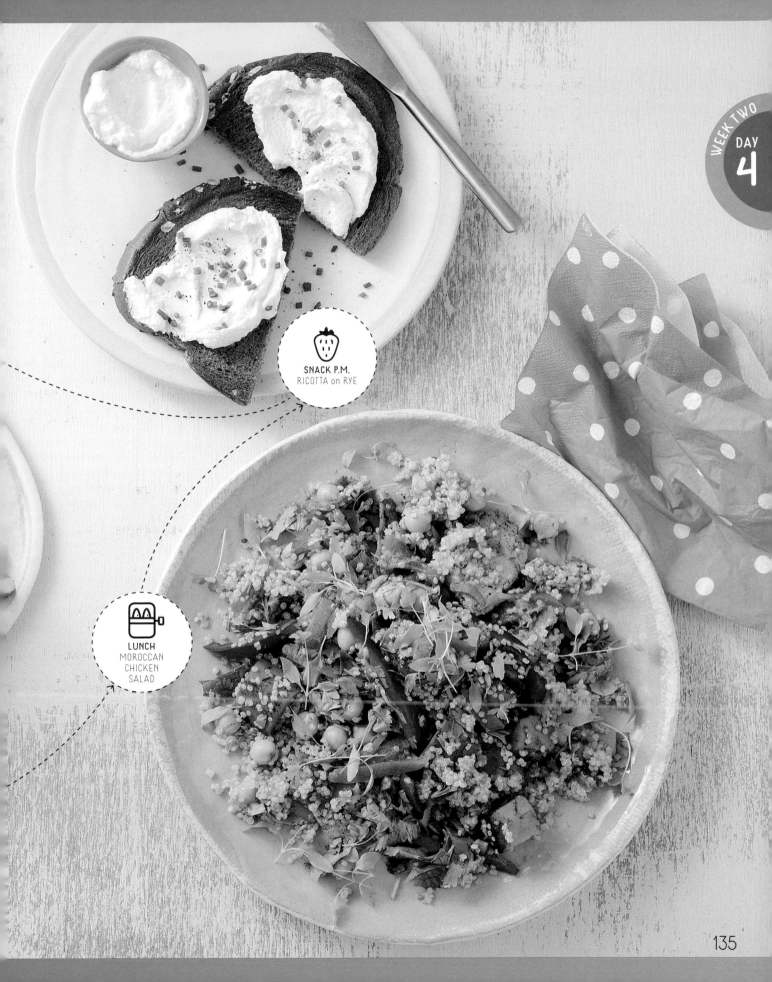

SNACK P.M.
RICOTTA on RYE

LUNCH
MOROCCAN
CHICKEN
SALAD

OVERNIGHT OATS with RASPBERRIES

| **SERVES** 1 | **PREP TIME** 5 MINUTES + OVERNIGHT CHILLING TIME | **DIFFICULTY** EASY

⅔ cup rolled oats

½ cup low-fat milk

1¾ oz low-fat plain yoghurt

1 teaspoon pure maple syrup

1 teaspoon chia seeds

3 oz frozen raspberries, thawed

1 tablespoon almonds, chopped

Place the oats, milk, yoghurt, maple syrup, chia seeds, and three-quarters of the raspberries in a bowl and mix until well combined.

Pour the oat mixture into a bowl or jar. Cover with plastic wrap and place in the refrigerator to chill overnight.

To serve, stir the overnight oats and top with the remaining raspberries and almonds.

PEACHY KEEN SMOOTHIE

SNACK A.M. | **SERVES** 1 | **PREP TIME** 5 MINUTES | **DIFFICULTY** EASY

1 oz rolled oats

1 large peach, with stone removed, chopped

½ medium banana, peeled and chopped

¾ cup low-fat milk

1¾ oz low-fat plain yoghurt

ice cubes

Place the oats, peach, banana, milk, yoghurt and ice cubes in a high-powered blender and blend until smooth.

To serve, pour into a glass or shaker.

MOROCCAN CHICKEN SALAD

LUNCH | **SERVES** 1 | **PREP TIME** 10 MINUTES | **COOKING TIME** 35 MINUTES | **DIFFICULTY** EASY

2 oz quinoa (about ⅓ cup)

2 oz pumpkin, peeled and cut into ½-in cubes

oil spray

3½ oz boneless skinless chicken breast sliced

1½ oz tinned chickpeas, drained and rinsed

¼ medium bell pepper, seeds removed and sliced

1 small handful fresh cilantro, chopped

finely grated zest of ½ lemon

juice of 1 lemon

sea salt and ground black pepper, to taste

MOROCCAN SEASONING

¼ teaspoon cayenne pepper

¼ teaspoon ground cinnamon

¼ teaspoon ground cumin

¼ teaspoon ground coriander

¼ teaspoon smoked paprika

1 teaspoon sea salt

½ garlic clove, crushed

juice of ½ lemon

To make the Moroccan seasoning, whisk the ground spices, salt, garlic, and lemon juice together in a small bowl.

Place the quinoa and ⅔ cup of water in a saucepan over high heat and bring to the boil, stirring occasionally. Cover and reduce the heat to low. Simmer for 10–12 minutes until the liquid is absorbed and the quinoa is tender. Set aside to cool.

Place the pumpkin in a small bowl with 1 teaspoon of the Moroccan seasoning and gently toss to combine. Ensure that all of the pumpkin cubes are lightly coated in the seasoning.

Heat a non-stick fry pan over medium heat and spray lightly with oil spray. Add the pumpkin and cook for 3–4 minutes or until all sides are lightly browned, turning occasionally. Add the chicken and cook for a further 3–4 minutes until both the pumpkin and chicken are cooked through. Set aside to cool.

To serve, place the pumpkin, chicken, quinoa, chickpeas, bell pepper, cilantro, lemon zest, and juice in a serving bowl. Season with salt and pepper, if desired, and toss gently to combine.

RICOTTA on RYE

SNACK P.M. **SERVES** 1 | **COOKING TIME** 5 MINUTES | **DIFFICULTY** EASY

1 slice rye bread

1 oz low-fat ricotta cheese

1 tablespoon chopped fresh chives

Toast the bread to your liking.

To serve, spread the ricotta over the toast and top with the chives.

ZUCCHINI PASTA BOLOGNESE

DINNER **SERVES** 2 | **PREP TIME** 20 MINUTES | **COOKING TIME** 45 MINUTES | **DIFFICULTY** EASY

1½ teaspoons olive oil

8 oz ground turkey or chicken (or 6 oz premium ground beef)

½ small brown onion, finely diced

1 garlic clove, crushed

½ medium carrot, grated

3½ oz mushrooms, chopped

2 tablespoons tomato paste

8 oz tinned crushed tomatoes

5¼ oz tinned brown lentils, drained and rinsed

2 medium zucchini

oil spray

1 small handful baby spinach leaves

sea salt and ground black pepper, to taste

1½ oz parmesan cheese, grated

chopped fresh basil, to serve

Heat the oil in a non-stick fry pan over medium heat. Add the ground meat and cook for 10 minutes or until browned, stirring frequently with a wooden spoon to break the meat up. Transfer to a heatproof bowl and set aside.

Add the onion and cook for 5 minutes or until soft and translucent. Add the garlic and cook for 1 minute, stirring frequently. Add the carrot and mushrooms and cook for a further 3–4 minutes or until soft. Add the tomato paste and cook for another 2 minutes or until the sauce is slightly thickened.

Add the tomatoes and bring to a boil. Reduce the heat to medium–low and simmer for 15–20 minutes, stirring occasionally. Add the lentils and simmer for a further 5 minutes or until the lentils are warmed through.

Meanwhile, spiralise the zucchini into large noodles. Heat a large non-stick fry pan over medium heat and spray lightly with oil spray. Add the zucchini and spinach and cook for 2–3 minutes or until the zucchini is soft and the spinach has wilted. Season with salt and pepper, if desired.

To serve, place the zucchini pasta in two serving bowls and top with the bolognese sauce. Sprinkle over the parmesan and basil.

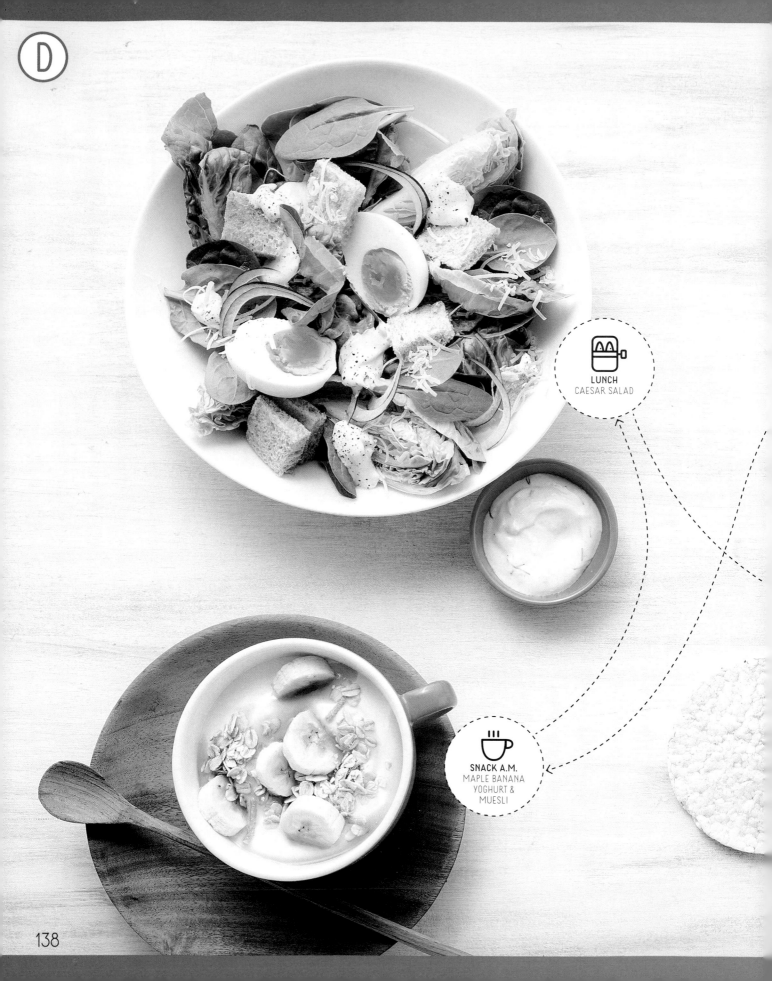

D

LUNCH
CAESAR SALAD

SNACK A.M.
MAPLE BANANA
YOGHURT &
MUESLI

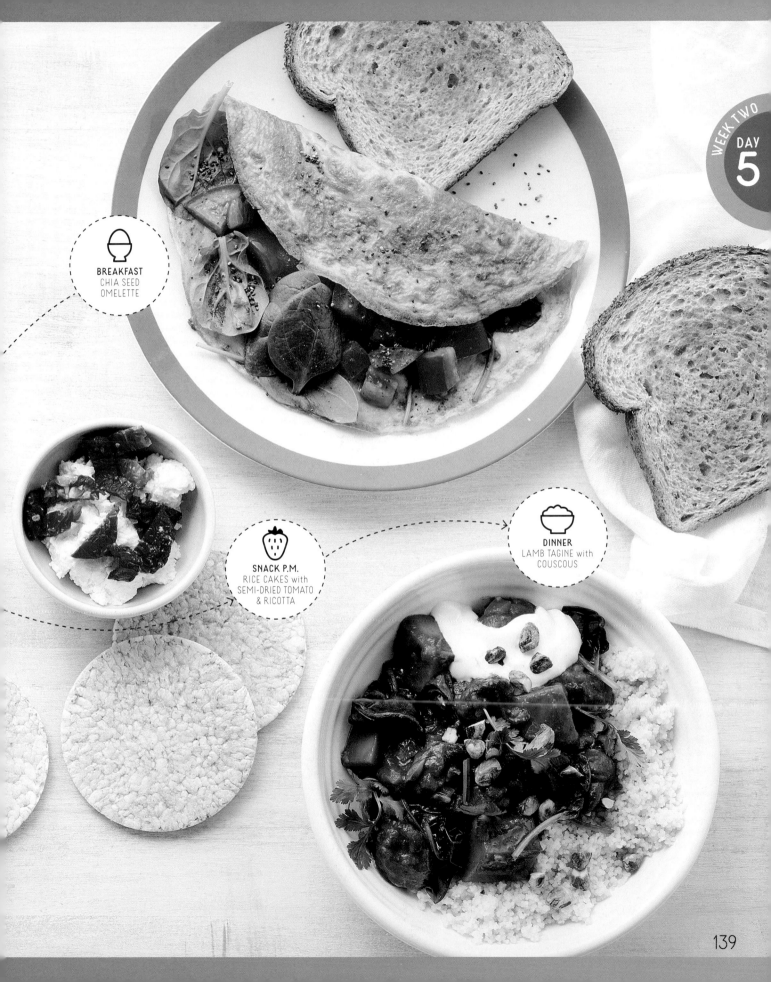

BREAKFAST
CHIA SEED
OMELETTE

SNACK P.M.
RICE CAKES with
SEMI-DRIED TOMATO
& RICOTTA

DINNER
LAMB TAGINE with
COUSCOUS

CHIA SEED OMELETTE

BREAKFAST | **SERVES** 1 | **PREP TIME** 10 MINUTES | **COOKING TIME** 5 MINUTES | **DIFFICULTY** EASY

2 large eggs

1 teaspoon chia seeds

sea salt and ground black pepper, to taste

¾ teaspoon olive oil

1 small handful baby spinach leaves

½ medium tomato, diced

⅔ oz reduced-fat cheddar cheese, grated

2 slices whole wheat bread

Whisk the eggs, chia seeds, salt, and pepper together in a small bowl.

Heat the oil in a non-stick fry pan over medium heat. Pour in the egg mixture and swirl to cover the base of the pan. Cook for 1–2 minutes or until the egg starts to set and the underside is golden in colour. Reduce the heat to medium–low.

Sprinkle the spinach, tomato, and cheese over the omelette. Cook for 1 minute or until the egg is set. Fold in half to cover the filling and transfer to a plate.

Toast the bread to your liking. Serve the omelette with the toast.

MAPLE BANANA YOGHURT & MUESLI

SNACK A.M. | **SERVES** 1 | **PREP TIME** 5 MINUTES | **DIFFICULTY** EASY

3½ oz low-fat plain yoghurt

½ teaspoon pure maple syrup

1 medium banana, peeled and sliced

1 oz natural muesli

Place the yoghurt, maple syrup, and three-quarters of the banana in a small bowl and mix until well combined

To serve, top with the muesli and the remaining banana.

CAESAR SALAD

LUNCH | **SERVES** 1 | **PREP TIME** 15 MINUTES | **COOKING TIME** 10 MINUTES | **DIFFICULTY** EASY

1 large egg

1 slice whole wheat bread

1¾ oz low-fat plain yoghurt

½ garlic clove, crushed

1 teaspoon Dijon mustard

lemon juice, to taste

1 teaspoon chopped fresh dill

1 large handful romaine lettuce leaves, chopped

1 small handful baby spinach leaves

¼ small red onion, finely sliced

⅓ oz parmesan cheese, grated

Place the egg in a saucepan and fill with cold water until it covers the egg by ¾ in. Bring to a boil over high heat. Reduce the heat to low and simmer, covered, for 5–6 minutes. Remove the egg with a slotted spoon and place in a bowl of iced water. Leave for 1 minute. Gently tap the egg on the bench to crack the shell and peel. Cut into halves.

Toast the bread to your liking. Cut into small squares.

Whisk the yoghurt, garlic, mustard, lemon juice, and dill together in a small bowl.

To serve, place the lettuce, spinach, half of the croutons, and half of the yoghurt dressing in a serving bowl and toss gently to combine. Top with the onion, egg halves, and remaining croutons. Drizzle over the remaining dressing and sprinkle with the parmesan.

RICE CAKES with SEMI-DRIED TOMATO & RICOTTA

SNACK P.M. **SERVES** 1 | **PREP TIME** 5 MINUTES | **DIFFICULTY** EASY

1¾ oz low-fat ricotta cheese

3 semi-dried tomatoes, thinly sliced

fresh basil leaves, torn, to taste (optional)

3 rice cakes

sea salt and ground black pepper, to taste

Place the ricotta, semi-dried tomato, and basil (if using) in a small bowl and mix until well combined.

To serve, spread the ricotta and semi-dried tomato mixture over the rice cakes. Season with salt and pepper, if desired.

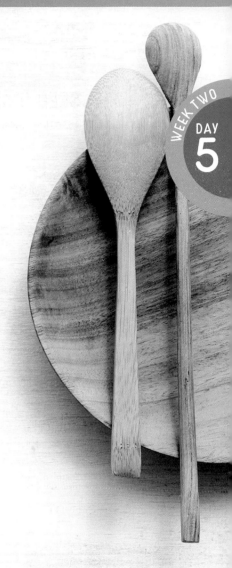

LAMB TAGINE with COUSCOUS

DINNER **SERVES** 2 | **PREP TIME** 15 MINUTES | **COOKING TIME** 40 MINUTES | **DIFFICULTY** EASY

oil spray

6 oz lean lamb leg steaks, cut into ¾-in cubes

½ small brown onion, diced

1 garlic clove, crushed

1 teaspoon sweet paprika

1 teaspoon ground coriander

1 teaspoon ground ginger

½ teaspoon chilli powder

¾ cup salt-reduced vegetable stock

5 oz tinned crushed tomatoes

1 sweet potato, peeled and cut into ½-in dice

8 dried apricot halves, sliced

finely grated zest and juice of 1 lemon

sea salt and ground black pepper, to taste

¼ teaspoon olive oil

2½ oz couscous

1 small handful fresh cilantro leaves, chopped

1 small handful baby spinach leaves

7 oz low-fat plain yoghurt

⅔ oz unsalted pistachio kernels, chopped

Heat a large saucepan over medium heat and spray lightly with oil spray. Add half of the lamb and cook for 2–3 minutes or until browned on all sides, stirring frequently. Transfer to a plate and set aside. Repeat with the remaining lamb.

Reheat the saucepan over medium heat. Add the onion and garlic and cook for 3–4 minutes, stirring frequently. Add the paprika, ground coriander, ginger, and chilli powder and cook for 1 minute or until fragrant, stirring constantly.

Return the lamb to the pan and add the stock, tomatoes, sweet potato, apricots, lemon zest, and juice. Season with salt and pepper, if desired, and stir to combine. Reduce the heat to low and simmer, covered, for 20–25 minutes or until the lamb is cooked through and the sweet potato is tender, stirring occasionally.

Meanwhile, in a small saucepan, bring the oil and ¾ cup of water to a boil. Add the couscous and remove from the heat. Leave to stand, covered, for 2–3 minutes before fluffing with a fork to help separate the grains. Stir through half of the cilantro and set aside.

Stir the spinach and half of the remaining cilantro through the tagine.

To serve, place the couscous in two serving bowls and top with the tagine and yoghurt. Sprinkle over the pistachios and remaining cilantro.

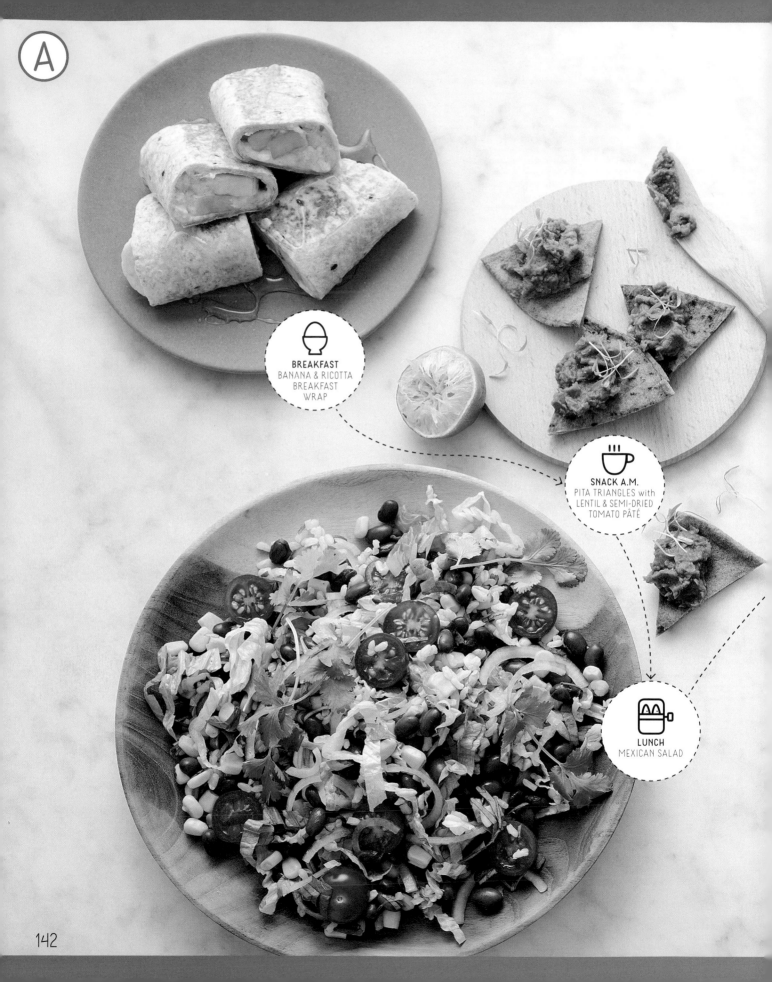

A

BREAKFAST
BANANA & RICOTTA
BREAKFAST
WRAP

SNACK A.M.
PITA TRIANGLES with
LENTIL & SEMI-DRIED
TOMATO PÂTÉ

LUNCH
MEXICAN SALAD

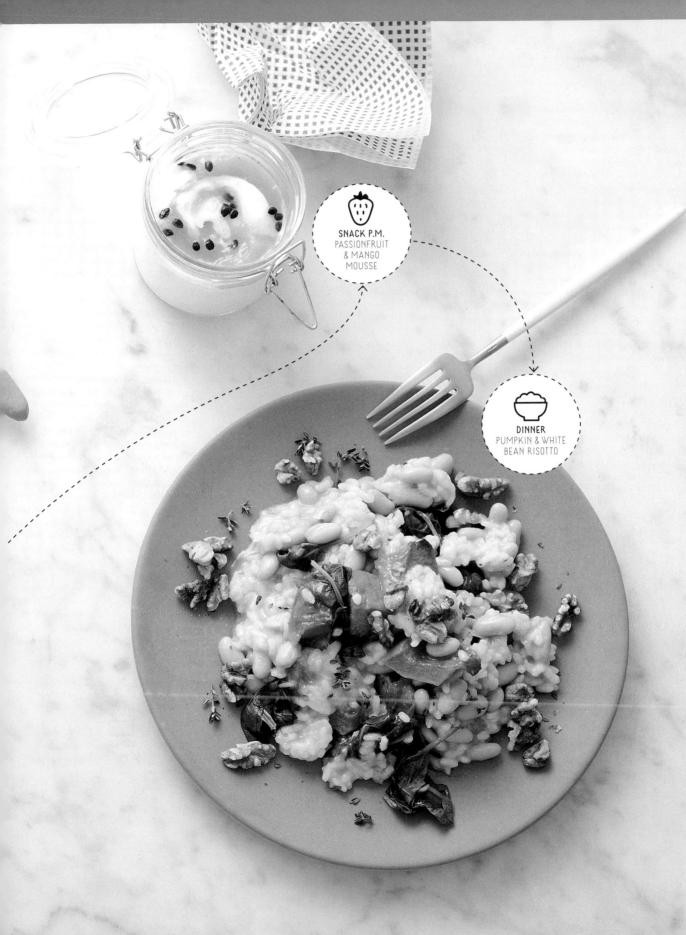

SNACK P.M.
PASSIONFRUIT
& MANGO
MOUSSE

DINNER
PUMPKIN & WHITE
BEAN RISOTTO

BANANA & RICOTTA BREAKFAST WRAP

SERVES 1 | **PREP TIME** 5 MINUTES | **COOKING TIME** 5 MINUTES | **DIFFICULTY** EASY

3½ oz low-fat ricotta cheese

¼ teaspoon ground cinnamon

1 whole wheat wrap

1 medium banana, peeled and sliced

2 teaspoons honey

Preheat a sandwich press.

Place the ricotta and cinnamon in a small bowl and mix until well combined.

Spread the ricotta over one-third of the wrap. Top with the banana, then roll up to enclose the filling.

Place the wrap in the sandwich press and toast for 3–4 minutes until the wrap is golden and the mixture is heated through.

To serve, cut the wrap into quarters and drizzle with honey.

PITA TRIANGLES with LENTIL & SEMI-DRIED TOMATO PÂTÉ

SERVES 1 | **PREP TIME** 10 MINUTES | **COOKING TIME** 20 MINUTES | **DIFFICULTY** EASY

½ whole wheat pita bread, cut into 4 wedges

oil spray

2¾ oz tinned lentils, drained and rinsed

4 semi-dried tomatoes, roughly chopped

¼ garlic clove, crushed

½ scallion, thinly sliced

¼ cup salt-reduced vegetable stock

½ teaspoon ground cumin

pinch of cayenne pepper

lemon juice, to taste

sea salt and ground black pepper, to taste

Preheat the oven to 400°F (350°F convection) and line a baking sheet with parchment paper.

Lay the pita wedges in a single layer on the lined baking sheet and spray lightly with oil spray. Bake in the oven for 5 minutes until they begin to colour. Turn over and bake for a further 5–8 minutes or until both sides are lightly coloured. Set aside to cool. To save time, the pita chips can be cooked the night before and stored in an airtight container.

Heat a small saucepan over medium–high heat. Add the lentils, semi-dried tomato, garlic, scallion, and stock and bring to a boil. Reduce the heat to medium–low and simmer for 5 minutes or until the tomato has softened. Remove from the heat and set aside to cool slightly.

Place the lentil and semi-dried tomato mixture, cumin, and cayenne in a food processor and pulse until smooth and creamy. Season with lemon juice, salt and black pepper, if desired.

To serve, place the lentil pâté in a small bowl and serve with the pita triangles.

MEXICAN SALAD

SERVES 1 | **PREP TIME** 10 MINUTES | **COOKING TIME** 25 MINUTES | **DIFFICULTY** EASY

2 tablespoons brown rice

¼ small red onion, sliced

5 cherry tomatoes, halved

1¾ oz frozen corn kernels, thawed

5¼ oz tinned red kidney beans, drained and rinsed

1 tablespoon chopped fresh cilantro

sea salt and ground black pepper, to taste

1 small handful lettuce leaves, shredded

lime juice, to taste

Place the rice and ½ cup of water in a small saucepan over high heat and bring to a boil, stirring occasionally. Cover and reduce the heat to medium–low. Simmer for 20–25 minutes or until the liquid is absorbed and the rice is tender. Remove from the heat and let stand, covered, for 5 minutes. Set aside to cool.

Place the rice, onion, tomatoes, corn, kidney beans, cilantro, salt, and pepper in a bowl and toss gently to combine.

To serve, place the shredded lettuce in a serving bowl and top with the rice salad. Squeeze over fresh lime juice.

PASSIONFRUIT & MANGO MOUSSE

SNACK P.M. | **SERVES** 1 | **PREP TIME** 5 MINUTES | **DIFFICULTY** EASY

½ medium mango, peeled
10¾ oz low-fat plain yoghurt
2½ passionfruit, halved

Place the mango and half of the yoghurt in a high-powered blender and blend until smooth.

To serve, place the remaining yoghurt in a serving bowl. Add the mango yoghurt and swirl through with a spoon. Top with the passionfruit pulp.

PUMPKIN & WHITE BEAN RISOTTO

DINNER | **SERVES** 2 | **PREP TIME** 10 MINUTES | **COOKING TIME** 50 MINUTES | **DIFFICULTY** MEDIUM

6⅓ oz pumpkin, peeled
and cut into ¾-in cubes
oil spray
sea salt and ground black
pepper, to taste
2 tablespoons walnuts
3 cups salt-reduced vegetable
stock
3 teaspoons olive oil
½ small brown onion,
finely chopped
1 garlic clove, crushed
4½ oz arborio rice
1 teaspoon fresh thyme leaves
2 large handfuls baby
spinach leaves
10¾ oz tinned cannellini
beans, drained and rinsed

Preheat the oven to 350°F (325°F convection) and line a baking sheet with parchment paper.

Place the pumpkin on the lined baking sheet and spray lightly with oil spray. Season with salt and pepper, if desired. Bake in the oven for 20–25 minutes or until it is lightly browned and tender.

Meanwhile, place the walnuts in a small dry non-stick fry pan over medium heat for 4–5 minutes or until lightly toasted and fragrant, stirring constantly. Set aside to cool. When cool enough to handle, roughly chop.

Heat the stock in a medium saucepan over medium heat.

Meanwhile, heat the oil in a large saucepan over medium heat. Add the onion and garlic and cook for 5 minutes until the onion is soft and translucent, stirring occasionally.

Add the rice and thyme and cook for 3–4 minutes until lightly toasted and fragrant.

Pour one-quarter of the warmed stock into the pan containing the rice and cook for 6–8 minutes or until most of the stock has been absorbed, stirring constantly.

Add the stock a ladleful at a time and allow the liquid to be absorbed before adding the next ladleful, stirring constantly. Cook for 20–25 minutes or until all the stock has been used and the rice is cooked but still al dente. If all the stock is used and the rice is not ready, add ¼ cup of hot water at a time until cooked.

Gently stir in the pumpkin, spinach, and cannellini beans and cook until heated through, stirring constantly.

To serve, place the risotto in two serving bowls and sprinkle over the walnuts.

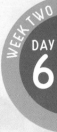

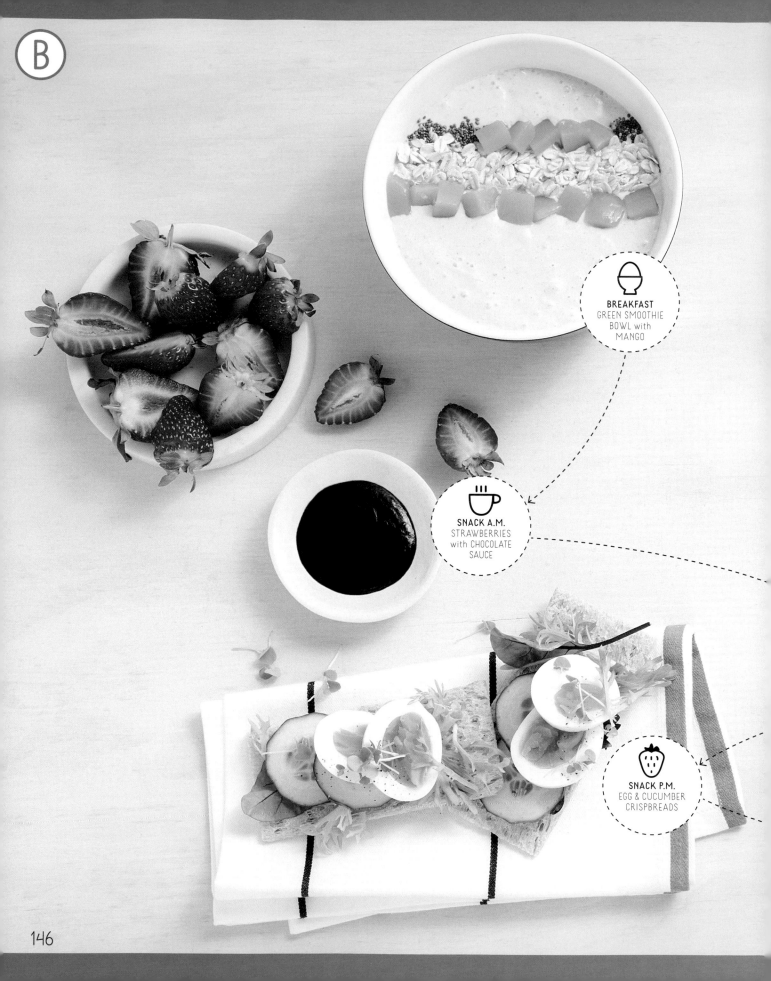

BREAKFAST
GREEN SMOOTHIE
BOWL with
MANGO

SNACK A.M.
STRAWBERRIES
with CHOCOLATE
SAUCE

SNACK P.M.
EGG & CUCUMBER
CRISPBREADS

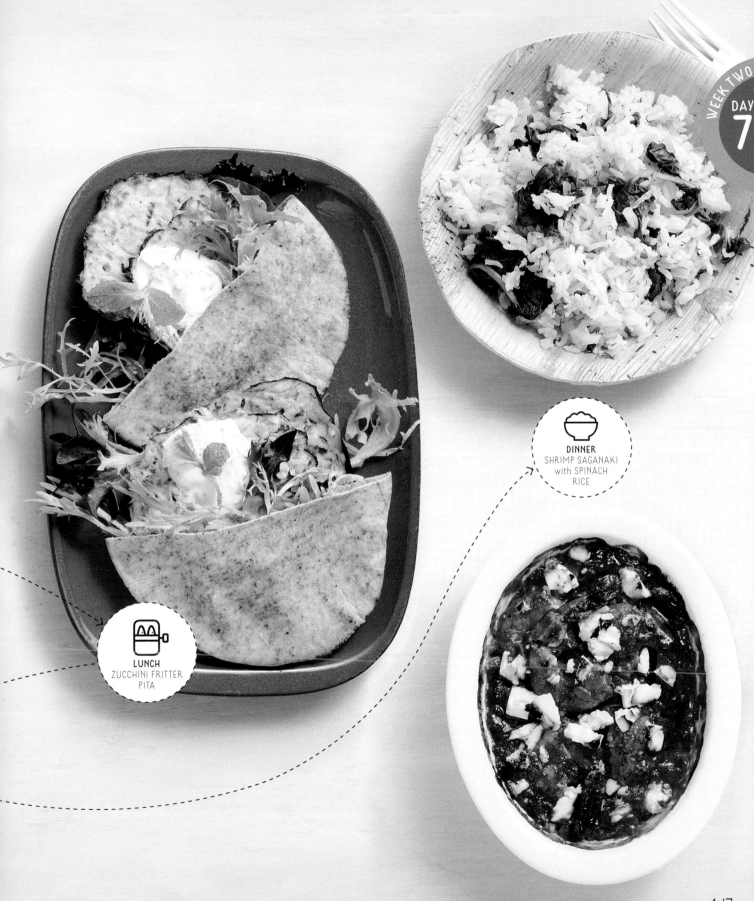

DINNER
SHRIMP SAGANAKI
with SPINACH
RICE

LUNCH
ZUCCHINI FRITTER
PITA

147

GREEN SMOOTHIE BOWL with MANGO

BREAKFAST | **SERVES** 1 | **PREP TIME** 5 MINUTES | **DIFFICULTY** EASY

1 frozen medium banana, chopped

1 small handful baby spinach leaves

7 oz low-fat plain yoghurt

½ cup low-fat milk

¼ medium mango, peeled and sliced

TOPPINGS

¼ cup natural muesli

¼ medium mango, peeled and sliced

2 teaspoons chia seeds

Place the banana, spinach, yoghurt, milk, and mango in a high-powered blender and blend until smooth.

To serve, pour into a serving bowl and top with the muesli, mango, and chia seeds.

STRAWBERRIES with CHOCOLATE SAUCE

SNACK A.M. | **SERVES** 1 | **PREP TIME** 5 MINUTES | **COOKING TIME** 5 MINUTES | **DIFFICULTY** EASY

1½ teaspoons coconut oil

1 teaspoon pure maple syrup

2 teaspoons raw cacao powder (see page 49)

4½ oz strawberries, halved

To make the chocolate sauce, heat the coconut oil and maple syrup in a small saucepan over low heat. Add the cacao powder and heat for 5 minutes until the sauce is warmed through and well combined, stirring constantly.

To serve, place the strawberries in a small bowl and serve the chocolate sauce alongside.

ZUCCHINI FRITTER PITA

LUNCH | **SERVES** 1 | **PREP TIME** 10 MINUTES + 30 MINUTES CHILLING TIME | **COOKING TIME** 20 MINUTES | **DIFFICULTY** EASY

1 medium zucchini, grated

2¾ oz tinned cannellini beans, drained and rinsed

½ oz salt-reduced low-fat feta cheese, crumbled

¼ small red onion, finely chopped

1 large egg, lightly beaten

sea salt and ground black pepper, to taste

oil spray

1¾ oz low-fat plain yoghurt

4 fresh mint leaves, finely chopped

1 small handful lettuce leaves

1 whole wheat pita bread, halved

Preheat the oven to 350°F (325°F convection) and line a baking sheet with parchment paper.

Using your hands, squeeze out as much liquid from the grated zucchini as possible. Transfer the zucchini to a mixing bowl.

Place the cannellini beans in a small bowl and mash with a fork until a smooth paste has formed. Place the cannellini bean paste, feta, onion, egg, salt, and pepper in the mixing bowl containing the zucchini and mix until well combined.

Shape the zucchini mixture into four even patties. Place on a plate, cover with plastic wrap and refrigerate for 30 minutes.

Place the patties on the lined baking sheet and spray lightly with oil spray. Bake in the oven for 10 minutes, then carefully turn and cook for a further 10 minutes or until golden.

Whisk the yoghurt and mint leaves together in a small bowl.

To serve, spread half of the minted yoghurt inside each pita half. Fill with the zucchini fritters and the lettuce. Drizzle over the remaining minted yoghurt.

EGG & CUCUMBER CRISPBREADS

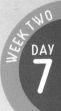

SNACK P.M. | **SERVES** 1 | **PREP TIME** 5 MINUTES | **COOKING TIME** 8 MINUTES | **DIFFICULTY** EASY

1 large egg

2 rye crispbreads

1 small handful lettuce leaves

½ Lebanese cucumber, sliced

Place the egg in a saucepan and fill with cold water until it covers the egg by ¾ in. Bring to a boil over high heat. Reduce the heat to low and simmer, covered, for 7–8 minutes. Remove the egg with a slotted spoon and place in a bowl of iced water. Leave for 1 minute. Gently tap the egg on the bench to crack the shell and peel. Slice into rounds.

To serve, top the crispbreads with the lettuce, cucumber, and egg.

SHRIMP SAGANAKI with SPINACH RICE

DINNER | **SERVES** 2 | **PREP TIME** 15 MINUTES | **COOKING TIME** 35 MINUTES | **DIFFICULTY** MEDIUM

oil spray

½ small brown onion, diced

1 garlic clove, crushed

½ fresh red chilli, finely diced

½ teaspoon dried oregano

20 medium raw shrimp, deveined, tails intact

1 tablespoon tomato paste

8 oz tinned crushed tomatoes

1 tablespoon chopped fresh parsley

2 oz salt-reduced low-fat feta cheese, crumbled

SPINACH RICE

oil spray

½ small brown onion, diced

1 large handful baby spinach leaves, finely chopped

2 teaspoons chopped fresh dill

2 teaspoons chopped fresh parsley

4¼ oz brown rice

lemon juice, to taste

sea salt and ground black pepper, to taste

To make the spinach rice, heat a saucepan over medium heat and spray lightly with oil spray. Add the onion and cook for 5 minutes or until soft and translucent, stirring occasionally. Add the spinach, half of the dill and parsley and cook for 5–10 minutes or until the spinach has wilted, stirring frequently. Add the rice and 1¼ cups of water and bring to a boil, stirring occasionally. Cover and reduce the heat to medium–low. Simmer for 20–25 minutes or until the liquid is absorbed and the rice is tender. Remove from the heat and let stand, covered, for 5 minutes. Stir in the remaining dill and parsley and season with lemon juice, salt and pepper, if desired.

Meanwhile, heat a non-stick fry pan over medium heat and spray lightly with oil spray. Add the onion and cook for 3–4 minutes or until soft, stirring occasionally. Add the garlic, chilli, oregano, and shrimp and cook for 2–3 minutes or until the shrimp are almost cooked through, stirring occasionally.

Add the tomato paste, crushed tomatoes, parsley, and ½ cup of water. Reduce the heat to medium–low and simmer for 7–10 minutes.

Preheat the broiler to high. Place the shrimp saganaki in a small baking dish and sprinkle over the feta. Broil for 3–5 minutes or until the feta is lightly browned.

Serve the shrimp saganaki with the spinach rice on the side.

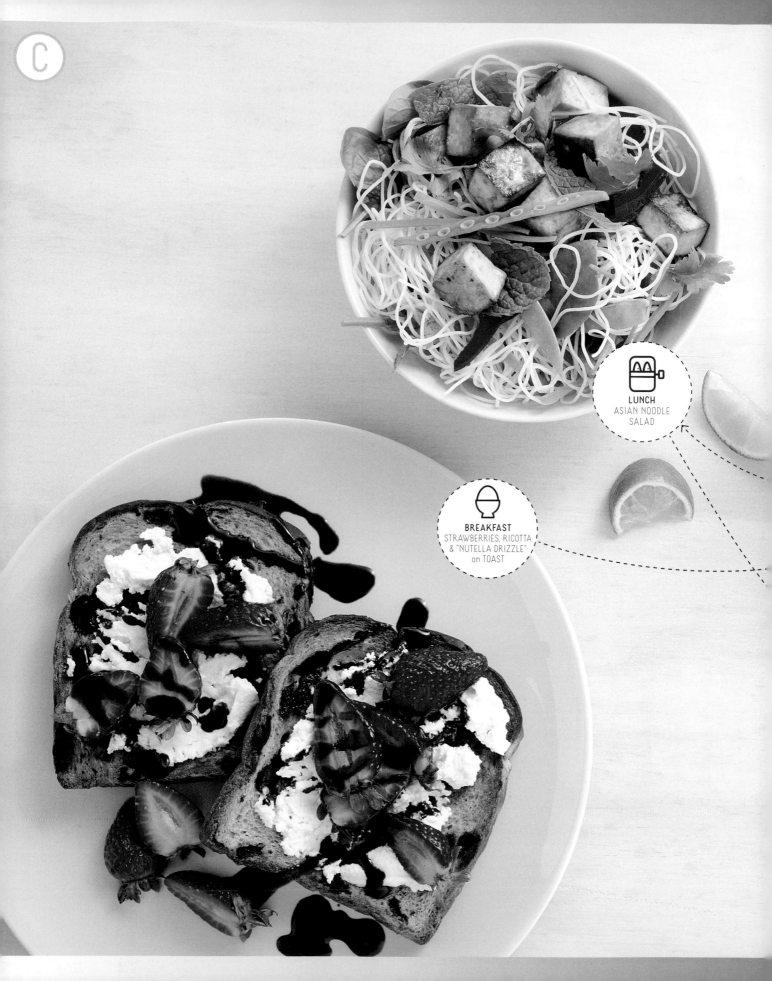

LUNCH
ASIAN NOODLE
SALAD

BREAKFAST
STRAWBERRIES, RICOTTA
& "NUTELLA DRIZZLE"
on TOAST

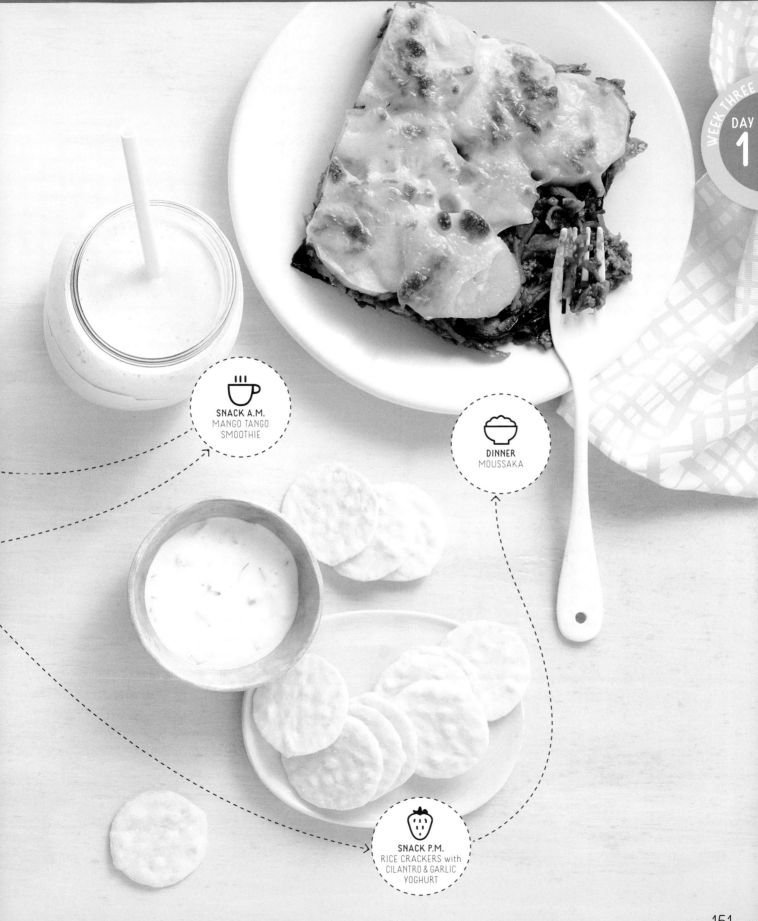

SNACK A.M.
MANGO TANGO
SMOOTHIE

DINNER
MOUSSAKA

SNACK P.M.
RICE CRACKERS with
CILANTRO & GARLIC
YOGHURT

STRAWBERRIES, RICOTTA & NUTELLA DRIZZLE on TOAST

SERVES 1 | **PREP TIME** 5 MINUTES + 30 MINUTES STANDING TIME | **COOKING TIME** 5 MINUTES | **DIFFICULTY** EASY

4½ oz strawberries, halved

juice of ¼ orange

1 teaspoon honey

2 slices raisin bread

2¾ oz low-fat ricotta cheese

NUTELLA DRIZZLE

1½ teaspoons coconut oil, melted

1 teaspoon pure maple syrup

2 teaspoons raw cacao powder
(see page 49)

1 teaspoon ground hazelnuts

Place the strawberries, orange juice, and honey in a small bowl and stir to combine. Set aside for 30 minutes at room temperature. This will cause the strawberries to soften a little and become syrupy.

To make the nutella drizzle, heat the coconut oil and maple syrup in a small saucepan over low heat. Add the cacao powder and ground hazelnuts and heat for 5 minutes until the sauce is warmed through and well combined, stirring constantly.

Toast the raisin bread to your liking.

To serve, spread the ricotta over the toast. Top with the strawberries and nutella drizzle.

MANGO TANGO SMOOTHIE

SERVES 1 | **PREP TIME** 5 MINUTES | **DIFFICULTY** EASY

1 oz rolled oats

1 medium mango, peeled
and sliced

3 oz pineapple, chopped

¾ cup low-fat milk

1¾ oz low-fat plain yoghurt

ice cubes

Place the oats, mango, pineapple, milk, yoghurt, and ice cubes in a high-powered blender and blend until smooth.

To serve, pour into a glass or shaker.

ASIAN NOODLE SALAD

SERVES 1 | **PREP TIME** 10 MINUTES + 10 MINUTES SOAKING TIME + 30 MINUTES MARINATING TIME | **COOKING TIME** 5 MINUTES | **DIFFICULTY** EASY

3½ oz rice vermicelli noodles

½ garlic clove, crushed

1 tablespoon salt-reduced
tamari or soy sauce

1 teaspoon lime juice,
or to taste

pinch of dried chilli flakes
(optional)

6 oz firm tofu, cut into
¾ in cubes

oil spray

¼ medium bell pepper,
seeds removed and
thinly sliced

1½ oz snow peas, trimmed
and sliced

¼ medium carrot, cut into
matchsticks (julienned)

1 small handful baby
spinach leaves

1 tablespoon chopped
fresh cilantro

1 tablespoon chopped
fresh mint

½ lime, cut into wedges

Place the noodles in a heatproof bowl and cover with boiling water. Leave for 10 minutes, then loosen the noodles with a fork. Drain and refresh under cool running water. Drain well and set aside to cool.

Meanwhile, whisk the garlic, tamari or soy sauce, lime juice, and chilli flakes (if using) together in a shallow bowl. Add the tofu and gently turn to coat. Cover with plastic wrap and refrigerate for 30 minutes to marinate.

Heat a non-stick fry pan over medium heat and spray lightly with oil spray. Add the tofu and cook for 4–5 minutes or until all sides are browned, turning occasionally. Transfer to a plate and set aside.

To serve, place the noodles, bell pepper, snow peas, carrot, spinach, cilantro, and mint in a bowl and toss gently to combine. Top with the tofu and serve with lime wedges on the side.

RICE CRACKERS with CILANTRO & GARLIC YOGHURT

SNACK P.M. | **SERVES** 1 | **PREP TIME** 5 MINUTES | **DIFFICULTY** EASY

12 plain rice crackers

CORIANDER & GARLIC YOGHURT

1¾ oz low-fat plain yoghurt

2 teaspoons chopped fresh cilantro

lemon juice, to taste

¼ garlic clove, crushed

sea salt and ground black pepper, to taste

To make the cilantro and garlic yoghurt, place the yoghurt, cilantro, lemon juice, garlic, salt, and pepper in a small bowl and mix until well combined. To save time, this can be made the night before and stored in an airtight container in the refrigerator.

Serve the rice crackers with the cilantro and garlic yoghurt.

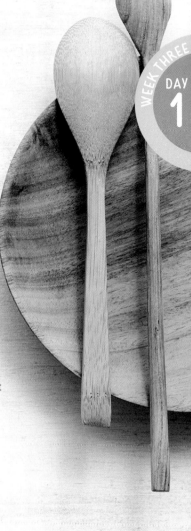

MOUSSAKA

DINNER | **SERVES** 2 | **PREP TIME** 15 MINUTES | **COOKING TIME** 1 HOUR 30 MINUTES | **DIFFICULTY** MEDIUM

1 medium eggplant, thinly sliced

oil spray

1½ teaspoons olive oil

½ small brown onion, finely chopped

1 garlic clove, crushed

1 medium carrot, grated

½ lb lean ground beef or lamb

1 teaspoon dried oregano

¼ teaspoon ground cinnamon

pinch of ground nutmeg

pinch of ground paprika

8 oz tinned crushed tomatoes

½ cup salt-reduced vegetable stock

1½ oz medium potato, peeled

1½ oz reduced-fat cheddar cheese, grated

Preheat the oven to 350°F (325°F convection) and line a baking sheet with parchment paper.

Lay the sliced eggplant in a single layer on the lined baking sheet and spray lightly with oil spray. Bake in the oven for 15–20 minutes until tender. Set aside.

Heat the oil in a large saucepan over medium heat. Add the onion, garlic, and carrot and cook for 5 minutes or until soft, stirring occasionally.

Add the ground meat and cook for 10–15 minutes or until browned, stirring frequently with a wooden spoon to help break up the mince. Add the oregano, cinnamon, nutmeg, paprika, tomatoes, and stock and stir to combine. Reduce the heat to medium–low and simmer, covered, for 15 minutes, stirring occasionally.

Meanwhile, place the potato in a saucepan. Add enough cold water to almost cover it and bring to the boil. Boil for 15 minutes or until the potato is tender. Drain and set aside to cool. When cool enough to handle, cut into ¼-in thick slices.

Spread a small ladleful of the meat mixture over the base of a 2-quart capacity dish. Layer half of the eggplant slices and half of the remaining meat mixture. Repeat the layers again, finishing with the meat mixture on top.

Arrange the potato slices over the meat mixture and sprinkle over the cheese.

Bake for 30 minutes or until the potato slices are golden and the cheese has melted. Let stand for 5 minutes and serve.

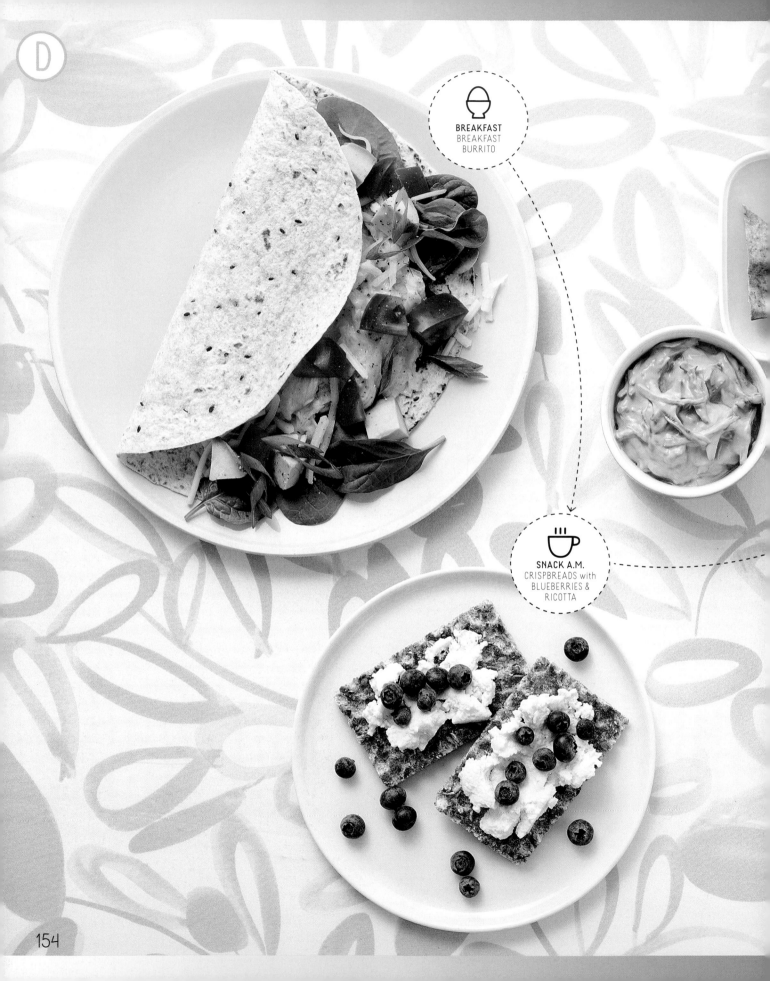

D

BREAKFAST
BREAKFAST
BURRITO

SNACK A.M.
CRISPBREADS with
BLUEBERRIES &
RICOTTA

154

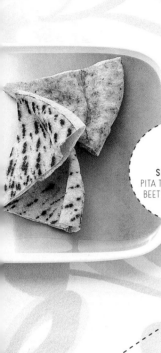

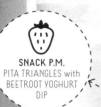

SNACK P.M.
PITA TRIANGLES with
BEETROOT YOGHURT
DIP

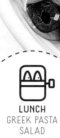

LUNCH
GREEK PASTA
SALAD

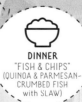

DINNER
"FISH & CHIPS"
(QUINOA & PARMESAN-
CRUMBED FISH
with SLAW)

155

BREAKFAST BURRITO

BREAKFAST **SERVES** 1 | **PREP TIME** 5 MINUTES | **COOKING TIME** 10 MINUTES | **DIFFICULTY** EASY

2 large eggs

sea salt and ground black pepper, to taste

1 whole wheat wrap

1 small handful baby spinach leaves

½ medium tomato, diced

½ scallion, thinly sliced

1 oz avocado, diced

⅔ oz reduced-fat cheddar cheese, grated

Whisk the eggs, salt, and pepper together in a small bowl. Heat a non-stick fry pan over medium heat and pour in the egg mixture. As the egg mixture begins to set, gently push it across the pan with a wooden spoon to form large folds. Ensure that you push from different directions and also include the mixture from around the edge of the pan. Do not stir constantly. Continue until no visible liquid egg remains and remove from the heat immediately.

To serve, place the wrap on a serving plate and place the scrambled egg, spinach, tomato, scallion, avocado, and cheese down the middle. Fold over the end and roll up to enclose the filling.

CRISPBREADS with BLUEBERRIES & RICOTTA

SNACK A.M. **SERVES** 1 | **PREP TIME** 2 MINUTES | **DIFFICULTY** EASY

1¾ oz low-fat ricotta cheese

2 rye crispbreads

3½ oz blueberries

To serve, spread the ricotta over the crispbreads and top with the blueberries.

GREEK PASTA SALAD

LUNCH **SERVES** 1 | **PREP TIME** 10 MINUTES | **COOKING TIME** 15 MINUTES | **DIFFICULTY** EASY

sea salt

1½ oz whole wheat pasta

2¾ oz tinned butter beans, drained and rinsed

½ Lebanese cucumber, sliced

5 cherry tomatoes, halved

2 kalamata olives, pitted and sliced

¼ small red onion, thinly sliced

1 oz salt-reduced low-fat feta cheese, crumbled

DRESSING

½ teaspoon finely chopped fresh oregano

½ garlic clove, crushed

2 teaspoons lemon juice

Fill a large saucepan with water, add a pinch of salt and bring to a boil. Add the pasta and cook until al dente (see the pasta packet for recommended cooking time). Drain and set aside to cool. To save time, the pasta can be made the night before and stored in an airtight container in the refrigerator.

To make the dressing, whisk the oregano, garlic, lemon juice, and 1 tablespoon of water together in a small bowl.

To serve, place the pasta, butter beans, cucumber, tomato, olives, and onion in a serving bowl and toss gently to combine. Sprinkle over the feta.

PITA TRIANGLES with BEETROOT YOGHURT DIP

SNACK P.M.   **SERVES** 1 | **PREP TIME** 5 MINUTES | **COOKING TIME** 15 MINUTES | **DIFFICULTY** EASY

½ whole wheat pita bread, cut into 4 wedges

oil spray

½ small beetroot, peeled and grated

pinch of ground cumin

pinch of ground coriander

lemon juice, to taste

3½ oz low-fat plain yoghurt

sea salt and ground black pepper, to taste

Preheat the oven to 400°F (350°F convection) and line a baking sheet with parchment paper.

Lay the pita wedges in a single layer on the lined baking sheet and spray lightly with oil spray. Bake in the oven for 5 minutes until they begin to colour. Turn the wedges over and bake for a further 5–8 minutes or until both sides are lightly coloured and set aside to cool.

Meanwhile, place the beetroot, cumin, coriander, lemon juice, yoghurt, salt, and pepper in a small bowl and mix until well combined.

Serve the pita triangles with the beetroot yoghurt dip.

"FISH & CHIPS" (QUINOA & PARMESAN–CRUMBED FISH with SLAW)

DINNER   **SERVES** 2 | **PREP TIME** 20 MINUTES | **COOKING TIME** 35 MINUTES | **DIFFICULTY** EASY

2 tablespoons quinoa flour or cornflour

1 large egg

2 oz quinoa flakes

finely grated zest of ½ lemon

⅔ oz parmesan cheese, finely grated

sea salt and ground black pepper, to taste

½ lb white fish fillet

1 medium sweet potato, washed, dried, and cut into ½-in thick chips

3 teaspoons olive oil

oil spray

½ lemon, cut into wedges

SLAW

3½ oz low-fat plain yoghurt

juice of ½ lemon

2 tablespoons finely chopped fresh parsley

3½ oz green cabbage, shredded

1 medium carrot, grated

2 medium green apples, cored and thinly sliced

Preheat the oven to 400°F (350°F convection) and line two baking sheets with parchment paper.

Place the quinoa flour or cornflour on a flat plate. Crack the egg into a small bowl and whisk until well combined. In a separate bowl, combine the quinoa flakes, lemon zest, parmesan, salt, and pepper.

Lightly coat the fish in the flour. Shake off any excess and then dip into the beaten egg. Coat the fish in the quinoa flake mixture, pressing firmly to ensure that it is evenly coated.

Place the sweet potato chips and oil in a mixing bowl and toss to combine. Ensure that all the chips are lightly coated.

Lay the chips in a single layer on one of the lined baking sheets and season with salt and pepper, if desired. Bake in the oven for 20 minutes or until tender and golden brown, turning once halfway through.

Place the crumbed fish on the second lined baking sheet and spray lightly with oil spray. Bake in the oven with the sweet potato chips for 10–15 minutes or until the fish is cooked through.

Meanwhile, to make the slaw, whisk the yoghurt, lemon juice, and parsley together in a small bowl. Place the cabbage, carrot, and apple in a mixing bowl. Drizzle over the yoghurt dressing and toss gently to combine.

To serve, place the crumbed fish, sweet potato chips, and slaw on two serving plates. Serve with lemon wedges on the side.

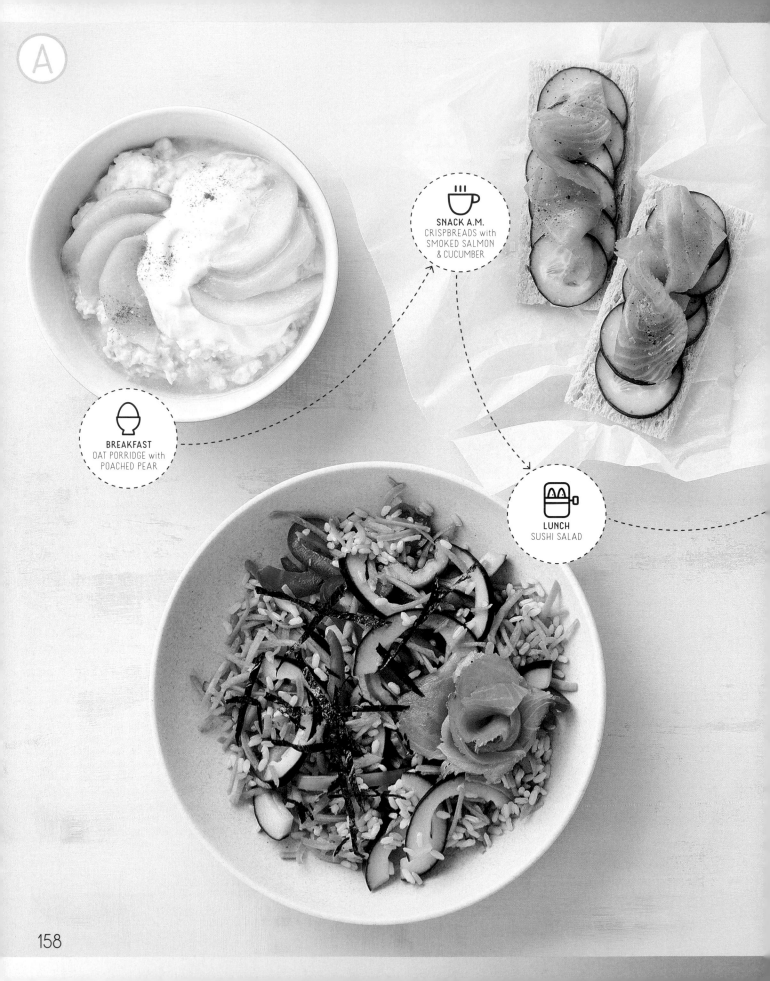

SNACK A.M.
CRISPBREADS with
SMOKED SALMON
& CUCUMBER

BREAKFAST
OAT PORRIDGE with
POACHED PEAR

LUNCH
SUSHI SALAD

SNACK P.M.
STICKY DATE
SMOOTHIE

DINNER
PAD THAI with
CHICKEN

WEEK THREE

DAY
3

159

OAT PORRIDGE with POACHED PEAR

SERVES 1 | **PREP TIME** 10 MINUTES | **COOKING TIME** 20 MINUTES | **DIFFICULTY** EASY

1 tablespoon honey

1 small pear, peeled, cored and halved

½ cup low-fat milk

2 oz rolled oats

3½ oz low-fat plain yoghurt

Bring the honey and 1 cup of water to a simmer in a small saucepan over medium–low heat. Add the pear halves and top up with a little water, if necessary (the pears should be completely covered). Cover with a lid and simmer for 10–15 minutes until the pear is just tender and the liquid is a little syrupy. Set aside to cool slightly. When cool enough to handle, cut into ¼-in thick slices. To save time, the pear can be poached the night before and stored in an airtight container in the refrigerator.

Bring 1 cup of water and ¼ cup of the milk to a boil over high heat. Stir in the oats and reduce the heat to medium–low. Simmer for 5 minutes or until thickened, stirring occasionally.

To serve, pour the porridge into a serving bowl. Top with the remaining milk, poached pear, and yoghurt. Drizzle over the poaching syrup.

CRISPBREADS with SMOKED SALMON & CUCUMBER

SERVES 1 | **PREP TIME** 2 MINUTES | **DIFFICULTY** EASY

2 rye crispbreads

1 Lebanese cucumber, thinly sliced

1¼ oz smoked salmon

sea salt and ground black pepper, to taste

To serve, top the crispbreads with the cucumber and smoked salmon. Season with salt and pepper, if desired.

SUSHI SALAD

SERVES 1 | **PREP TIME** 10 MINUTES | **COOKING TIME** 25 MINUTES | **DIFFICULTY** EASY

2 tablespoons brown rice

½ medium carrot, grated

¼ medium red bell pepper, seeds removed and thinly sliced

¼ medium green bell pepper, seeds removed and thinly sliced

½ Lebanese cucumber, thinly sliced

2½ oz smoked salmon, thinly sliced

2 nori sheets, cut into thin strips

DRESSING

2 teaspoons rice wine vinegar

1 teaspoon salt-reduced tamari or soy sauce

pinch of dried chilli flakes

juice of ¼ lime

Place the rice and ½ cup of water in a small saucepan over high heat and bring to a boil, stirring occasionally. Cover and reduce the heat to medium–low. Simmer for 20–25 minutes or until the liquid is absorbed and the rice is tender. Remove from the heat and let stand, covered, for 5 minutes. Set aside to cool.

To make the dressing, whisk the rice wine vinegar, tamari or soy sauce, chilli flakes, and lime juice together in a small bowl.

To serve, place the rice, carrot, bell peppers, cucumber, smoked salmon, and nori in a bowl. Drizzle over the dressing and toss gently to combine.

STICKY DATE SMOOTHIE

SNACK P.M. | **SERVES** 1 | **PREP TIME** 5 MINUTES + 30 MINUTES SOAKING TIME | **DIFFICULTY** EASY

3 medjool dates, pitted

1 cup low-fat milk

3½ oz low-fat plain yoghurt

Place the dates in a heatproof bowl, cover with boiling water, and leave to soak for 30 minutes to soften. Drain.

Place the dates, milk, and yoghurt in a high-powered blender and blend until smooth.

To serve, pour into a glass or shaker.

PAD THAI with CHICKEN

DINNER | **SERVES** 2 | **PREP TIME** 15 MINUTES + 10 MINUTES SOAKING TIME | **COOKING TIME** 15 MINUTES
DIFFICULTY MEDIUM

7 oz rice vermicelli or flat rice noodles

3 teaspoons sesame oil

3½ oz bonless skinless chicken breast, thinly sliced

1 medium carrot, cut into matchsticks (julienned)

2 scallions, thinly sliced

3 oz snow peas, trimmed and halved

2 large eggs, lightly beaten

1 large handful bean sprouts

1 small handful fresh cilantro, chopped

⅔ oz unsalted peanuts, chopped

sliced fresh red chilli, to serve (optional)

lime wedges, to serve

SAUCE

½ teaspoon finely chopped fresh red chilli

2 tablespoons salt-reduced tamari or soy sauce

juice of ½ lime

1 tablespoon honey

Place the noodles in a heatproof bowl and cover with boiling water. Leave for 10 minutes, then loosen the noodles with a fork. Drain and refresh under cool running water. Drain well and set aside.

To make the sauce, whisk the chilli, tamari or soy sauce, lime juice, honey, and 2 teaspoons of hot water together in a small bowl.

Heat a wok over high heat until hot. Add half the oil and carefully swirl it around to coat the sides of the wok. Heat until very hot.

Add half of the chicken and stir-fry for 2–3 minutes or until browned and just cooked through. Transfer to a plate. Repeat with the remaining chicken.

Reheat the wok over high heat. Add the remaining oil and carefully swirl it around to coat the sides of the wok. Add the carrot and scallions and stir-fry for 1 minute. Add the snow peas and stir-fry for 1 minute or until tender-crisp.

Make a well in the centre of the vegetables. Add the egg and stir-fry for 1 minute or until the egg is almost cooked. Add the noodles, chicken, and sauce and stir-fry for 1 minute or until heated through. Add the bean sprouts and toss to combine.

To serve, place the pad Thai on two serving plates and sprinkle over the cilantro, peanuts, and chilli (if using). Serve with lime wedges on the side.

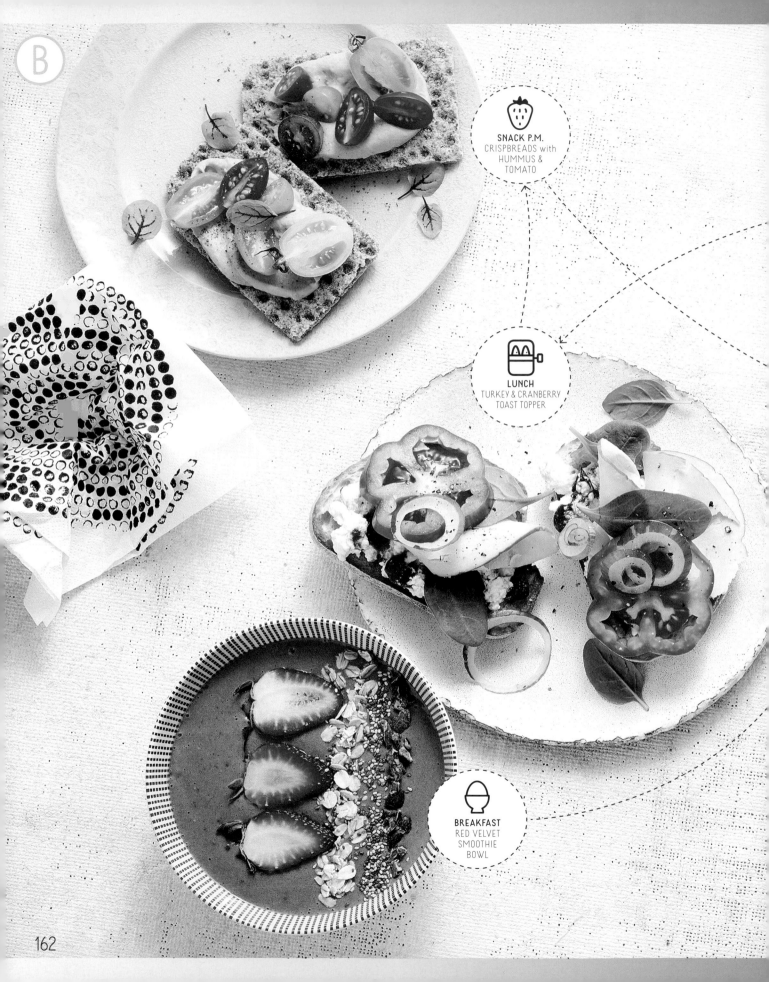

B

SNACK P.M.
CRISPBREADS with
HUMMUS &
TOMATO

LUNCH
TURKEY & CRANBERRY
TOAST TOPPER

BREAKFAST
RED VELVET
SMOOTHIE
BOWL

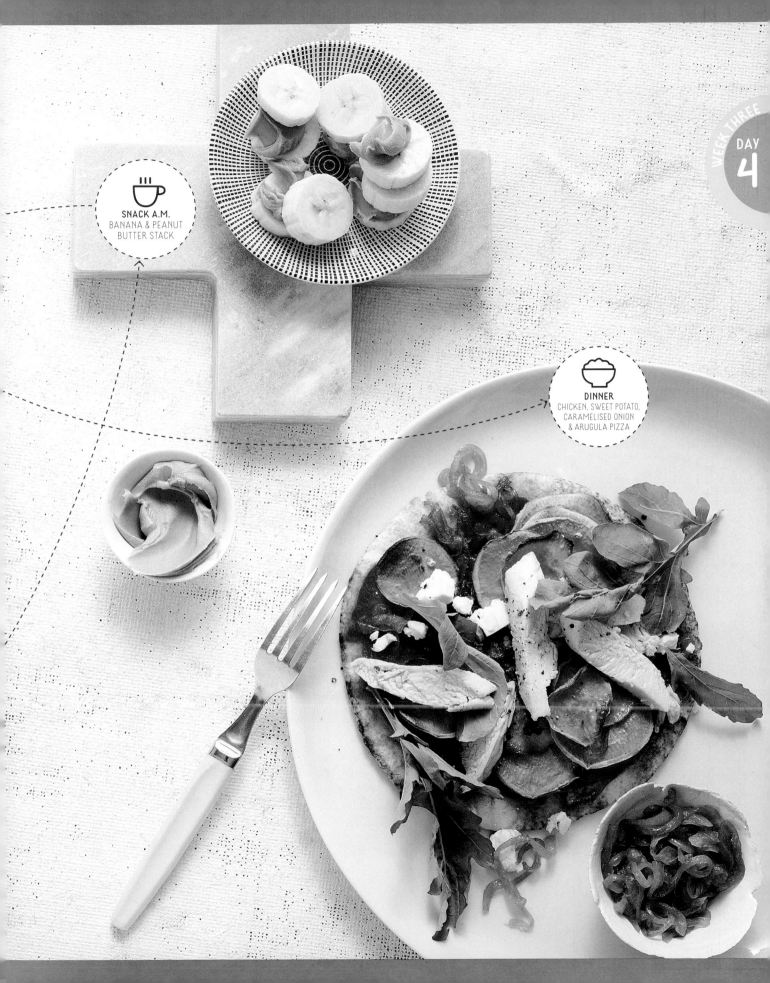

SNACK A.M.
BANANA & PEANUT
BUTTER STACK

DINNER
CHICKEN, SWEET POTATO,
CARAMELISED ONION
& ARUGULA PIZZA

RED VELVET SMOOTHIE BOWL

SERVES 1 | **PREP TIME** 5 MINUTES + 30 MINUTES SOAKING TIME | **DIFFICULTY** EASY

3 medjool dates, pitted

4½ oz strawberries, hulled

½ small beetroot, peeled and chopped

2 tablespoons carob powder or 1 tablespoon raw cacao powder (see page 49)

7 oz low-fat plain yoghurt

½ cup low-fat milk

TOPPINGS

1 oz natural muesli

2 teaspoons chia seeds

1 tablespoon raw cacao nibs

Place the dates in a heatproof bowl, cover with boiling water, and let soak for 30 minutes to soften. Drain.

Place the dates, strawberries (reserve one as a garnish, if desired), beetroot, carob or cacao powder, yoghurt, and milk in a high-powered blender and blend until smooth.

To serve, pour the smoothie mixture into a bowl and top with the muesli, chia seeds, cacao nibs, and reserved strawberry.

BANANA & PEANUT BUTTER STACK

SERVES 1 | **PREP TIME** 2 MINUTES | **DIFFICULTY** EASY

2 teaspoons 100% natural peanut butter

½ medium banana, peeled and cut into ½-in thick slices

Spread a small amount of peanut butter in between each of the banana slices to make a stack.

Repeat until all the peanut butter and banana is used.

TURKEY & CRANBERRY TOAST TOPPER

SERVES 1 | **PREP TIME** 5 MINUTES | **COOKING TIME** 2 MINUTES | **DIFFICULTY** EASY

1¾ oz low-fat ricotta cheese

1 teaspoon cranberry sauce

2 slices whole wheat bread

3 oz cooked turkey breast, sliced

¾ medium tomato, sliced

¼ small red onion, thinly sliced

1 small handful baby spinach leaves

sea salt and ground black pepper, to taste

Place the ricotta and cranberry sauce in a small bowl and mix until well combined.

Toast the bread to your liking.

To serve, spread the cranberry-ricotta mixture over the toast. Top with the turkey, tomato, onion, and spinach. Season with salt and pepper, if desired.

CRISPBREADS with HUMMUS & TOMATO

SNACK P.M. **SERVES** 1 | **PREP TIME** 5 MINUTES | **DIFFICULTY** EASY

2¾ hummus (see page 254)

2 rye crispbreads

1 medium tomato or 10 cherry tomatoes, sliced or halved

ground black pepper, to taste

To serve, spread the hummus over the crispbreads. Top with tomato and season with pepper, if desired.

CHICKEN, SWEET POTATO, CARAMELISED ONION & ARUGULA PIZZA

DINNER

SERVES 2 | **PREP TIME** 15 MINUTES | **COOKING TIME** 40 MINUTES | **DIFFICULTY** EASY

1 medium sweet potato, peeled and thinly sliced

oil spray

7 oz boneless skinless chicken breast, thinly sliced

2 whole wheat pita breads

2¾ oz tomato passata (tomato puree)

2 oz salt-reduced low-fat feta cheese, crumbled

1 small handful arugula leaves

sea salt and ground black pepper, to taste

CARAMELISED ONION

oil spray

1 small brown onion, thinly sliced

2 teaspoon pure maple syrup

1 teaspoon balsamic vinegar

Preheat the oven to 425°F (400°F convection) and line three baking sheets with parchment paper.

To caramelise the onion, heat a small non-stick fry pan over low heat and spray lightly with oil spray. Add the onion and cook slowly for 15–20 minutes or until soft and golden, stirring occasionally. Don't be tempted to increase the heat as this can cause the onion to burn. Add the maple syrup and balsamic vinegar and cook for a further 5–10 minutes or until sticky and caramelised, stirring occasionally. Set aside to cool. To save time, the onion can be caramelised the night before and stored in an airtight container in the refrigerator.

Meanwhile, place the sweet potato on one of the lined baking sheets and spray lightly with oil spray. Roast in the oven for 8–10 minutes until tender and lightly browned. Set aside.

Reduce the oven temperature to 350°F (325°F convection).

Heat a non-stick fry pan over medium heat and spray lightly with oil spray. Cook the chicken for 3–4 minutes until just cooked through, stirring occasionally. Set aside.

Lay the pita breads on a clean work surface and spread over the passata. Scatter over the caramelised onion and top with the sweet potato, chicken, and feta.

Place the pizzas on the lined baking sheets and bake for 8–10 minutes or until the toppings are hot and the edges are golden brown.

To serve, top the pizzas with the arugula and season with salt and pepper, if desired.

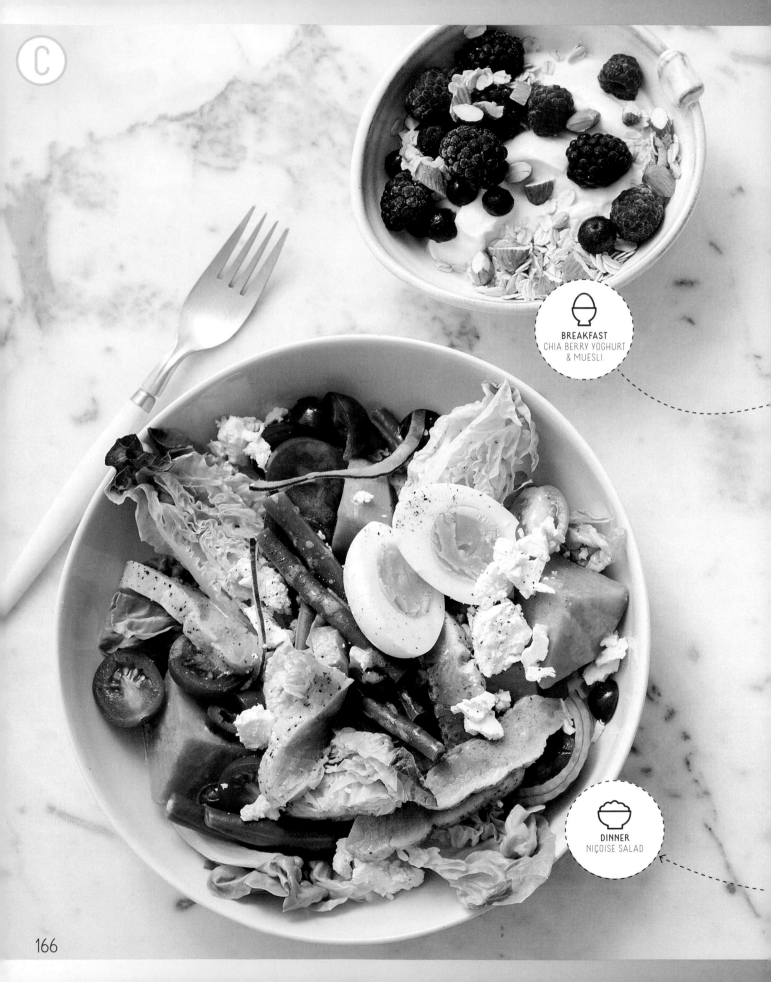

BREAKFAST
CHIA BERRY YOGHURT
& MUESLI

DINNER
NIÇOISE SALAD

SNACK A.M.
PEACHY KEEN
SMOOTHIE

LUNCH
VEGETARIAN
SALAD WRAP

SNACK P.M.
RICE CRACKERS
with MINTED
YOGHURT

167

CHIA BERRY YOGHURT & MUESLI

BREAKFAST | **SERVES** 1 | **PREP TIME** 5 MINUTES | **DIFFICULTY** EASY

5¼ oz low-fat plain yoghurt

1 teaspoon chia seeds

3 oz frozen mixed berries, thawed

2 oz natural muesli

1 tablespoon almonds, chopped

Place the yoghurt, chia seeds, and three-quarters of the berries in a small bowl and mix until well combined.

To serve, top with the muesli, almonds, and remaining berries.

PEACHY KEEN SMOOTHIE

SNACK A.M. | **SERVES** 1 | **PREP TIME** 5 MINUTES | **DIFFICULTY** EASY

¼ cup rolled oats

1 large peach, with stone removed, chopped

½ medium banana, peeled and chopped

¾ cup low-fat milk

1¾ oz low-fat plain yoghurt

ice cubes

Place the oats, peach, banana, milk, yoghurt, and ice cubes in a high-powered blender and blend until smooth.

To serve, pour into a glass or shaker.

VEGETARIAN SALAD WRAP

LUNCH | **SERVES** 1 | **PREP TIME** 10 MINUTES | **DIFFICULTY** EASY

1 whole wheat wrap

1½ oz hummus (see page 254)

4 oz tinned four-bean mix, drained and rinsed

1 small handful baby spinach leaves

¼ medium carrot, grated

¼ small beetroot, peeled and grated

½ medium tomato, sliced

1 small handful fresh parsley, chopped

To serve, place the wrap on a serving plate and spread over the hummus. Place the four-bean mix, spinach, carrot, beetroot, tomato, and parsley down the middle of the wrap. Fold over the end and roll up to enclose the filling.

RICE CRACKERS with MINTED YOGHURT

SNACK P.M. | **SERVES** 1 | **PREP TIME** 5 MINUTES | **DIFFICULTY** EASY

12 plain rice crackers

MINTED YOGHURT

1¾ oz low-fat plain yoghurt

2 tablespoons chopped
fresh mint

¼ garlic clove, crushed

lemon juice, to taste

sea salt and ground black
pepper, to taste

To make the minted yoghurt, whisk the yoghurt, mint, garlic, lemon juice, salt, and pepper together in a small bowl. To save time, the minted yoghurt can be made the night before and stored in an airtight container in the refrigerator.

Serve the rice crackers with the minted yoghurt.

NIÇOISE SALAD

DINNER | **SERVES** 2 | **PREP TIME** 10 MINUTES | **COOKING TIME** 25 MINUTES | **DIFFICULTY** EASY

2 large eggs

oil spray

Two 3-oz salmon fillets,
skin removed, deboned

1 sweet potato, peeled
and cut into 1-in cubes

15 green beans, trimmed
and halved

10 cherry tomatoes, halved

½ small red onion,
thinly sliced

4 kalamata olives, pitted
and sliced

2 large handfuls lettuce
leaves

sea salt and ground black
pepper, to taste

2 oz salt-reduced low-fat feta
cheese, crumbled

DRESSING

1½ teaspoons olive oil

2 teaspoons red wine vinegar

½ teaspoon Dijon mustard

Place the eggs in a saucepan and fill with cold water until it covers the eggs by ¾ in. Bring to a boil over high heat. Reduce the heat to low and simmer, covered, for 7–8 minutes. Remove the eggs with a slotted spoon and place in a bowl of iced water. Leave for 1 minute. Gently tap the eggs gently on the bench to crack the shell and peel.

Heat a non-stick fry pan over medium heat and spray lightly with oil spray. Add the salmon and cook for 5–6 minutes or until cooked to your liking, turning occasionally. Transfer to a plate and set aside to rest for 2 minutes. Flake the salmon into bite-sized pieces using two forks and set aside.

To make the dressing, whisk the oil, vinegar, and mustard together in a small bowl.

Fill a saucepan with water until 2 in deep and insert a steamer basket. Cover with a lid and bring the water to a boil over high heat, then reduce the heat to medium. Add the sweet potato and steam for 7 minutes or until tender. Set aside to cool.

Add the beans and steam, covered, for 2–3 minutes or until tender-crisp. Refresh under cool running water and drain well.

Place the sweet potato, beans, tomato, onion, olives, and lettuce in a large mixing bowl. Drizzle over the dressing, season with salt and pepper, if desired, and toss gently to combine.

To serve, place the salad on two serving plates and top with the salmon, egg, and feta.

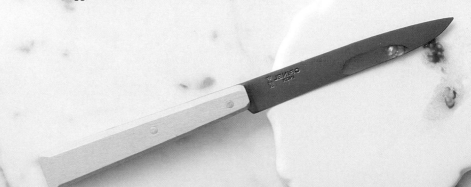

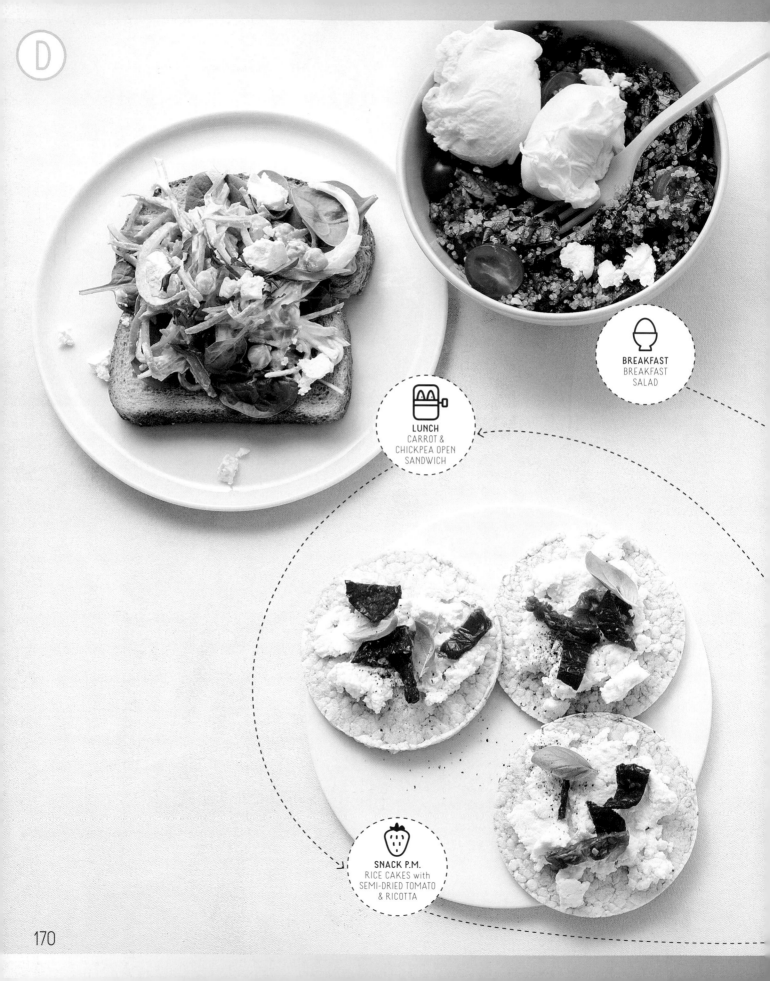

D

BREAKFAST
BREAKFAST
SALAD

LUNCH
CARROT &
CHICKPEA OPEN
SANDWICH

SNACK P.M.
RICE CAKES with
SEMI-DRIED TOMATO
& RICOTTA

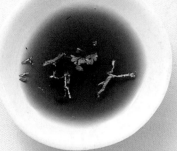

DINNER
BROWN RICE,
CHICKEN & ORANGE
SALAD

SNACK A.M.
APRICOT & PLUM
PARFAIT

171

BREAKFAST SALAD

SERVES 1 | **PREP TIME** 5 MINUTES | **COOKING TIME** 20 MINUTES | **DIFFICULTY** EASY

2 oz quinoa

1½ teaspoons olive oil

1 garlic clove, crushed

1 small handful kale, stalks removed and leaves roughly chopped

sea salt and ground black pepper, to taste

1 teaspoon white vinegar

2 large eggs

5 cherry tomatoes, halved

1 oz salt-reduced low-fat feta cheese, crumbled

Place the quinoa and 1 cup of water in a saucepan over high heat and bring to a boil, stirring occasionally. Cover and reduce the heat to low. Simmer for 10–12 minutes or until the liquid is absorbed and the quinoa is tender.

Heat the oil in a large non-stick fry pan over medium heat. Add the garlic and cook for 1–2 minutes or until fragrant, stirring constantly. Add the quinoa and stir to combine. Add the kale and cook for 1–2 minutes or until wilted, stirring constantly. Season with salt and pepper, if desired.

Fill a saucepan with water until 3 in deep. Add the vinegar and bring to a boil over medium heat, then reduce the heat to medium–low. The water should just be simmering. Break the eggs into the water and cook for 2–3 minutes for a semi-soft yolk or 3–4 minutes for a firm yolk. Remove the eggs with a slotted spoon and allow to drain on paper towel.

To serve, place the quinoa and kale mixture in a large serving bowl. Top with the tomato and poached eggs and sprinkle over the feta.

APRICOT & PLUM PARFAIT

SERVES 1 | **PREP TIME** 5 MINUTES + 10 MINUTES CHILLING TIME | **DIFFICULTY** EASY

3½ oz low-fat plain yoghurt

2½ small apricots, with stones removed, chopped

1½ plums, with stones removed, chopped

¼ cup natural muesli

honey, to drizzle

Layer the yoghurt, apricot, and plums in a glass.

Place in the refrigerator to chill for 10 minutes.

To serve, top with the muesli and drizzle with honey.

CARROT & CHICKPEA OPEN SANDWICH

SERVES 1 | **PREP TIME** 10 MINUTES | **DIFFICULTY** EASY

1 medium carrot, grated

⅔ oz salt-reduced low-fat feta cheese, crumbled

2¾ oz tinned chickpeas, drained and rinsed

¼ small red onion, thinly sliced

2 teaspoons chopped fresh parsley

2 tablespoons low-fat plain yoghurt

lemon juice, to taste

1 slice whole wheat bread

1 small handful baby spinach leaves

Place the carrot, feta, chickpeas, onion, parsley, yoghurt, and lemon juice in a medium bowl and toss gently to combine.

To serve, place the bread on a serving plate and top with the spinach and the carrot and chickpea mixture.

RICE CAKES with SEMI-DRIED TOMATO & RICOTTA

SNACK P.M. | **SERVES** 1 | **PREP TIME** 5 MINUTES | **DIFFICULTY** EASY

1¾ oz low-fat ricotta cheese

3 semi-dried tomatoes, finely sliced

fresh basil leaves, torn, to taste

3 rice cakes

sea salt and ground black pepper, to taste

Place the ricotta cheese, semi-dried tomato, and basil in a small bowl and mix until well combined.

To serve, spread the ricotta and semi-dried tomato mixture over the rice cakes. Season with salt and pepper, if desired.

BROWN RICE, CHICKEN & ORANGE SALAD

DINNER | **SERVES** 2 | **PREP TIME** 15 MINUTES | **COOKING TIME** 25 MINUTES | **DIFFICULTY** MEDIUM

2 oz brown rice

2 cups salt-reduced chicken stock

½ garlic clove, finely chopped

1 sprig fresh thyme

7 oz boneless skinless chicken breast

1 medium carrot, grated

½ medium red bell pepper, seeds removed and thinly sliced

1 medium orange, peeled and segmented

1 large handful baby spinach leaves

2 scallions, thinly sliced

2 tablespoons raisins

2 tablespoons unsalted pistachio kernels, chopped

sea salt and ground black pepper, to taste

1¾ oz soft goat's cheese, crumbled

ORANGE & CILANTRO DRESSING

1 teaspoon honey

2 teaspoons balsamic vinegar

freshly squeezed orange juice, to taste

1 tablespoon finely chopped fresh cilantro

Place the rice and 1 cup of water in a small saucepan over high heat and bring to a boil, stirring occasionally. Cover and reduce the heat to medium–low. Simmer for 20–25 minutes or until the liquid is absorbed and the rice is tender. Remove from the heat and leave to stand, covered, for 5 minutes. Set aside to cool.

Meanwhile, place the stock, garlic, and thyme in a medium saucepan over medium–high heat and bring to a boil. Add the chicken and return to a boil. Reduce the heat to low and simmer, covered, for 15 minutes or until the chicken is cooked through. Remove from the heat and leave the chicken to stand in the stock for 5 minutes. Transfer to a plate and set aside to cool. Slice the chicken into thin strips.

To make the dressing, whisk the honey, vinegar, orange juice, cilantro, and 1 tablespoon of water together in a small bowl.

Place the rice, carrot, bell pepper, orange segments, spinach, scallions, raisins, and pistachios in a medium bowl. Drizzle over the dressing, season with salt and pepper, if desired, and toss gently to combine.

To serve, place the rice salad on two serving plates and top with the chicken and goat's cheese.

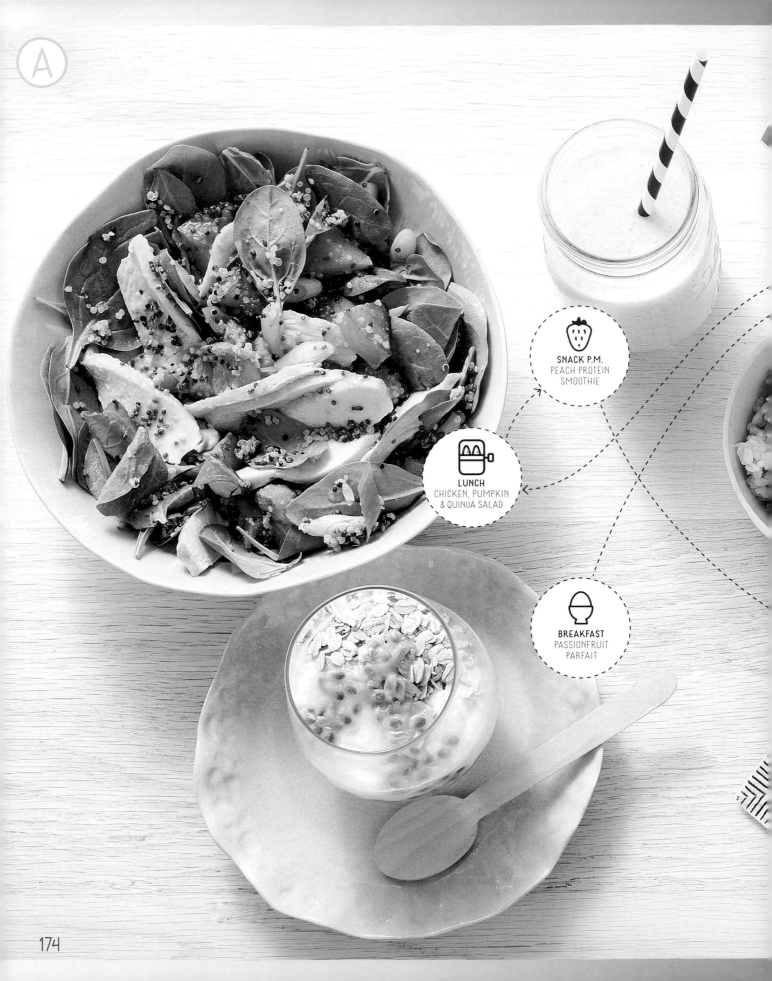

SNACK P.M.
PEACH PROTEIN
SMOOTHIE

LUNCH
CHICKEN, PUMPKIN
& QUINUA SALAD

BREAKFAST
PASSIONFRUIT
PARFAIT

A

174

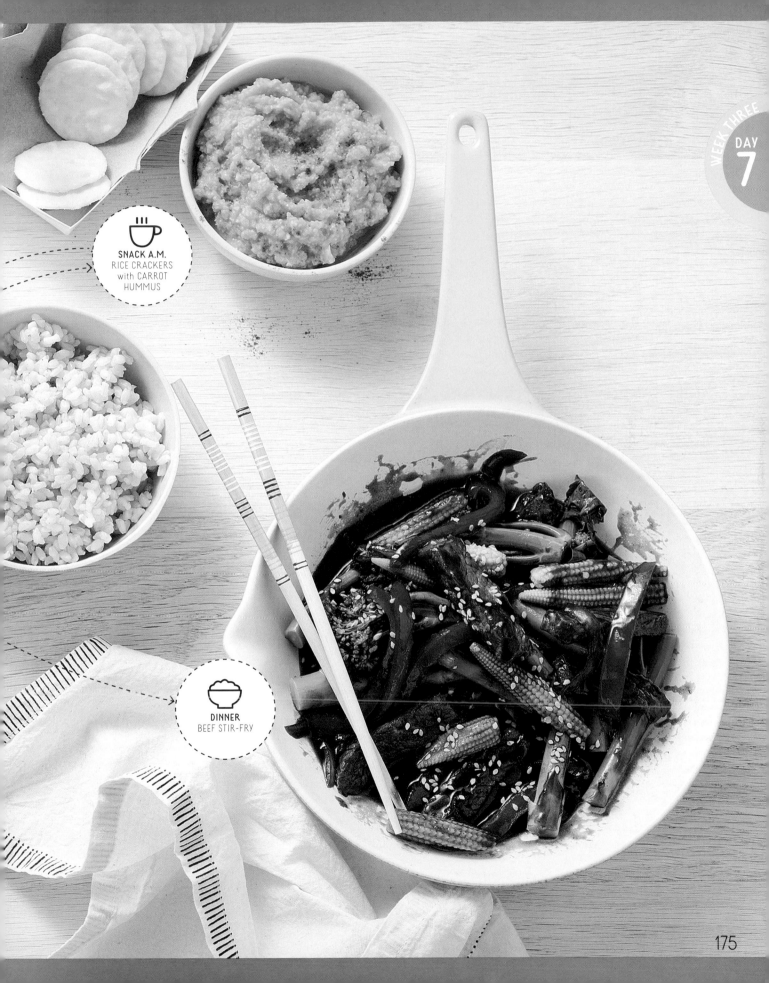

SNACK A.M.
RICE CRACKERS
with CARROT
HUMMUS

DINNER
BEEF STIR-FRY

175

PASSIONFRUIT PARFAIT

BREAKFAST | **SERVES** 1 | **PREP TIME** 5 MINUTES + 10 MINUTES CHILLING TIME | **DIFFICULTY** EASY

7 oz low-fat plain yoghurt

2 oz natural muesli

5 passionfruit, halved

Layer the yoghurt, muesli, and passionfruit in a glass.

Place in the refrigerator to chill for 10 minutes. Serve.

RICE CRACKERS with CARROT HUMMUS

SNACK A.M. | **SERVES** 1 | **PREP TIME** 5 MINUTES | **COOKING TIME** 20 MINUTES | **DIFFICULTY** EASY

12 plain rice crackers

CARROT HUMMUS

1 medium carrot,
roughly chopped

2¾ oz tinned chickpeas,
drained and rinsed

¼ garlic clove, crushed

lemon juice, to taste

pinch of smoked paprika

sea salt, to taste

To make the carrot hummus, place the carrot in a small saucepan and fill with cold water until it just covers the carrots. Bring the water to a boil then reduce the heat to medium–low. Simmer for 15–20 minutes until tender. Drain and set aside to cool.

Place the carrot, chickpeas, garlic, lemon juice, paprika, and salt in a food processor and pulse until smooth and creamy. To save time, the carrot hummus can be made the night before and stored in an airtight container in the refrigerator.

Serve the rice crackers with the carrot hummus.

CHICKEN, PUMPKIN & QUINOA SALAD

LUNCH | **SERVES** 1 | **PREP TIME** 10 MINUTES | **COOKING TIME** 25 MINUTES | **DIFFICULTY** EASY

4¼ oz pumpkin, peeled
and cut into 1-in cubes

oil spray

sea salt and ground black
pepper, to taste

3½ oz boneless skinless
chicken breast fillet

1 oz quinoa

1 scallion, thinly sliced

1 small handful baby
spinach leaves

**HONEY MUSTARD
DRESSING**

juice of ½ orange

1 teaspoon honey

1 teaspoon wholegrain
mustard

Preheat the oven to 350°F (325°F convection) and line two baking sheets with parchment paper.

Place the pumpkin on one of the lined baking sheets. Lightly spray with oil spray and season with salt and pepper, if desired.

Place the chicken on the other lined baking sheet. Lightly spray with oil spray and season with salt and pepper, if desired.

Roast the pumpkin and chicken in the oven for 20–25 minutes or until the pumpkin is tender and the chicken is cooked through, turning the pumpkin with tongs every 10–12 minutes. Set aside to cool slightly. When cool enough to handle, cut the chicken into ¼-in thick slices.

Meanwhile, place the quinoa and ½ cup of water in a saucepan over high heat and bring to the boil, stirring occasionally. Cover and reduce the heat to low. Simmer for 10–12 minutes until the quinoa is tender. Drain off any excess liquid.

To save time, the pumpkin, chicken, and quinoa can be cooked the night before and stored in an airtight container in the refrigerator.

To make the honey mustard dressing, whisk the orange juice, honey, and mustard together in a small bowl.

To serve, place the quinoa, pumpkin, chicken, scallion, and spinach in a serving bowl. Drizzle over the dressing and toss gently to combine.

PEACH PROTEIN SMOOTHIE

SNACK P.M. | **SERVES** 1 | **PREP TIME** 5 MINUTES | **DIFFICULTY** EASY

1 large peach, stone removed, cut into bite-sized pieces

3½ oz low-fat plain yoghurt

1 cup low-fat milk

1 scoop 1 oz protein powder (optional)

Place the peach, yoghurt, milk, and protein powder (if using) in a high-powered blender and blend until smooth.

To serve, pour into a glass or shaker.

BEEF STIR-FRY

DINNER | **SERVES** 2 | **PREP TIME** 10 MINUTES | **COOKING TIME** 25 MINUTES | **DIFFICULTY** EASY

4¼ oz brown rice

3 teaspoons sesame oil

6 oz lean beef strips

½ small brown onion, sliced

½ medium red bell pepper, seeds removed and thinly sliced

2 oz baby corn

4¾ oz broccolini, sliced

2 garlic cloves, crushed

2 tablespoons oyster sauce

2½ tablespoons salt-reduced tamari or soy sauce

1 tablespoon sesame seeds

Place the rice and 1¼ cups of water in a small saucepan over high heat and bring to the boil, stirring occasionally. Cover and reduce the heat to medium–low. Simmer for 20–25 minutes or until the liquid is absorbed and the rice is tender. Remove from the heat and leave to stand, covered, for 5 minutes.

Meanwhile, heat a large wok over high heat until hot. Add half of the oil and carefully swirl it around to coat the sides of the wok. Heat until very hot.

Add half of the beef and stir-fry for 1–2 minutes or until browned and just cooked. Transfer to a plate and set aside to rest. Reheat the wok and repeat with the remaining beef.

Heat the remaining oil in the wok over high heat. Add the onion, bell pepper, baby corn, broccolini, and garlic and stir-fry for 2 minutes. Add 1 tablespoon of water and cook, covered, for 30–60 seconds until the vegetables are tender-crisp.

Add the oyster sauce and tamari or soy sauce and toss until well combined. Add the sesame seeds and beef and stir-fry for 1 minute or until heated through.

To serve, place the rice in two serving bowls and top with the beef stir-fry.

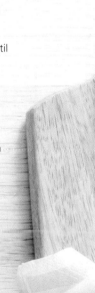

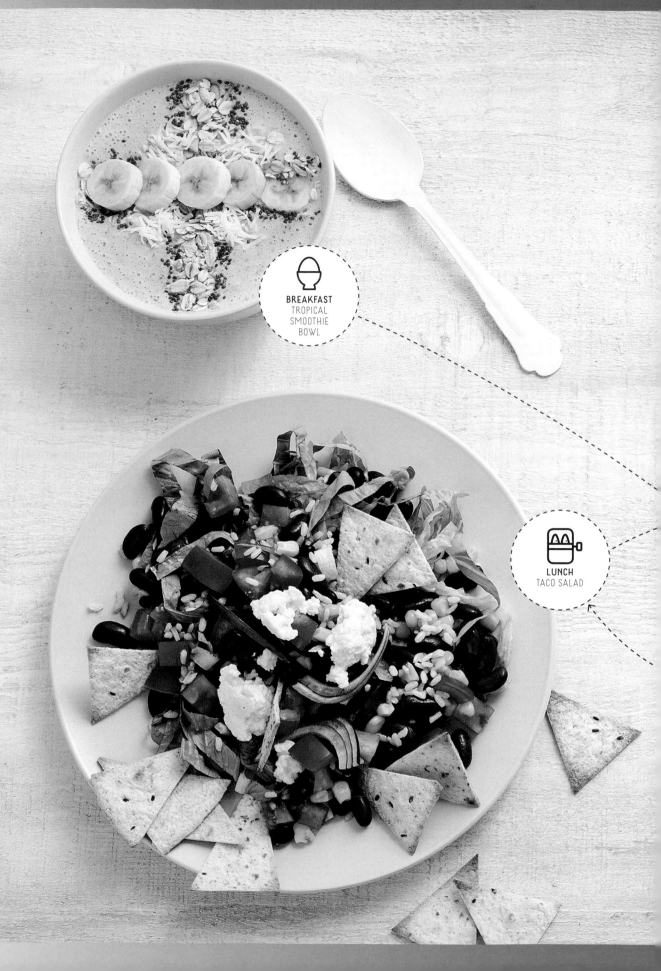

B

BREAKFAST
TROPICAL
SMOOTHIE
BOWL

LUNCH
TACO SALAD

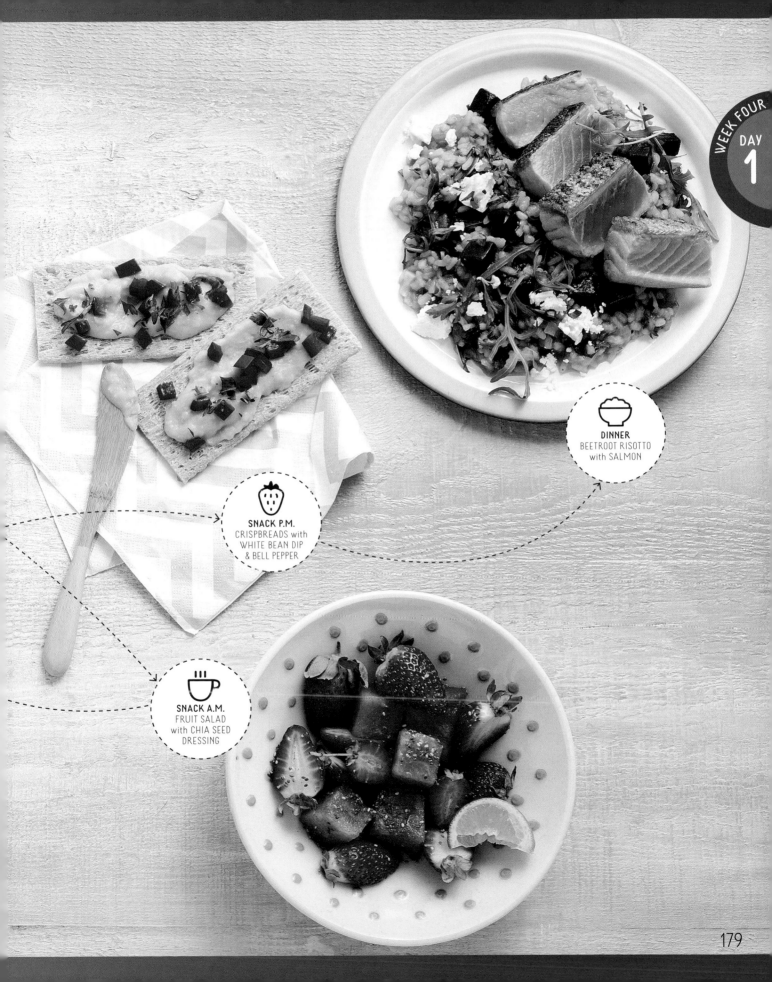

WEEK FOUR

DAY 1

DINNER
BEETROOT RISOTTO
with SALMON

SNACK P.M.
CRISPBREADS with
WHITE BEAN DIP
& BELL PEPPER

SNACK A.M.
FRUIT SALAD
with CHIA SEED
DRESSING

TROPICAL SMOOTHIE BOWL

BREAKFAST **SERVES** 1 | **PREP TIME** 5 MINUTES | **DIFFICULTY** EASY

4¾ oz pineapple, chopped

½ frozen medium banana, chopped

1 small handful kale, stalks removed and leaves roughly chopped

7 oz low-fat plain yoghurt

½ cup low-fat milk

TOPPINGS

¼ cup natural muesli

¼ medium banana, peeled and sliced

1 teaspoon chia seeds

2 teaspoons shredded coconut

Place the pineapple, banana, kale, yoghurt, and milk in a high-powered blender and blend until smooth.

To serve, pour the smoothie mixture into a bowl and top with the muesli, banana, chia seeds, and shredded coconut.

FRUIT SALAD with CHIA SEED DRESSING

SNACK A.M. **SERVES** 1 | **PREP TIME** 5 MINUTES | **DIFFICULTY** EASY

2⅓ oz watermelon, diced

2⅓ oz strawberries, halved

CHIA SEED DRESSING

2 teaspoons chia seeds

1 teaspoon honey

juice of ½ lime

To make the chia seed dressing, whisk the chia seeds, honey, and lime juice together in a small bowl.

To serve, place the watermelon and strawberries in a serving bowl. Drizzle over the dressing and toss gently to combine.

TACO SALAD

LUNCH **SERVES** 1 | **PREP TIME** 10 MINUTES | **COOKING TIME** 30 MINUTES | **DIFFICULTY** EASY

2 tablespoons brown rice

½ whole wheat wrap, cut into 4 wedges

1 small handful lettuce leaves, shredded

¼ small red onion, thinly sliced

½ medium tomato, diced

2 tablespoons tinned corn kernels, drained and rinsed

5¼ oz tinned kidney beans, drained and rinsed

1¾ oz low-fat ricotta cheese

CILANTRO & HONEY DRESSING

1 tablespoon chopped fresh cilantro

2 teaspoons lime juice

½ teaspoon honey

Place the rice and ½ cup of water in a small saucepan over high heat and bring to the boil, stirring occasionally. Cover and reduce the heat to medium–low. Simmer for 20–25 minutes or until the liquid is absorbed and the rice is tender. Remove from the heat and leave to stand, covered, for 5 minutes.

Preheat the broiler to high and line a baking sheet with parchment paper.

Place the wrap wedges on the lined baking sheet and broil for 2 minutes or until toasted. Set aside to cool.

To make the dressing, whisk the cilantro, lime juice, and honey together in a small bowl.

To serve, place the lettuce on the bottom of a large shallow bowl. Top with the rice, onion, tomato, corn, kidney beans, and ricotta. Drizzle over the dressing. Serve with the toasted triangles on the side.

CRISPBREADS with WHITE BEAN DIP & BELL PEPPER

SNACK P.M. | **SERVES** 1 | **PREP TIME** 5 MINUTES | **DIFFICULTY** EASY

2 rye crispbreads

½ medium red bell pepper, seeds removed and diced

chopped fresh parsley, to garnish (optional)

WHITE BEAN DIP

2¾ oz tinned cannellini beans, drained and rinsed

¼ garlic clove, crushed

lemon juice, to taste

2 teaspoons chopped fresh parsley

sea salt and ground black pepper, to taste

To make the white bean dip, place the cannellini beans, garlic, lemon juice, parsley, salt, pepper, and 1 tablespoon of water in a food processor and pulse until smooth and creamy. To save time, the white bean dip can be made the night before and stored in an airtight container in the refrigerator.

To serve, spread the dip over the crispbreads and top with the bell pepper and parsley (if using).

BEETROOT RISOTTO with SALMON

DINNER | **SERVES** 2 | **PREP TIME** 10 MINUTES | **COOKING TIME** 1 HOUR 20 MINUTES | **DIFFICULTY** MEDIUM

2½ small beetroots

3 cups salt-reduced vegetable stock

oil spray

½ small brown onion, finely chopped

1 garlic clove, crushed

4¼ oz arborio rice

2 teaspoons fresh thyme leaves

Two 3-oz salmon fillets, skin removed and deboned

1 large handful arugula leaves

2⅛ oz salt-reduced low-fat feta cheese, crumbled

2 tablespoons chopped fresh parsley

Preheat the oven to 350°F (320°F convection).

Wrap the beetroot in foil with 1 tablespoon of water (this helps the beetroot to steam). Place in a small roasting pan and bake in the oven for 30–40 minutes or until tender. Test the beetroot with a skewer—it is cooked if a skewer pierces the flesh easily. Set aside to cool. When cool enough to handle, peel and dice into cubes. To save time, the beetroot can be roasted the night before and stored in an airtight container in the refrigerator.

Heat the stock in a medium saucepan over medium heat.

Heat a saucepan over medium heat and spray lightly with oil spray. Add the onion and garlic and cook for 5 minutes or until the onion is soft and translucent, stirring occasionally. Add the rice and thyme and cook for 3–4 minutes or until lightly toasted and fragrant, stirring constantly. Pour one-quarter of the warmed stock into the pan containing the rice and cook until most of the stock has been absorbed, stirring constantly.

Add the stock a ladleful at a time and allow the liquid to be absorbed before adding the next ladleful, stirring constantly. Cook for 20–25 minutes or until all the stock has been used and the rice is cooked but still al dente. If all the stock is used and the rice is not ready, add ¼ cup of hot water at a time until cooked.

Meanwhile, heat a medium non-stick fry pan over medium heat and spray lightly with oil spray. Add the salmon and cook for 5–6 minutes or until cooked to your liking, turning occasionally. Transfer to a plate and set aside to rest for 2 minutes. Cut into thick slices.

Stir the beetroot and arugula through the risotto. Cook until the beetroot is heated through and the arugula has wilted, stirring constantly.

To serve, place the risotto in two serving bowls and top with the salmon. Sprinkle over the feta and parsley.

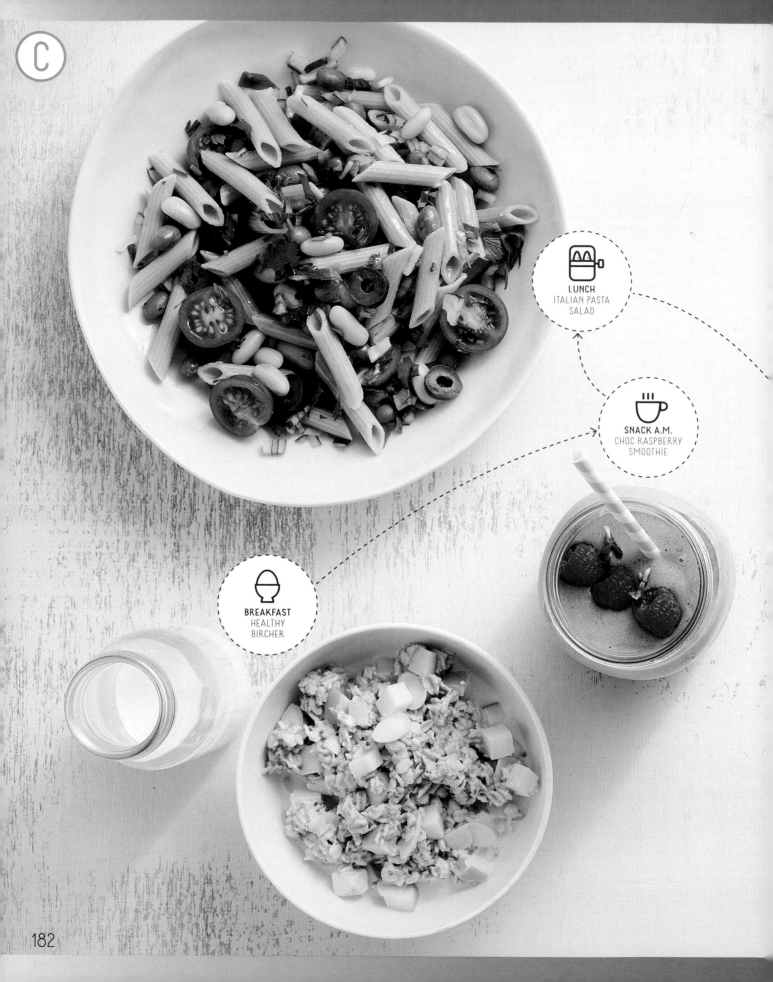

C

LUNCH
ITALIAN PASTA
SALAD

SNACK A.M.
CHOC RASPBERRY
SMOOTHIE

BREAKFAST
HEALTHY
BIRCHER

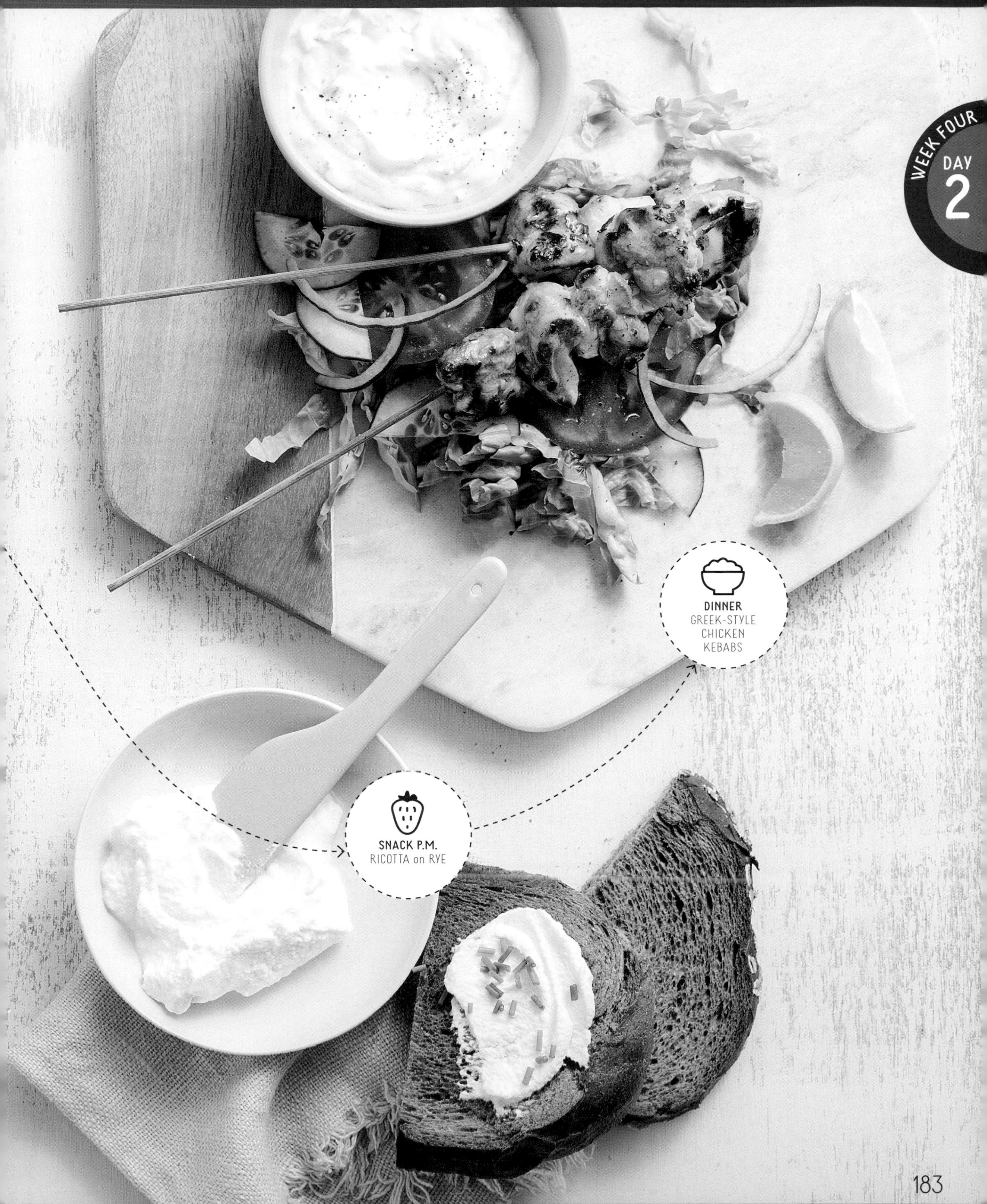

DINNER
GREEK-STYLE
CHICKEN
KEBABS

SNACK P.M.
RICOTTA on RYE

HEALTHY BIRCHER

BREAKFAST   **SERVES** 1 | **PREP TIME** 5 MINUTES + OVERNIGHT CHILLING TIME | **DIFFICULTY** EASY

2 oz rolled oats

1 teaspoon chia seeds

¾ cup low-fat milk

1 teaspoon pure maple syrup

1 teaspoon pure vanilla extract

1 tablespoon flaked almonds

½ medium apple

Place the oats, chia seeds, milk, maple syrup, vanilla, and almonds in a bowl and stir until well combined.

Cover with plastic wrap and place in the refrigerator to soak overnight.

The next morning, roughly dice the apple.

To serve, transfer the bircher to a serving bowl or jar and stir through the apple.

CHOC RASPBERRY SMOOTHIE

SNACK A.M.   **SERVES** 1 | **PREP TIME** 5 MINUTES + 30 MINUTES SOAKING TIME | **DIFFICULTY** EASY

1½ medjool dates, pitted

1 oz rolled oats

5¾ oz raspberries

1 tablespoon carob powder or 2 teaspoons cacao powder (see page 49)

¾ cup low-fat milk

1¾ oz low-fat plain yoghurt

ice cubes

Place the dates in a heatproof bowl, cover with boiling water and let soak for 30 minutes to soften. Drain.

Place the dates, oats, and 5 oz of the raspberries, carob or cacao powder, milk, yoghurt, and ice cubes in a high-powered blender and blend until smooth.

To serve, pour into a glass or shaker and garnish with the remaining raspberries.

ITALIAN PASTA SALAD

LUNCH   **SERVES** 1 | **PREP TIME** 10 MINUTES | **COOKING TIME** 15 MINUTES | **DIFFICULTY** EASY

sea salt

3 oz whole wheat pasta

2¾ oz tinned cannellini beans, drained and rinsed

2¾ oz tinned borlotti beans, drained and rinsed

8 cherry tomatoes, halved

4 kalamata olives, pitted and chopped

¼ small red onion, finely chopped

½ garlic clove, crushed

1 small handful fresh parsley, chopped

sea salt and ground black pepper, to taste

Fill a large saucepan with water, add a pinch of salt, and bring to a boil. Add the pasta and cook until al dente (see the pasta packet for recommended cooking time). Drain and set aside to cool. To save time, the pasta can be cooked the night before and stored in an airtight container in the refrigerator.

To serve, place the beans, tomatoes, olives, onion, garlic, parsley, and pasta in a serving bowl. Season with salt and pepper, if desired, and toss gently to combine.

RICOTTA on RYE

SNACK P.M. | **SERVES** 1 | **PREP TIME** 5 MINUTES | **DIFFICULTY** EASY

1 slice rye bread

1 oz low-fat ricotta cheese

1 tablespoon chopped
fresh chives

Toast the bread to your liking.

To serve, spread the ricotta over the toast
and top with the chives.

 ## GREEK-STYLE CHICKEN KEBABS

DINNER | **SERVES** 2 | **PREP TIME** 15 MINUTES + 30 MINUTES MARINATING TIME | **COOKING TIME** 10 MINUTES | **DIFFICULTY** EASY

⅔ lb boneless skinless
chicken breast (or ¾ lb lean
lamb fillets), cut into 1½-in
cubes

3 large handfuls lettuce
leaves

2 medium tomatoes, sliced

½ small red onion, sliced

1½ Lebanese cucumbers,
halved lengthways
and thinly sliced

7 oz tzatziki (see page 254)

DRESSING

juice of ½ lemon

1½ teaspoons olive oil

¼ teaspoon chopped
fresh oregano

MARINADE

½ garlic clove, crushed

1 teaspoon lemon juice

½ teaspoon chopped
fresh rosemary

½ teaspoon chopped
fresh oregano

sea salt and ground black
pepper, to taste

To make the marinade, whisk the garlic, lemon juice,
rosemary, oregano, salt, and pepper together in a small
bowl. Pour the marinade into a large, shallow baking dish.

Place the chicken in the dish and turn to coat. Ensure
that all the chicken is coated. Cover with plastic wrap and
place in the refrigerator for 30 minutes to marinate.

Meanwhile, soak 4 wooden skewers in cold water for
30 minutes. This will help stop the skewers from burning
when cooking the kebabs.

Preheat a barbecue grill-plate or chargrill pan over
high heat.

Thread the chicken onto the skewers and grill for
8–10 minutes or until the chicken is cooked through,
turning frequently.

To make the dressing, whisk the lemon juice, oil, and
oregano together in a small bowl.

Place the lettuce, tomato, onion, and cucumber in
a large bowl. Drizzle over the dressing and toss gently
to combine.

To serve, place the kebabs and salad on two serving
plates. Serve with the tzatziki on the side.

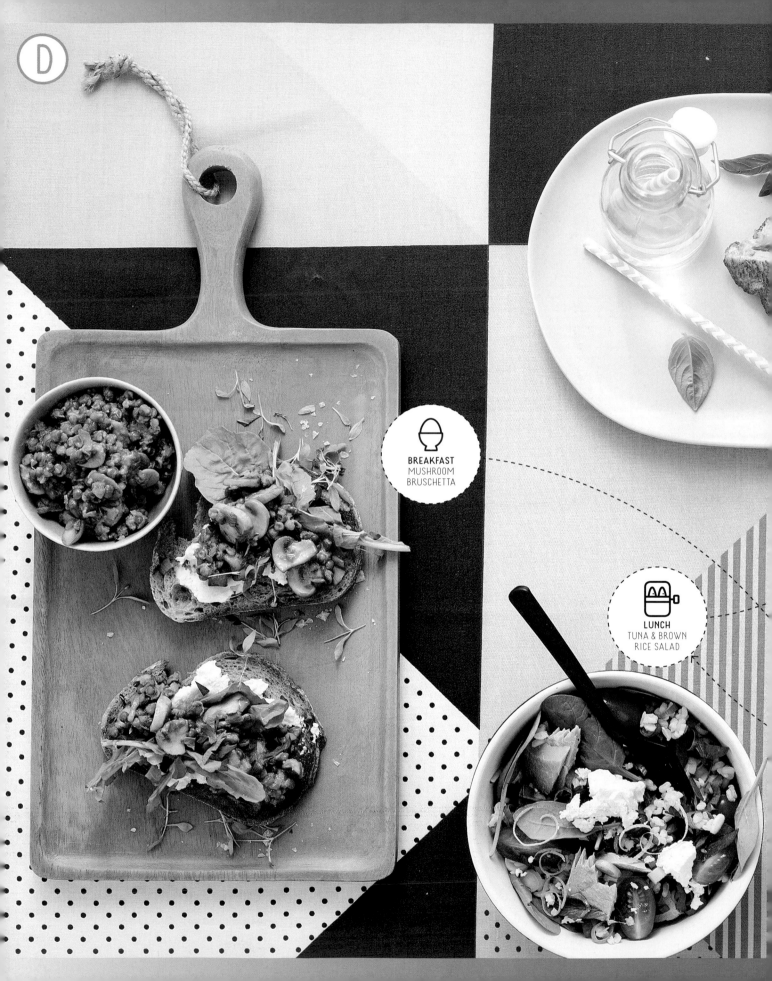

D

BREAKFAST
MUSHROOM
BRUSCHETTA

LUNCH
TUNA & BROWN
RICE SALAD

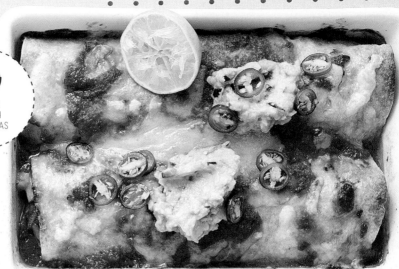

DINNER
CHICKEN
ENCHILADAS

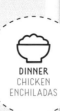

SNACK P.M.
TOMATO & CHEESE
TOASTIE

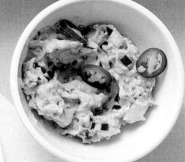

SNACK A.M.
CRISPBREADS with
BLUEBERRIES &
RICOTTA

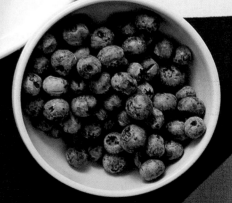

187

MUSHROOM BRUSCHETTA

BREAKFAST | **SERVES** 1 | **PREP TIME** 10 MINUTES | **COOKING TIME** 20 MINUTES | **DIFFICULTY** EASY

1½ teaspoons olive oil

½ garlic clove, crushed

2¾ oz button mushrooms, sliced

1 sprig fresh thyme, leaves picked

5¼ oz tinned brown lentils, drained and rinsed

¼ cup low-fat milk

sea salt and ground black pepper, to taste

2 slices whole wheat bread

1 oz low-fat ricotta cheese

1 small handful arugula leaves

1 tablespoon chopped fresh parsley

Heat the oil in a non-stick fry pan over medium heat. Add the garlic, mushrooms, and thyme and cook for 6–7 minutes or until the mushrooms are tender and juicy.

Add the lentils and milk and bring to the boil. Reduce the heat to low and simmer for 10 minutes or until the milk has reduced and thickened. Season with salt and pepper, if desired.

Meanwhile, toast the bread to your liking.

To serve, spread the ricotta over the toast and top with the arugula and mushroom mixture. Sprinkle over the parsley.

CRISPBREADS with BLUEBERRIES & RICOTTA

SNACK A.M. | **SERVES** 1 | **PREP TIME** 2 MINUTES | **DIFFICULTY** EASY

1¾ oz low-fat ricotta cheese

2 rye crispbreads

3½ oz blueberries

To serve, spread the ricotta over the crispbreads and top with the blueberries.

TUNA & BROWN RICE SALAD

LUNCH | **SERVES** 1 | **PREP TIME** 10 MINUTES | **COOKING TIME** 25 MINUTES | **DIFFICULTY** EASY

2 tablespoons brown rice

1¾ oz tinned tuna in springwater, drained

1 scallion, thinly sliced

1 small handful baby spinach leaves

5 cherry tomatoes, halved

2 kalamata olives, pitted and sliced

finely grated zest and juice of ½ lemon

2 teaspoons chopped fresh parsley

⅔ oz salt-reduced low-fat feta cheese, crumbled

Place the rice and ½ cup of water in a small saucepan over high heat and bring to a boil, stirring occasionally. Cover and reduce the heat to medium–low. Simmer for 20–25 minutes or until the liquid is absorbed and the rice is tender. Remove from the heat and let stand, covered, for 5 minutes. Set aside to cool.
To save time, the rice can be cooked the night before and stored in an airtight container in the refrigerator.

To serve, place the rice, tuna, scallion, spinach, tomatoes, olives, lemon zest, and juice and parsley in a serving bowl and toss gently to combine. Sprinkle over the feta.

TOMATO & CHEESE TOASTIE

SNACK P.M. | **SERVES** 1 | **PREP TIME** 5 MINUTES | **COOKING TIME** 5 MINUTES | **DIFFICULTY** EASY

1 slice whole wheat bread, halved

½ medium tomato, sliced

⅔ oz reduced-fat cheddar cheese, sliced

sea salt and ground black pepper, to taste

fresh basil leaves, to serve

Preheat a sandwich press.

Place one half of the bread on a clean chopping board and top with the tomato and cheese. Season with salt and pepper, if desired. Top with the other half of the bread.

Place the sandwich on the sandwich press and gently press down the lid. Toast for 3–5 minutes or until the cheese is melted and the sandwich is golden. Garnish with basil and serve.

CHICKEN ENCHILADAS

DINNER | **SERVES** 4 | **PREP TIME** 15 MINUTES | **COOKING TIME** 45 MINUTES | **DIFFICULTY** MEDIUM

oil spray

1 small brown onion, finely chopped

1 medium red bell pepper, seeds removed and chopped

1 garlic clove, crushed

½ fresh green chilli, chopped (optional)

1 teaspoon chilli powder

½ teaspoon ground cumin

¼ teaspoon smoked paprika

pinch of dried oregano

sea salt and ground black pepper, to taste

21 oz tinned crushed tomatoes

1 lb bonless skinless chicken breast, cut into 2-in cubes

12 oz pineapple, diced

1¾ oz dried mango, diced

2 tablespoons tinned corn kernels, drained

2 whole wheat wraps

3 oz reduced-fat cheddar cheese, grated

GUACAMOLE

3½ oz avocado

lime juice, to taste

finely chopped fresh green chilli, to taste

½ small red onion, finely chopped

1 tablespoon chopped fresh cilantro

sea salt and ground black pepper, to taste

Preheat the oven to 400°F (350°F convection).

Heat a large saucepan over medium heat and spray lightly with oil spray. Add the onion and bell pepper and cook for 5–7 minutes or until the onion is translucent and the pepper is soft. Add the garlic, green chilli (if using), chilli powder, cumin, paprika, oregano, salt, and pepper and cook for 1 minute or until fragrant, stirring constantly.

Remove from the heat and stir in the tomatoes. Using a stick blender, carefully blend until smooth. Transfer half the blended tomato mixture to a bowl and set aside.

Return the pan with the remaining tomato mixture to a simmer over medium–low heat. Add the chicken and cook, covered, for 10–15 minutes or until the chicken is cooked through, stirring occasionally. Remove from the heat and stir through the pineapple, dried mango, and corn.

Place the wraps on a clean chopping board and top with the chicken and tomato mixture. Roll up each wrap to enclose the filling. Place in the baking dish seam-side down.

Spoon over the reserved tomato mixture and sprinkle over the cheese. Bake in the oven for 20 minutes or until the cheese has melted and the filling is heated through.

Meanwhile, to make the guacamole, scoop the avocado out into a small bowl and roughly mash with a fork. Add the lime juice, chilli, onion, and cilantro and gently mix to combine. Season with salt and pepper, if desired.

To serve, cut the enchiladas in half and place on four serving plates. Top with the guacamole.

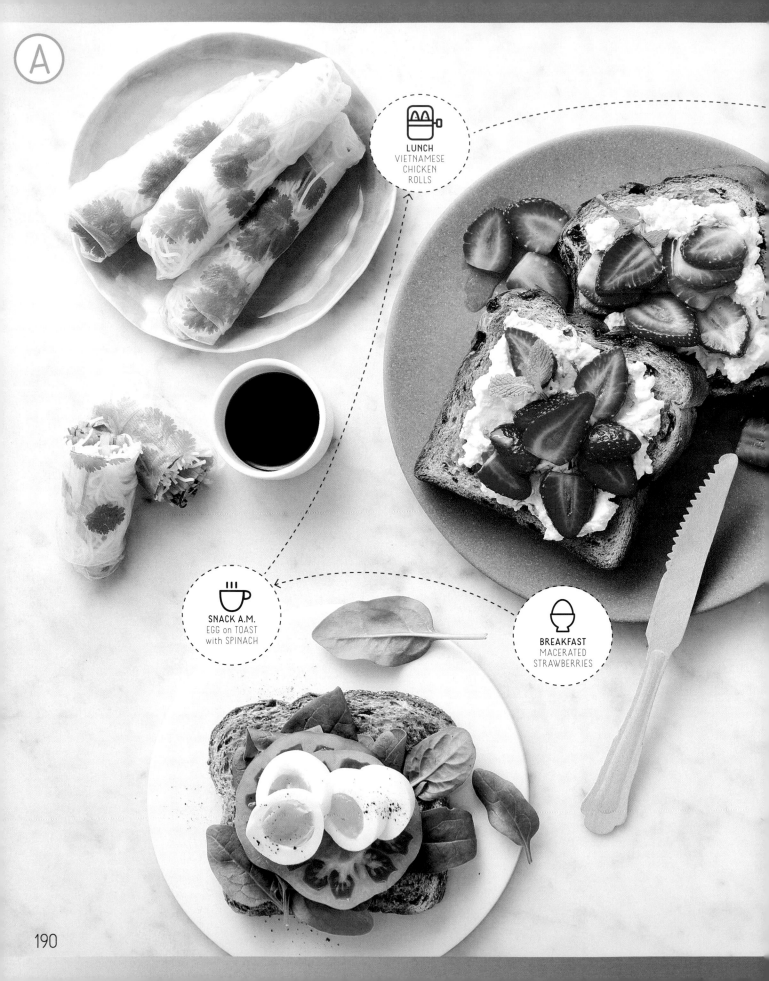

A

LUNCH
VIETNAMESE
CHICKEN
ROLLS

SNACK A.M.
EGG on TOAST
with SPINACH

BREAKFAST
MACERATED
STRAWBERRIES

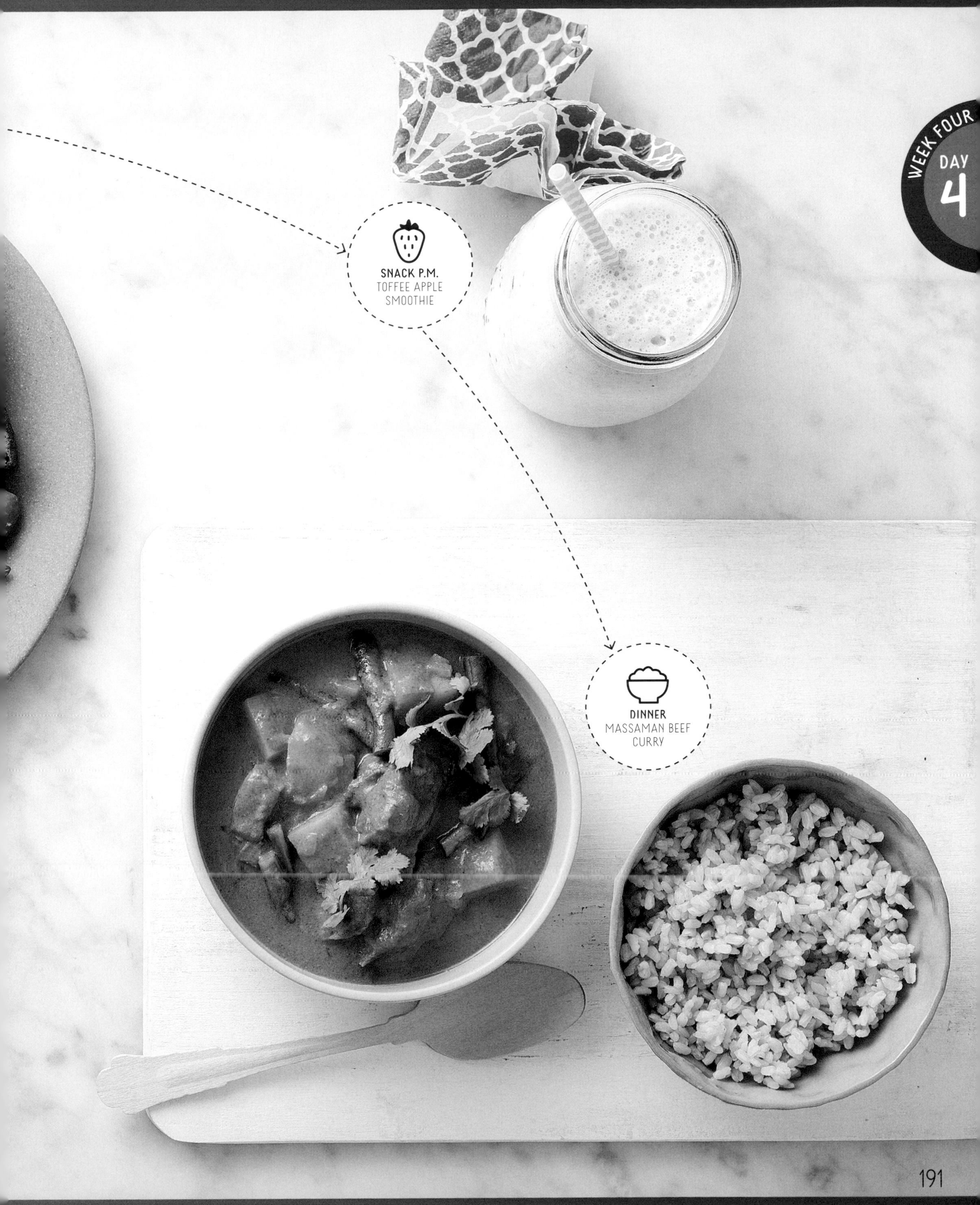

SNACK P.M.
TOFFEE APPLE
SMOOTHIE

DINNER
MASSAMAN BEEF
CURRY

MACERATED STRAWBERRIES

BREAKFAST | **SERVES** 1 | **PREP TIME** 5 MINUTES + 30 MINUTES STANDING TIME | **COOKING TIME** 2 MINUTES | **DIFFICULTY** EASY

9 oz strawberries, hulled
and sliced

juice of ¼ orange

1 teaspoon honey

3½ oz low-fat ricotta cheese

3 fresh mint leaves,
finely chopped

2 slices raisin bread

Place the strawberries, orange juice, and honey in a small bowl and stir
to combine. Set aside for 30 minutes at room temperature. This will
cause the strawberries to soften a little and become syrupy.

Place the ricotta and mint in a small bowl and mix until well combined.

Toast the raisin bread to your liking.

To serve, spread the ricotta mixture over the toast and top with the
macerated strawberries.

EGG on TOAST with SPINACH

SNACK A.M. | **SERVES** 1 | **PREP TIME** 5 MINUTES | **COOKING TIME** 10 MINUTES | **DIFFICULTY** EASY

1 large egg

1 slice whole wheat bread

1 small handful baby spinach
leaves

½ medium tomato, sliced

Place the egg in a saucepan and fill with cold water until it covers the egg by ¾ in.
Bring to a boil over high heat. Reduce the heat to low and simmer, covered, for
7–8 minutes. Remove the egg with a slotted spoon and place in a bowl of iced water.
Leave for 1 minute. Gently tap the egg on the bench to crack the shell and peel.
Slice into rounds.

Toast the bread to your liking.

To serve, top the toast with the spinach, tomato, and egg.

VIETNAMESE CHICKEN ROLLS

LUNCH | **SERVES** 1 | **PREP TIME** 15 MINUTES + 10 MINUTES SOAKING TIME | **DIFFICULTY** EASY

1 oz rice vermicelli noodles

4 small rice paper wrappers

½ Lebanese cucumber,
thinly sliced

1 small handful bean sprouts

½ medium carrot, thinly sliced

¼ medium red bell peppers,
seeds removed and
thinly sliced

3½ oz boneless skinless
chicken breast, cooked and
shredded (see page 272)

fresh cilantro leaves,
to serve (optional)

salt-reduced tamari or
soy sauce, to serve

Place the noodles in a heatproof bowl and cover with boiling water. Leave for 10 minutes,
then loosen the noodles with a fork. Drain and refresh under cool running water.
Drain well and set aside to cool. When cool enough to handle, cut into shorter lengths.

Place the rice paper wrappers, prepared vegetables, chicken, and noodles on the clean
work surface, ready to roll.

Fill a large bowl with warm water for the wrappers. Working with one wrapper at a time,
dip into the water for 1 second to soften. Do not soak as the wrappers can become too
soft and tear.

Place the wrapper on a chopping board and place one-quarter of the noodles,
vegetables, and chicken on the bottom third, adding a few cilantro leaves, if desired.
Bring the bottom of the wrapper up and over the filling, fold in the sides and then roll up.
Set the roll aside, seam-side down, while you prepare the remaining rolls. Repeat with
the remaining ingredients to make four rolls in total.

Serve the rolls with a small dish of tamari or soy sauce for dipping.

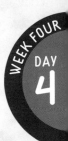

TOFFEE APPLE SMOOTHIE

SNACK P.M. SERVES 1 | **PREP TIME** 5 MINUTES + 30 MINUTES SOAKING TIME | **DIFFICULTY** EASY

1½ medjool dates, pitted

1¾ oz unsweetened apple sauce

1 tablespoon pure maple syrup

pinch of ground cinnamon

1 cup low-fat milk

3½ oz low-fat plain yoghurt

ice cubes

Place the dates in a heatproof bowl, cover with boiling water and let soak for 30 minutes to soften. Drain.

Place the dates, apple sauce, maple syrup, cinnamon, milk, yoghurt, and ice cubes in a high-powered blender and blend until smooth.

To serve, pour into a glass or shaker.

MASSAMAN BEEF CURRY

DINNER SERVES 2 | **PREP TIME** 10 MINUTES | **COOKING TIME** 1 HOUR 20 MINUTES | **DIFFICULTY** EASY

4¼ oz brown rice

3 teaspoons olive oil

½ small brown onion, finely chopped

6 oz lean beef shank, cut into 1-in cubes

1 tablespoon massaman curry paste

1 cup salt-reduced vegetable stock

5 oz tinned crushed tomatoes

½ cup light coconut milk

1 medium potato, cut into ½-in cubes

8 green beans, trimmed and halved

sea salt and ground black pepper, to taste

fresh cilantro leaves, to garnish

Place the rice and 1¼ cups of water in a small saucepan over high heat and bring to a boil, stirring occasionally. Cover and reduce the heat to medium–low. Simmer for 20–25 minutes or until the liquid is absorbed and the rice is tender. Remove from the heat and let stand, covered, for 5 minutes.

Meanwhile, heat the oil in a saucepan over medium heat. Add the onion and cook for 4–5 minutes or until soft and translucent, stirring occasionally. Add the beef and cook for 5 minutes or until lightly browned, stirring frequently.

Add the curry paste and cook for 1 minute or until fragrant, stirring constantly. Stir in the stock, tomatoes, and coconut milk and reduce the heat to medium–low. Simmer for 45 minutes, covered, or until the beef is tender, stirring occasionally.

Add the potato and simmer, covered, for 15–20 minutes or until tender. Add the beans and simmer for a further 5 minutes or until tender. Season with salt and pepper, if desired.

To serve, place the rice in two serving bowls and top with the massaman curry. Sprinkle over the cilantro.

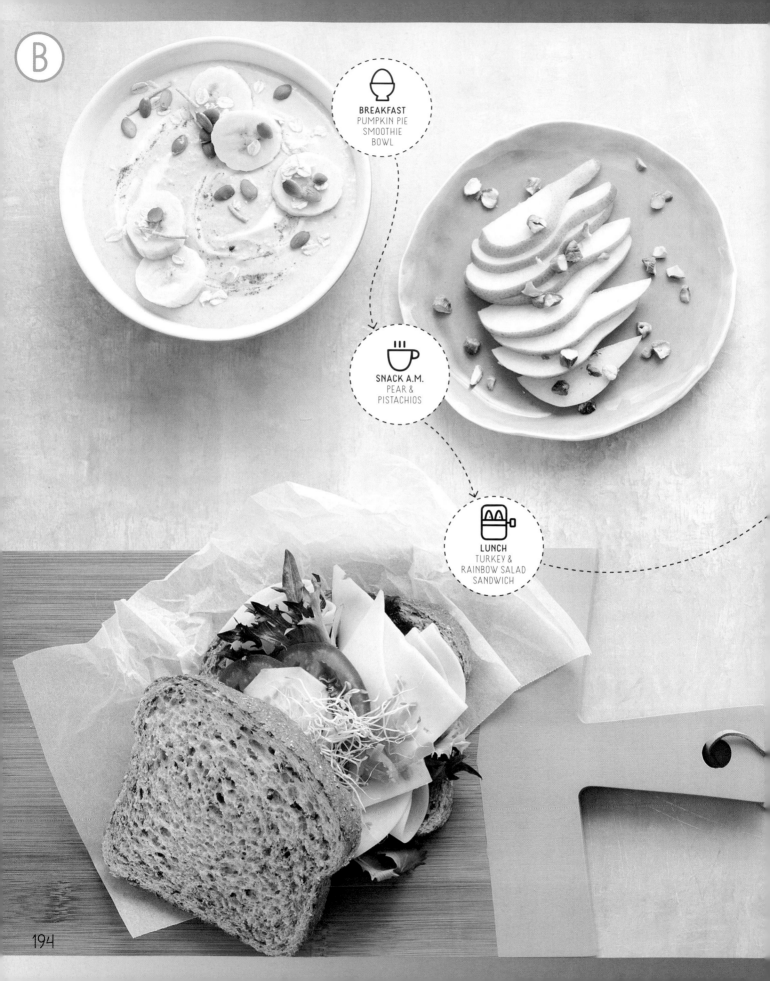

BREAKFAST
PUMPKIN PIE
SMOOTHIE
BOWL

SNACK A.M.
PEAR &
PISTACHIOS

LUNCH
TURKEY &
RAINBOW SALAD
SANDWICH

194

SNACK P.M.
RICE CAKES with
HUMMUS, TOMATO
& SPINACH

DINNER
SPAGHETTI
MARINARA

PUMPKIN PIE SMOOTHIE BOWL

BREAKFAST **SERVES** 1 | **PREP TIME** 5 MINUTES | **COOKING TIME** 15 MINUTES | **DIFFICULTY** EASY

2 oz pumpkin, cut into small cubes

1 frozen medium banana, chopped

7 oz low-fat plain yoghurt

½ cup low-fat milk

2 teaspoons pure maple syrup

pinch of ground cinnamon

pinch of ground nutmeg

pinch of ground ginger

TOPPINGS

1 oz natural muesli

⅓ oz pumpkin seeds (pepitas)

½ medium banana, peeled and sliced

Fill a saucepan with water until 2 in deep and insert a steamer basket. Cover with a lid and bring the water to the boil over high heat, then reduce the heat to medium. Add the pumpkin and steam, covered, for 12–15 minutes or until soft. Alternatively, microwave on high for 8–10 minutes. Set aside to cool.

Place the pumpkin, banana, yoghurt, milk, maple syrup, cinnamon, nutmeg, and ginger in a high-powered blender and blend until smooth.

To serve, pour the smoothie mixture into a bowl and top with the muesli, pumpkin seeds, and banana.

PEAR & PISTACHIOS

SNACK A.M. **SERVES** 1 | **PREP TIME** 2 MINUTES | **DIFFICULTY** EASY

½ small pear, sliced

1 tablespoon unsalted pistachio kernels, chopped

To serve, place the pear in a small serving bowl and top with the pistachios.

TURKEY & RAINBOW SALAD SANDWICH

LUNCH **SERVES** 1 | **PREP TIME** 10 MINUTES | **DIFFICULTY** EASY

1 teaspoon cranberry sauce or Dijon mustard, to taste

2 slices whole wheat bread

3 oz cooked turkey breast, sliced

⅔ oz Swiss cheese, sliced

1 small handful lettuce leaves

¼ medium carrot, coarsely grated

¼ Lebanese cucumber, thinly sliced

½ medium tomato, sliced

1 small handful alfalfa sprouts

Spread the cranberry sauce or mustard on one slice of bread. Layer the turkey, cheese, lettuce, carrot, cucumber, tomato, and alfalfa.

Top with the other slice of bread.

To serve, place on a serving plate and cut in half.

RICE CAKES with HUMMUS, TOMATO & SPINACH

SNACK P.M.   **SERVES** 1 | **PREP TIME** 5 MINUTES | **DIFFICULTY** EASY

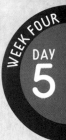
2¾ oz hummus (see page 254)

3 rice cakes

1 small handful baby
spinach leaves

5 cherry tomatoes, halved

To serve, spread the hummus over the rice cakes.
Top with the spinach and tomatoes.

SPAGHETTI MARINARA

DINNER   **SERVES** 2 | **PREP TIME** 15 MINUTES | **COOKING TIME** 20 MINUTES | **DIFFICULTY** MEDIUM

5¾ oz whole wheat spaghetti

oil spray

½ small brown onion,
finely diced

2 garlic cloves, crushed

8 black mussels, scrubbed
and beards removed

15 cherry tomatoes, halved

½ fresh red chilli, seeds
removed and finely chopped

4 fresh basil leaves,
thinly sliced

2¼ oz white fish fillet,
cut into ¾-in pieces

5 raw prawns, peeled and
deveined, tails intact

10¾ oz tinned crushed
tomatoes

lemon juice, to taste

sea salt and ground black
pepper, to taste

1 large handful fresh parsley,
finely chopped

1½ oz parmesan cheese,
grated

Fill a large saucepan with water, add a pinch of salt
and bring to a boil. Add the pasta and cook until
al dente (see the pasta packet for recommended
cooking time). Drain and set aside.

Meanwhile, heat a large non-stick fry pan over
medium heat and spray lightly with oil spray. Add the
onion and garlic and cook for 3–4 minutes or until the
onion is soft and translucent, stirring frequently.

Add the mussels, cherry tomatoes, chilli, basil, and
2 tablespoons of water. Increase the heat to high and
cook, covered, for 2–3 minutes or until the mussels
have opened.

Move the mussels to the side of the pan and reduce
the heat to medium. Add the fish and prawns and
cook for 1–2 minutes, then carefully turn over and
cook for a further 1–2 minutes.

Add the crushed tomatoes and cook for 5–7 minutes
or until the seafood is tender and the tomatoes are
heated through. Season with lemon juice, salt, and
pepper, if desired.

Add the spaghetti and parsley and toss gently
to combine.

To serve, place the spaghetti marinara in two bowls
and sprinkle over the parmesan.

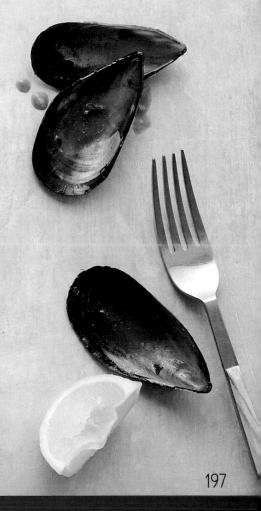

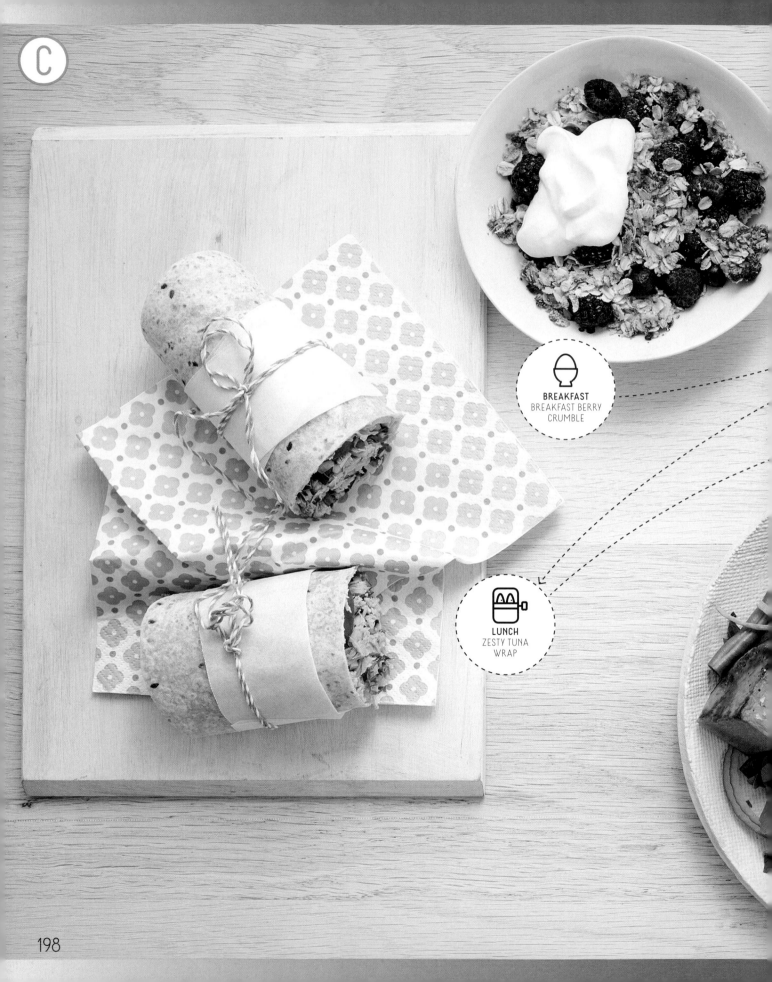

BREAKFAST
BREAKFAST BERRY CRUMBLE

LUNCH
ZESTY TUNA WRAP

198

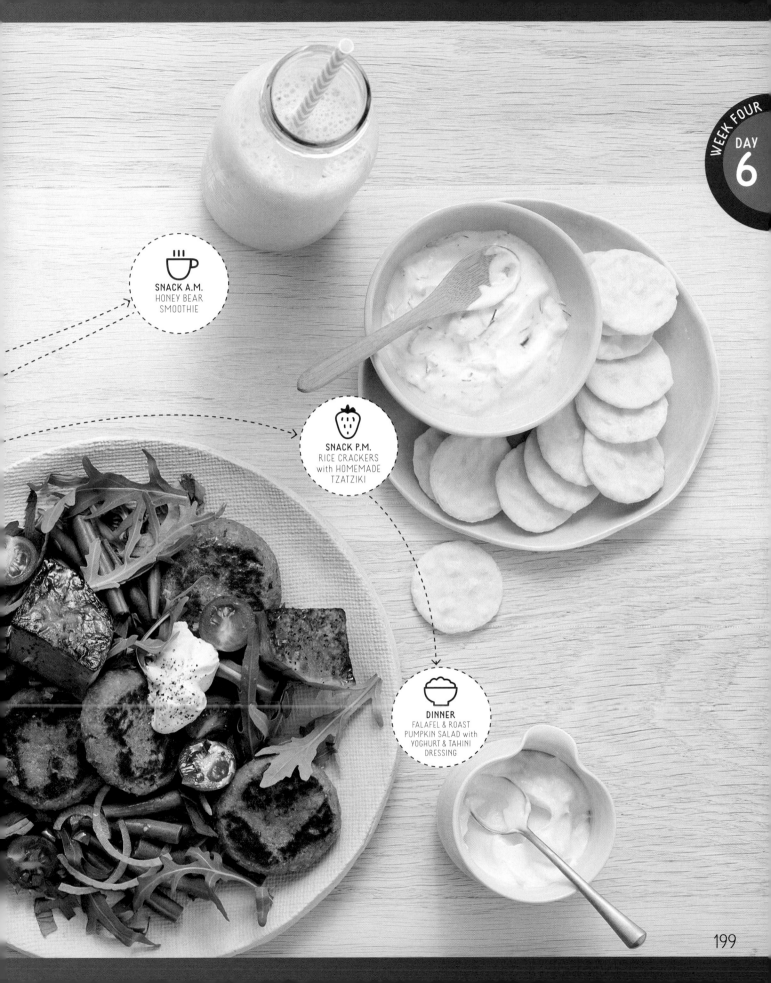

SNACK A.M.
HONEY BEAR
SMOOTHIE

SNACK P.M.
RICE CRACKERS
with HOMEMADE
TZATZIKI

DINNER
FALAFEL & ROAST
PUMPKIN SALAD with
YOGHURT & TAHINI
DRESSING

BREAKFAST BERRY CRUMBLE

BREAKFAST | **SERVES** 1 | **PREP TIME** 10 MINUTES + 3 MINUTES STANDING TIME | **COOKING TIME** 35 MINUTES | **DIFFICULTY** EASY

1¾ oz rolled oats

1¾ tablespoons plain wholemeal flour

1½ teaspoons coconut oil, melted

1 teaspoon ground almonds

3 oz frozen mixed berries, thawed

5¼ oz low-fat plain yoghurt

Preheat the oven to 350°F (325°F convection).

Place the oats, flour, coconut oil, and ground almonds in a bowl and mix until well combined.

Place the berries in an ovenproof ramekin and top with the oat mixture.

Bake for 30–35 minutes or until the crumble is golden. Leave to stand for a few minutes then transfer to a bowl.

Serve the crumble topped with the yoghurt.

HONEY BEAR SMOOTHIE

SNACK A.M. | **SERVES** 1 | **PREP TIME** 5 MINUTES | **DIFFICULTY** EASY

1 oz rolled oats

1½ medium bananas, peeled and chopped

¾ cup low-fat milk

1¾ oz low-fat plain yoghurt

2 teaspoons honey

¼ teaspoon ground cinnamon

ice cubes

Place the oats, banana, milk, yoghurt, honey, cinnamon, and ice cubes in a high-powered blender and blend until smooth.

To serve, pour into a glass or shaker.

ZESTY TUNA WRAP

LUNCH | **SERVES** 1 | **PREP TIME** 10 MINUTES | **DIFFICULTY** EASY

3½ oz tinned tuna in springwater, drained

¼ small red onion, finely chopped

1 small handful fresh parsley, finely chopped

sea salt and ground black pepper, to taste

1 small handful mixed lettuce leaves

finely grated zest and juice of ¼ lemon

1 whole wheat wrap

2 kalamata olives, pitted and sliced

½ medium tomato, sliced

Place the tuna, onion, and parsley in a small bowl and mix until well combined. Season with salt and pepper, if desired.

Place the lettuce, lemon zest, and juice in another small bowl and toss gently to combine.

To serve, place the wrap on a serving plate and place the tuna mixture, lettuce mixture, olives, and tomato down the middle. Fold over the end and roll up to enclose the filling.

RICE CRACKERS with TZATZIKI

SNACK P.M. | **SERVES** 1 | **PREP TIME** 5 MINUTES | **DIFFICULTY** EASY

12 plain rice crackers

1¾ oz tzatziki (see page 254)

Serve the rice crackers with the tzatziki.

FALAFEL & ROAST PUMPKIN SALAD
with YOGHURT & TAHINI DRESSING

DINNER | **SERVES** 2 | **PREP TIME** 15 MINUTES + 30 MINUTES CHILLING TIME | **COOKING TIME** 35 MINUTES | **DIFFICULTY** MEDIUM

¾ lb pumpkin, peeled and cut into ¼-in cubes

oil spray

sea salt and ground black pepper, to taste

15 green beans, trimmed and halved

10 cherry tomatoes, halved

½ small red onion, sliced

1 large handful arugula leaves

1 small handful fresh mint, roughly chopped

1 small handful fresh parsley, roughly chopped

FALAFEL

½ small brown onion, finely chopped

2 garlic cloves, crushed

15 oz tinned chickpeas, drained and rinsed

1 teaspoon ground cumin

1 teaspoon ground coriander

½ teaspoon sweet paprika

1½ tablespoons whole wheat plain flour

lemon juice, to taste

sea salt and ground black pepper, to taste

oil spray

YOGHURT & TAHINI DRESSING

7 oz low-fat plain yoghurt

2 teaspoons tahini

1 teaspoon honey

lime juice, to taste

Preheat the oven to 350°F (325°F convection) and line two baking sheets with parchment paper.

Place the pumpkin on one of the lined baking sheets and spray lightly with oil spray. Season with salt and pepper, if desired. Roast in the oven for 20–25 minutes or until the pumpkin is tender and lightly browned, turning with tongs every 10 minutes. Set aside to cool.

To make the falafel, place the onion, garlic, chickpeas, cumin, coriander, paprika, flour, lemon juice, salt, and pepper in a food processor and process until almost smooth. Shape the mixture into eight even patties. Place on a plate, cover with plastic wrap, and refrigerate for 30 minutes.

Place the falafels on the second baking sheet and spray lightly with oil spray. Bake in the oven for 15 minutes or until golden and cooked through, carefully turning halfway through.

Meanwhile, to make the yoghurt and tahini dressing, whisk the yoghurt, tahini, honey, and lime together in a small bowl.

Place the pumpkin, beans, tomatoes, onion, arugula, mint, and parsley in a large bowl and toss gently to combine.

To serve, place the roast pumpkin salad on two serving plates. Top with four falafels each and drizzle over the yoghurt and tahini dressing.

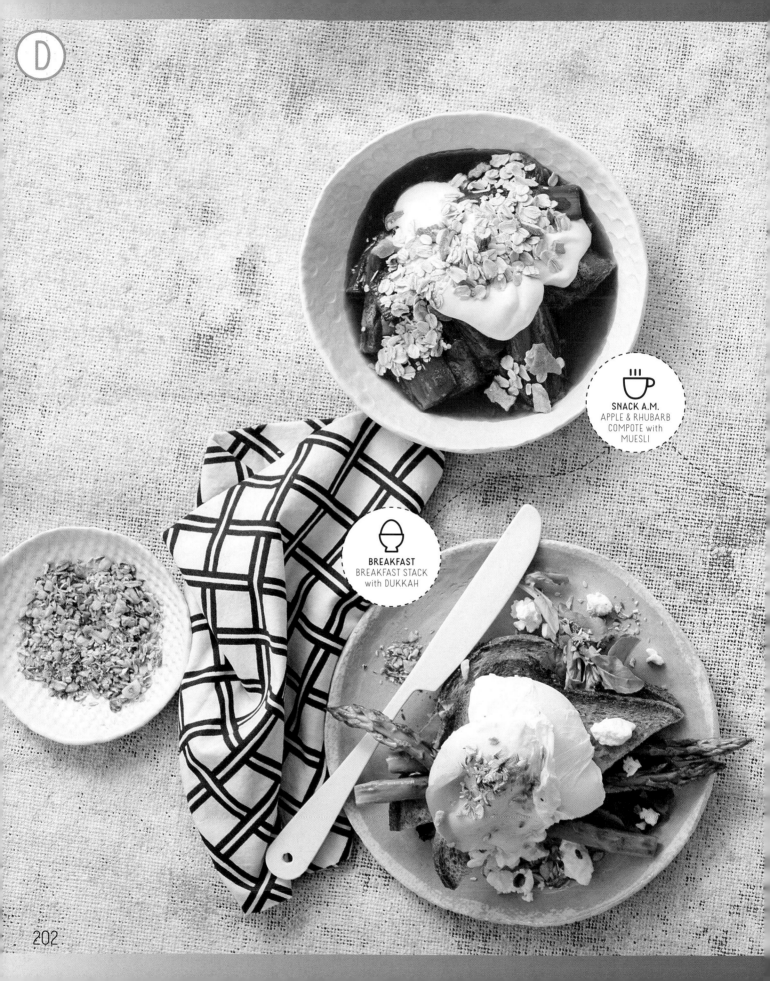

SNACK A.M.
APPLE & RHUBARB
COMPOTE with
MUESLI

BREAKFAST
BREAKFAST STACK
with DUKKAH

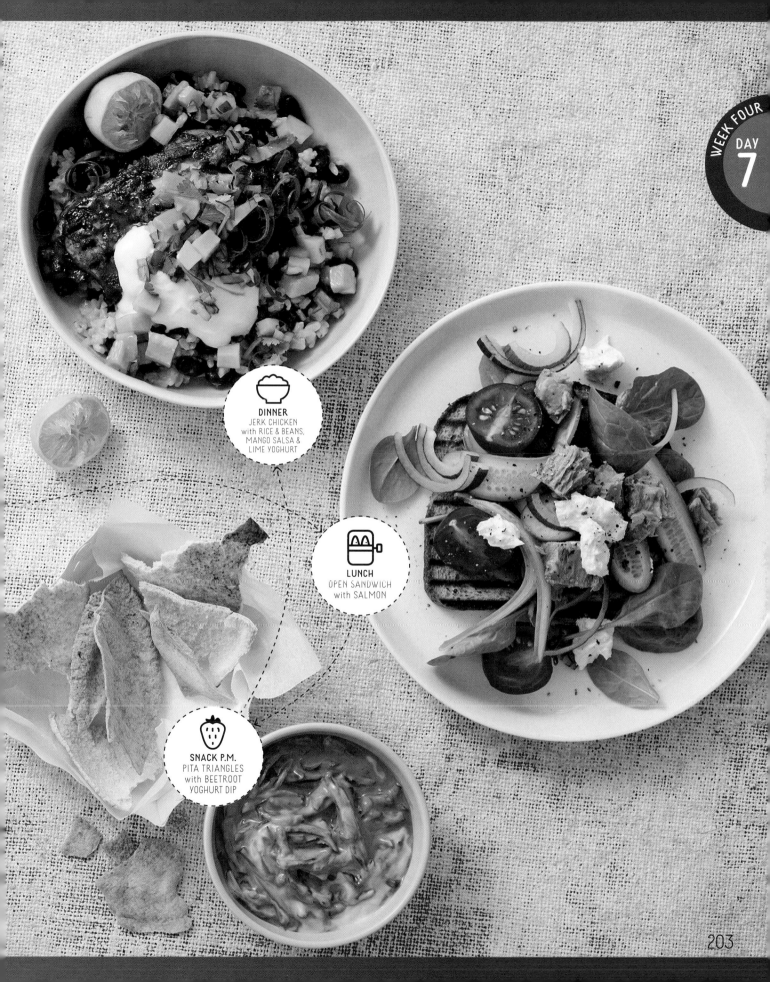

DINNER
JERK CHICKEN
with RICE & BEANS,
MANGO SALSA &
LIME YOGHURT

LUNCH
OPEN SANDWICH
with SALMON

SNACK P.M.
PITA TRIANGLES
with BEETROOT
YOGHURT DIP

BREAKFAST STACK with DUKKAH

SERVES 1 | **PREP TIME** 10 MINUTES | **COOKING TIME** 20 MINUTES | **DIFFICULTY** EASY

3 asparagus spears, trimmed

1 teaspoon white vinegar

2 large eggs

1½ slices whole wheat bread

1 small handful arugula leaves

1 oz salt-reduced low-fat feta cheese, crumbled

DUKKAH

1 teaspoon hazelnuts, chopped

1 teaspoon sesame seeds

2 tablespoons rolled oats

¼ teaspoon coriander seeds

¼ teaspoon cumin seeds

sea salt and ground black pepper, to taste

To make the dukkah, heat a non-stick fry pan over medium heat. Add the hazelnuts and cook for 5–10 minutes or until fragrant and lightly toasted, stirring constantly. Transfer to a bowl and set aside to cool. Add the sesame seeds and toast for 2 minutes or until fragrant. Transfer to the bowl that contains the hazelnuts and set aside to cool. Place the hazelnuts, sesame seeds, oats, coriander seeds, cumin seeds, salt, and pepper in a mortar and grind into a coarse powder with the pestle. Alternatively, you can use an electric coffee grinder.

Heat a non-stick fry pan over medium–high heat. Add the asparagus spears and cook for 3–5 minutes or until they start to change colour and reach the desired tenderness.

Fill a saucepan with water until 3 in deep. Add the vinegar and bring to a boil over medium heat, then reduce the heat to medium–low. The water should just be simmering. Break the eggs into the water and cook for 2–3 minutes for a semi-soft yolk or 3–4 minutes for a firm yolk. Remove the eggs with a slotted spoon and allow to drain on paper towel.

Toast the bread to your liking and cut into three triangles.

To serve, place one toasted triangle on a serving plate and top with the arugula. Top with another toasted triangle followed by the asparagus. Finally, top with the third toasted triangle and the poached eggs. Sprinkle over the feta and dukkah.

APPLE & RHUBARB COMPOTE with MUESLI

SERVES 1 | **PREP TIME** 10 MINUTES | **COOKING TIME** 10 MINUTES | **DIFFICULTY** EASY

½ medium apple, peeled, cored and sliced

7 oz rhubarb, trimmed and sliced

1 tablespoon honey

½ teaspoon pure vanilla extract

½ star anise

1 cardamom pod, bruised

3½ oz low-fat plain yoghurt

1 oz natural muesli

Place the apple, rhubarb, honey, vanilla, star anise, and cardamom pod and ½ cup of water in a medium saucepan and bring to a simmer over medium heat, stirring occasionally. Reduce the heat to low and simmer for 8–10 minutes or until the rhubarb and apple are soft and the sauce has thickened.

Remove and discard the star anise and cardamom pod and set the compote aside to cool.

To serve, place the apple and rhubarb compote in a serving bowl and top with the yoghurt and muesli.

OPEN SANDWICH with SALMON

SERVES 1 | **PREP TIME** 5 MINUTES | **COOKING TIME** 2 MINUTES | **DIFFICULTY** EASY

1 slice whole wheat bread

1 small handful baby spinach leaves

½ Lebanese cucumber, sliced

¼ small red onion, thinly sliced

3 cherry tomatoes, halved

1¼ oz tinned salmon, drained

¾ oz soft goat's cheese

ground black pepper, to taste

Toast the bread to your liking.

To serve, place the bread on a serving plate and top with the spinach, cucumber, onion, tomato, salmon, and goat's cheese. Season with pepper, if desired.

PITA TRIANGLES with BEETROOT YOGHURT DIP

SNACK P.M. | **SERVES** 1 | **PREP TIME** 5 MINUTES | **COOKING TIME** 15 MINUTES | **DIFFICULTY** EASY

½ whole wheat pita bread, cut into 4 wedges

½ small beetroot, peeled and grated

pinch of ground cumin

pinch of ground coriander

lemon juice, to taste

3½ oz low-fat plain yoghurt

sea salt and ground black pepper, to taste

oil spray

Preheat the oven to 400°F (350°F convection) and line a baking sheet with parchment paper.

Lay the pita wedges in a single layer on the lined baking sheet and spray lightly with oil spray. Bake in the oven for 5 minutes until they begin to colour. Turn the wedges over and bake for a further 5–8 minutes or until both sides are lightly coloured and set aside to cool.

Meanwhile, place the beetroot, cumin, coriander, lemon juice, yoghurt, salt, and pepper in a small bowl and mix until well combined.

Serve the pita triangles with the beetroot yoghurt dip.

JERK CHICKEN with RICE & BEANS, MANGO SALSA & LIME YOGHURT

DINNER

SERVES 2 | **PREP TIME** 30 MINUTES + 4 HOURS OR OVERNIGHT MARINATING TIME | **COOKING TIME** 45 MINUTES | **DIFFICULTY** MEDIUM

7 oz boneless skinless chicken breast

oil spray

lime wedges, to serve

JERK MARINADE

½ small brown onion, finely chopped

1 scallion, finely chopped

½ fresh red chilli, seeds removed and chopped

1 garlic clove, chopped

2 teaspoons grated fresh ginger

2 teaspoons fresh thyme leaves, finely chopped

1 tablespoon salt-reduced tamari or soy sauce

2 teaspoons honey

pinch of ground cinnamon

pinch of ground nutmeg

½ teaspoon ground allspice

2 teaspoons lime juice

RICE & BEANS

2 oz brown rice

½ cup light coconut milk

1 scallion, thinly sliced

1 garlic clove, crushed

¼ teaspoon finely chopped fresh thyme

5¼ oz tinned kidney beans, drained and rinsed

MANGO SALSA

2 medium mangoes, peeled, seed removed and diced

½ small red onion, finely chopped

1 tablespoon chopped fresh cilantro

1 tablespoon lime juice

1 tablespoon orange juice

sea salt and ground black pepper, to taste

LIME YOGHURT

7 oz low-fat plain yoghurt

finely grated lime zest and juice, to taste

To make the jerk marinade, place the onion, scallion, chilli, garlic, ginger, thyme, tamari or soy sauce, honey, cinnamon, nutmeg, allspice, and lime juice in a food processor and process into a smooth paste. Pour into a shallow baking dish. Wearing disposable kitchen gloves, place the chicken in the baking dish and rub with the marinade. Cover with plastic wrap and refrigerate for at least 4 hours or overnight to marinate.

To make the rice and beans, bring the rice, coconut milk, scallion, garlic, thyme, and ⅓ cup of water to the boil over high heat. Reduce the heat to low and cook, covered, for 20–25 minutes or until the liquid is absorbed and the rice is tender. Remove from the heat, stir through the kidney beans, then leave to stand, covered, for 5 minutes.

Meanwhile, to make the salsa, place the mango, onion, cilantro, lime juice, orange juice, salt, and pepper in a small bowl and gently stir to combine. Set aside.

Heat a barbecue grill plate or chargrill pan over high heat. Place the chicken on the grill-plate and brush with the marinade. Grill for 5–6 minutes, then turn over and cook for a further 5–6 minutes or until cooked through. Transfer to a plate and set aside to rest.

To make the lime yoghurt, place the yoghurt, lime zest, and juice in a small bowl and mix until well combined.

To serve, place the rice and bean mixture in two serving bowls. Top with the chicken and mango salsa. Drizzle over the yoghurt sauce.

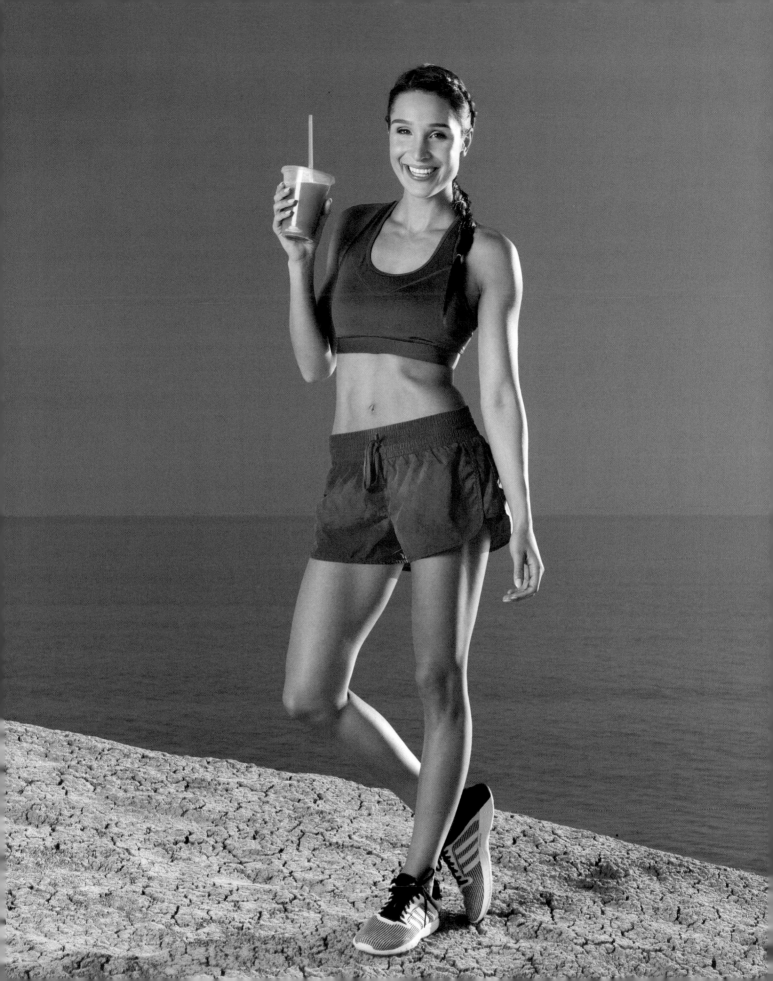

3 PART

SWAP-OUT RECIPES

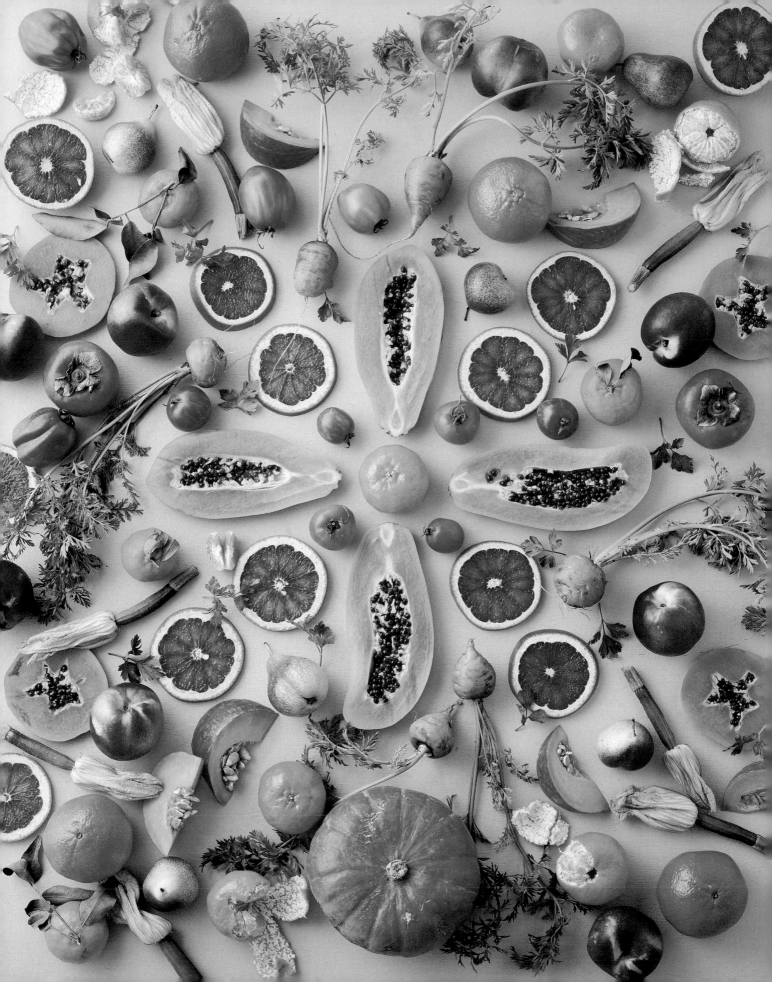

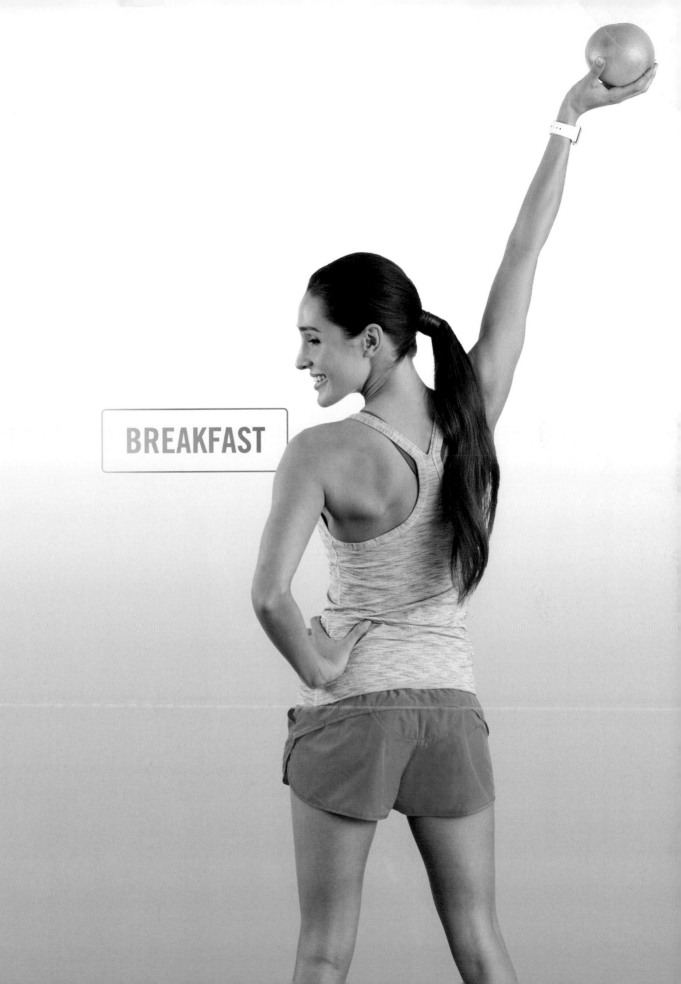

(D) EGGS with AVOCADO & FETA SMASH

SERVES 1
PREP TIME 10 MINUTES
COOKING TIME 5 MINUTES
DIFFICULTY EASY

This is my go-to breakfast on weekends. This recipe is just as good as the one served at my favourite local cafe.

1 oz avocado

¼ small red onion, finely chopped

1 oz salt-reduced low-fat feta cheese, crumbled

3 cherry tomatoes, quartered

lemon juice, to taste

sea salt and ground black pepper, to taste

1 teaspoon white vinegar

2 large eggs

2 slices whole wheat bread

1 small handful baby spinach leaves

Place the avocado in a small bowl and roughly mash using a fork. Add the onion, feta, tomato, lemon juice, salt, and pepper and mix until well combined.

Fill a saucepan with water until 3 in deep. Add the vinegar and bring to a boil over medium heat, then reduce the heat to medium–low. The water should just be simmering. Break the eggs into the water and cook for 2–3 minutes for a semi-soft yolk or 3–4 minutes for a firm yolk. Remove the eggs with a slotted spoon and allow to drain on paper towel.

Toast the bread to your liking.

To serve, place the toast on a serving plate and top with the spinach, avocado, and feta smash and the eggs.

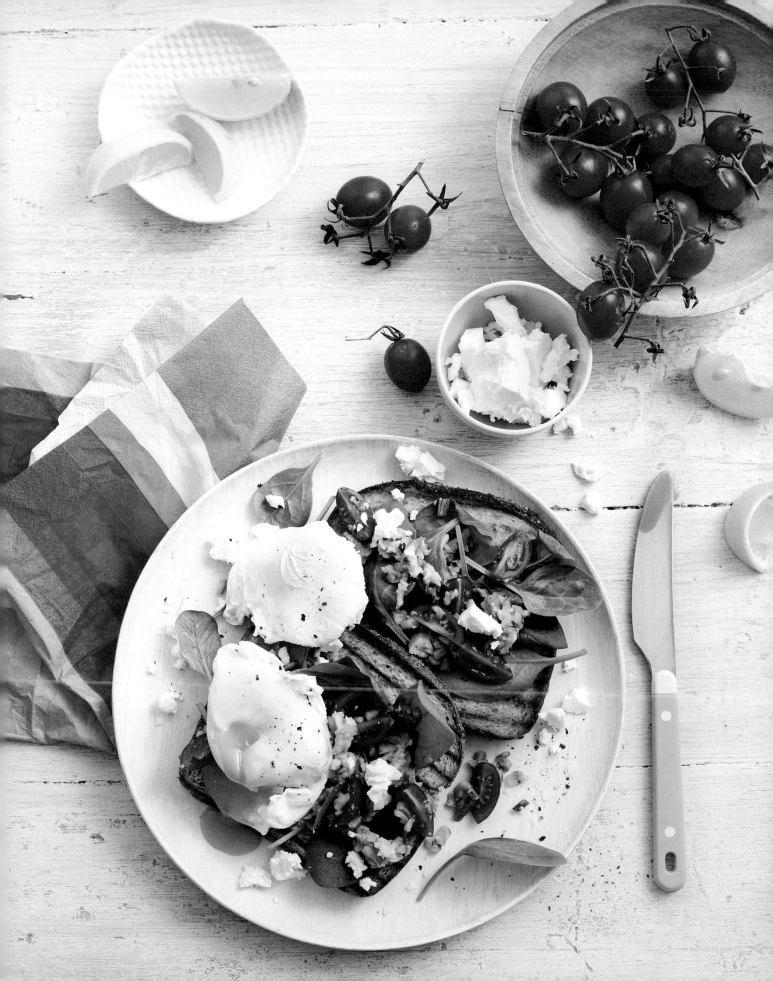

(C) FIG & RICOTTA TOAST TOPPER

SERVES 1
PREP TIME 5 MINUTES
COOKING TIME 2 MINUTES
DIFFICULTY EASY

A little bit of decadence on toast!

2 slices whole wheat bread
2¾ oz low-fat ricotta cheese
1 medium fig, sliced

1 heaping tablespoon walnuts, roughly chopped
honey, to drizzle

Toast the bread to your liking.

To serve, place the toast on a serving plate. Spread the ricotta over the toast and top with the fig. Sprinkle over the walnuts and drizzle with honey.

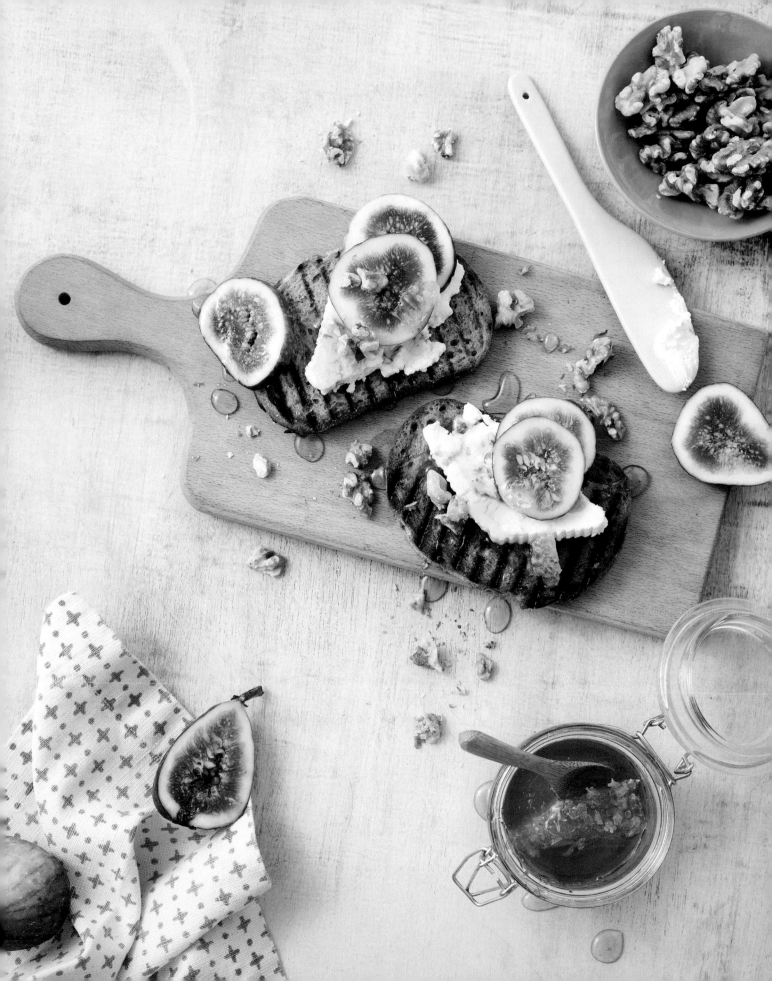

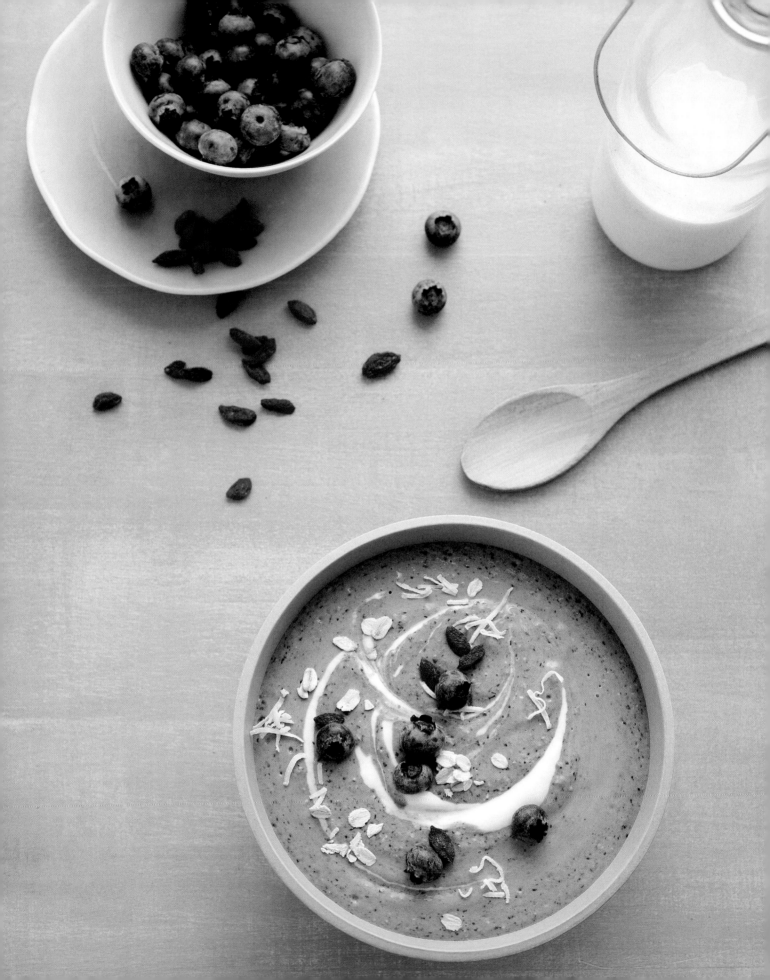

Ⓑ BLUEBERRY SMOOTHIE BOWL

SERVES 1
PREP TIME 5 MINUTES
DIFFICULTY EASY

Say hello to your new favourite summer breakfast! This bowl of blueberry goodness will go down a treat on warm mornings.

5¾ oz frozen blueberries

1 oz tinned chickpeas, drained and rinsed

7 oz low-fat plain yoghurt

½ cup low-fat milk

TOPPINGS

1 oz natural muesli

1½ oz or 8 frozen blueberries, thawed

1½ teaspoons goji berries

1 tablespoon shredded coconut

Place the blueberries, chickpeas, yoghurt, and milk in a blender and blend until smooth.

To serve, pour the smoothie mixture into a bowl and top with the muesli, blueberries, goji berries, and shredded coconut.

APPLE & STRAWBERRY CREPE

SERVES 1
PREP TIME 5 MINUTES
COOKING TIME 7 MINUTES
DIFFICULTY EASY

Dessert for breakfast? Yes, please!

½ medium apple, cored
and cut into bite-sized pieces

2 teaspoons pure maple syrup

4½ oz strawberries, hulled
and quartered

3½ oz low-fat ricotta cheese

1 whole wheat lavash

Heat a small saucepan over medium heat. Add the apple, maple syrup, and
2 tablespoons of water and cook, covered, for 5 minutes or until the apple
is soft, stirring occasionally. Add the strawberries and cook, covered, for
1 minute.

Transfer the apple and strawberries to a bowl. Add the ricotta and stir
until well combined. Set aside to cool slightly.

Warm the lavash in a dry pan over medium heat for 30 seconds.
Remove from the heat and cut in half.

To serve, place the lavash halves on a serving plate and place the apple
mixture down the middle of each. Fold over the ends and roll up to enclose
the filling.

Ⓓ LENTIL & TOMATO BRUSCHETTA

SERVES 1
PREP TIME 5 MINUTES
COOKING TIME 10 MINUTES
DIFFICULTY EASY

If you're more of a savoury bruschetta kind of person, then this recipe is for you. Try using yellow cherry tomatoes for some added colour, if you like.

8 cherry tomatoes, halved

¾ teaspoon olive oil

½ garlic clove, crushed

¼ teaspoon dried oregano

1 small handful baby spinach leaves, thinly sliced

5¼ oz tinned brown lentils, drained and rinsed

lemon juice, to taste

sea salt and ground black pepper, to taste

2 slices whole wheat bread

1 oz salt-reduced low-fat feta cheese, crumbled

1 teaspoon pine nuts

1 tablespoon sliced fresh basil

Preheat the oven to 400°F (350°F convection) and line a baking sheet with parchment paper.

Place the cherry tomatoes and ¼ teaspoon of the oil in a small bowl and toss gently to combine. Place the cherry tomatoes on the lined baking sheet and roast in the oven for 5 minutes or until they begin to soften. Set aside.

Heat the remaining oil in a non-stick fry pan over medium heat. Add the garlic and oregano and cook for 1 minute or until fragrant, stirring occasionally. Add the spinach and cook for 1 minute or until wilted.

Add the lentils, lemon juice, salt, and pepper and cook for 1 minute or until the lentils are warmed through, stirring occasionally.

Toast the bread to your liking.

To serve, place the toast on a serving plate. Top with the lentil and spinach mixture and roasted tomatoes. Sprinkle over the feta, pine nuts, and basil.

(D) SPINACH & FETA BREAKFAST MUFFIN

MAKES 2
PREP TIME 5 MINUTES
COOKING TIME 20 MINUTES
DIFFICULTY EASY

These savoury muffins are great for breakfast on the go! They freeze really well too, so you can make a big batch and then thaw and reheat them as you like.

oil spray

2 large handfuls baby spinach leaves, finely chopped

1 oz salt-reduced low-fat feta cheese, crumbled

5 oz whole wheat flour

1 teaspoon baking powder

pinch of sweet paprika

4 large eggs

½ cup low-fat milk

sea salt and ground black pepper, to taste

1 tablespoon pine nuts

Preheat the oven to 350°F (325°F convection) and place 6 cupcake liners in a 6 cup muffin tin. Lightly spray the liners with oil spray.

Place the spinach and feta in each of the cupcake liners.

Sift the flour, baking powder, and paprika over a large mixing bowl and stir until well combined.

Whisk the eggs, milk, salt, and pepper together in a mixing bowl. Add the egg mixture to the flour mixture and stir gently to combine. Do not over-mix.

Spoon the batter evenly into the cupcake liners and press the pine nuts into the top of each. Bake in the oven for 15–20 minutes or until firm and golden.

Leave to cool for 2 minutes and serve. Allow the remaining muffins to cool completely and keep in the refrigerator for up to 5 days or in the freezer for up to 2 months.

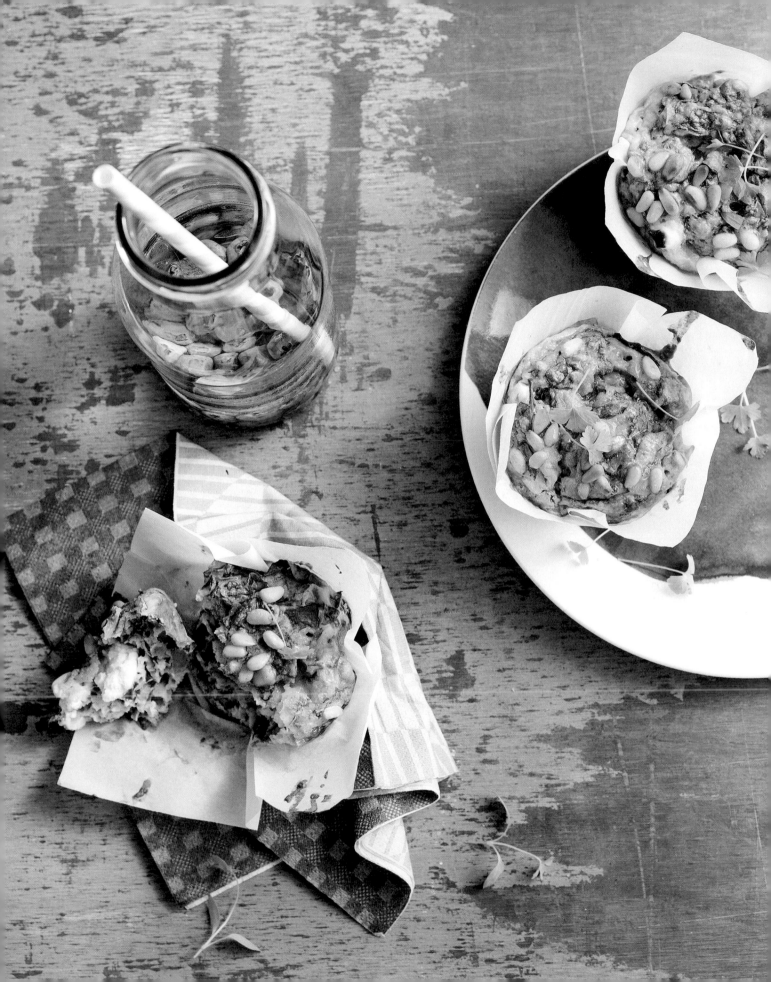

ⓓ HOMEMADE BAKED BEANS

SERVES 1
PREP TIME 10 MINUTES
COOKING TIME 15 MINUTES
DIFFICULTY EASY

Throw away the tinned baked beans! Once you've tried this recipe, you won't go back. The flavours are amazing and so satisfying—perfect to enjoy after a big morning workout.

1½ teaspoons olive oil

¼ small brown onion, finely chopped

¼ garlic clove, crushed

¼ teaspoon dried mixed herbs

4 oz tinned crushed tomatoes

3½ oz tinned cannellini beans, drained and rinsed

1 teaspoon Worcestershire sauce

1 teaspoon pure maple syrup

2 slices whole wheat bread

⅔ oz reduced-fat cheddar cheese, grated

1 tablespoon chopped fresh parsley

Heat the oil in a small saucepan over medium heat. Add the onion, garlic, and mixed herbs and cook for 3–4 minutes or until the onion is soft and translucent, stirring occasionally.

Add the crushed tomatoes, cannellini beans, Worcestershire sauce, and maple syrup. Reduce the heat to medium–low and cook for 5–10 minutes or until heated through, stirring occasionally.

Meanwhile, toast the bread to your liking.

To serve, place the toast on a serving plate and top with the baked beans. Sprinkle over the grated cheese and parsley.

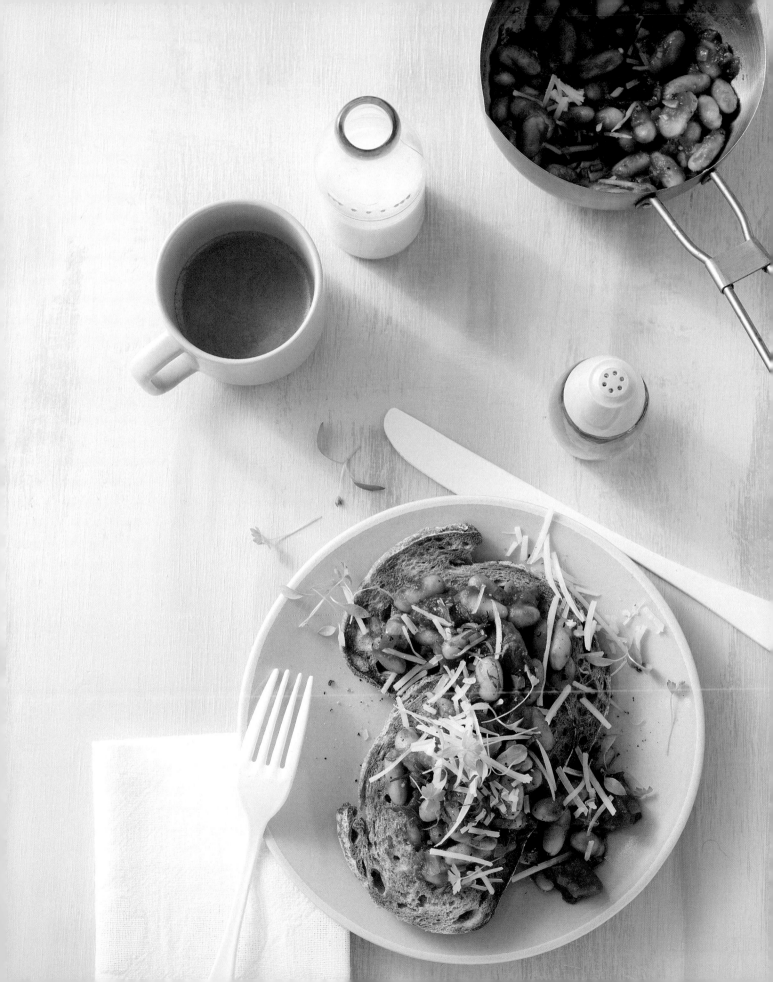

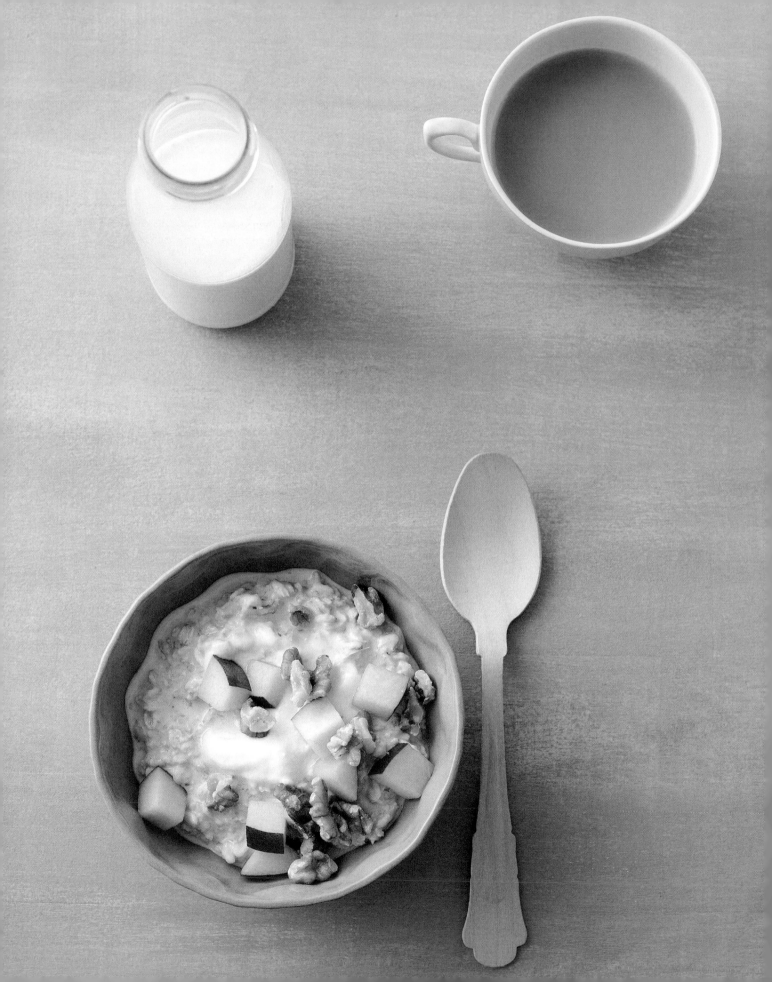

Ⓒ GINGER & PEACH OVERNIGHT OATS

SERVES 1

PREP TIME 5 MINUTES +
OVERNIGHT CHILLING TIME

DIFFICULTY EASY

Sick of your regular overnight oats? Then you need to try this combo! The zing of fresh ginger works so well with peach. This recipe is perfect for cool autumn mornings.

2 oz rolled oats (about ⅔ cup)

½ cup low-fat milk

1¾ oz low-fat plain yoghurt

1 teaspoon finely grated fresh ginger

½ large peach, with stone removed, diced

1 heaping tablespoon walnuts, roughly chopped

Place the oats, milk, yoghurt, ginger, and peach in a bowl and mix until well combined.

Pour the oat mixture into a bowl or jar. Cover with plastic wrap and place in the refrigerator to chill overnight.

To serve, stir the overnight oats and sprinkle over the walnuts.

ⓒ STEWED APPLE OVERNIGHT OATS

SERVES 1

PREP TIME 5 MINUTES +
OVERNIGHT CHILLING TIME

COOKING TIME 4 MINUTES

DIFFICULTY EASY

This is a great combo to help warm you up on a cold winter's morning! If you prefer a tarter flavour I suggest using a Granny Smith apple, or if you like a little more sweetness go for a pink lady.

½ medium apple, cored
and cut into bite-sized pieces

lemon juice, to taste

¼ teaspoon ground cinnamon,
plus extra to dust (optional)

2 oz rolled oats

½ cup low-fat milk

1¾ oz low-fat plain yoghurt

3 teaspoons chia seeds

Heat a small saucepan over medium heat. Add the apple, lemon juice, cinnamon, and 1 tablespoon of water and cook, covered, for 4 minutes or until the apple is soft, stirring occasionally. Set aside to cool.

Place the oats, milk, yoghurt, cooked apple, and chia seeds in a bowl and mix until well combined.

Pour the oat mixture into a bowl or jar. Cover with plastic wrap and place in the refrigerator to chill overnight.

To serve, stir the overnight oats and dust with cinnamon, if desired.

Ⓒ BANANA & PECAN OVERNIGHT OATS

SERVES 1
PREP TIME 5 MINUTES +
OVERNIGHT CHILLING TIME
DIFFICULTY EASY

Don't stress if you don't have pecans in your pantry for this—you can just use walnuts instead.

2 oz rolled oats (about ⅔ cup)
½ cup low-fat milk
1¾ oz low-fat plain yoghurt

1 heaping tablespoon pecans, roughly chopped
1 teaspoon ground cinnamon
½ medium banana, peeled

Place the oats, milk, yoghurt, pecans, and cinnamon in a bowl and mix until well combined.

Pour the oat mixture into a bowl or jar. Cover with plastic wrap and place in the refrigerator to chill overnight.

To serve, mash the banana and stir through the overnight oats.

Ⓓ MUSHROOM, SPINACH & WHITE BEAN CREPE

SERVES 1

PREP TIME 5 MINUTES

COOKING TIME 10 MINUTES

DIFFICULTY EASY

Treat yourself with this delicious savoury crepe. You won't be disappointed!

1½ teaspoons olive oil

¼ small red onion, finely chopped

1¾ oz mushrooms, thinly sliced

1 small handful baby spinach leaves

5 oz tinned cannellini beans, drained and rinsed

1¾ oz low-fat ricotta cheese

sea salt and ground black pepper, to taste

1 whole wheat lavash

Heat the oil in a non-stick fry pan over medium heat. Add the onion and mushrooms and cook for 5 minutes or until the onion is soft and translucent, stirring occasionally.

Add the spinach, cannellini beans, and ricotta and cook for another 1–2 minutes or until the spinach has wilted and the beans and ricotta are warmed through, stirring occasionally. Season with salt and pepper, if desired.

Warm the lavash in a dry pan over medium heat for 30 seconds. Remove from the heat and cut in half.

To serve, place the lavash halves on a serving plate and place the mushroom and cannellini bean mixture down the middle of each. Fold over the ends and roll up to enclose the filling.

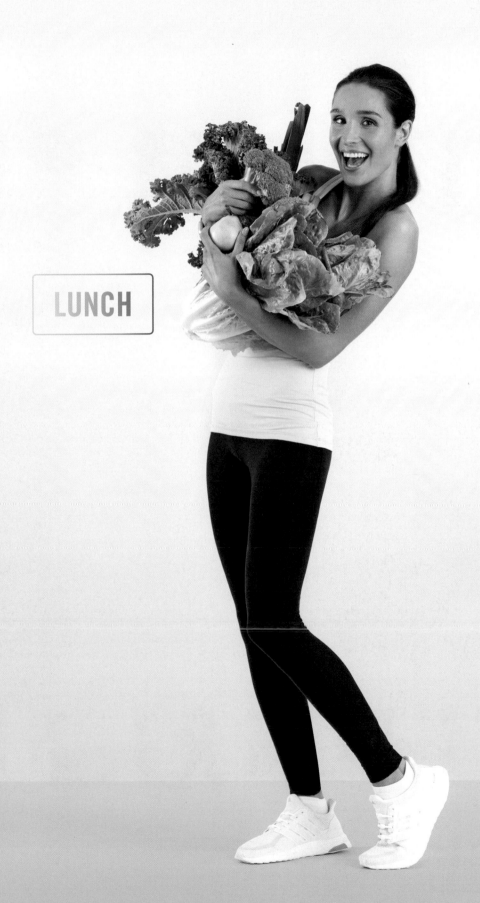

LUNCH

⒟ MEDITERRANEAN NACHOS

SERVES 1

PREP TIME 10 MINUTES +
30 MINUTES MARINATING TIME

COOKING TIME 10 MINUTES

DIFFICULTY EASY

This recipe is a healthier—and more delicious—version of traditional nachos! It is packed full of colour and flavour. To save time, the pita bread can be cooked the night before, then cooled and stored in an airtight container overnight.

½ whole wheat pita bread,
cut into wedges

oil spray

5 cherry tomatoes, halved

½ Lebanese cucumber, finely chopped

¼ small red onion, finely chopped

2 teaspoons fresh mint leaves

½ teaspoon balsamic vinegar

lemon juice, to taste

sea salt and ground black pepper,
to taste

2 kalamata olives, pitted and chopped

2¾ oz hummus (see page 254)

MINTED YOGHURT

3½ oz low-fat plain yoghurt

½ garlic clove, crushed

1 tablespoon chopped fresh mint

finely grated lemon zest and juice,
to taste

sea salt and ground black pepper,
to taste

Preheat the oven to 400°F (350°F convection) and line a baking sheet with parchment paper.

Lay the pita wedges in a single layer on the lined baking sheet and spray lightly with oil spray. Bake in the oven for 5 minutes until they begin to colour. Turn the wedges over and bake for a further 5–8 minutes or until both sides are lightly coloured and set aside to cool.

Place the tomato, cucumber, onion, mint, vinegar, lemon juice, salt, and pepper in a bowl and toss gently to combine. Cover with plastic wrap and refrigerate for 30 minutes to marinate.

To make the minted yoghurt, whisk the yoghurt, garlic, mint, lemon zest and juice, salt, and pepper together in a small bowl.

To serve, place the pita triangles on the bottom of a serving bowl or plate. Top with the tomato and cucumber salad. Sprinkle over the olives and top with the hummus and minted yoghurt.

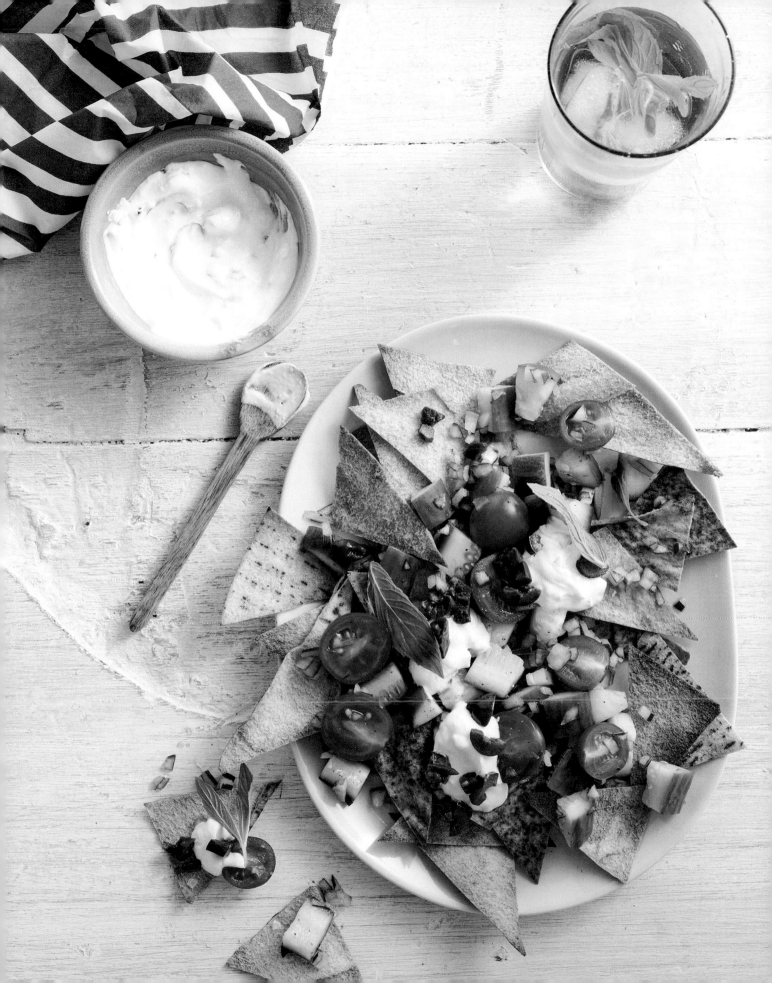

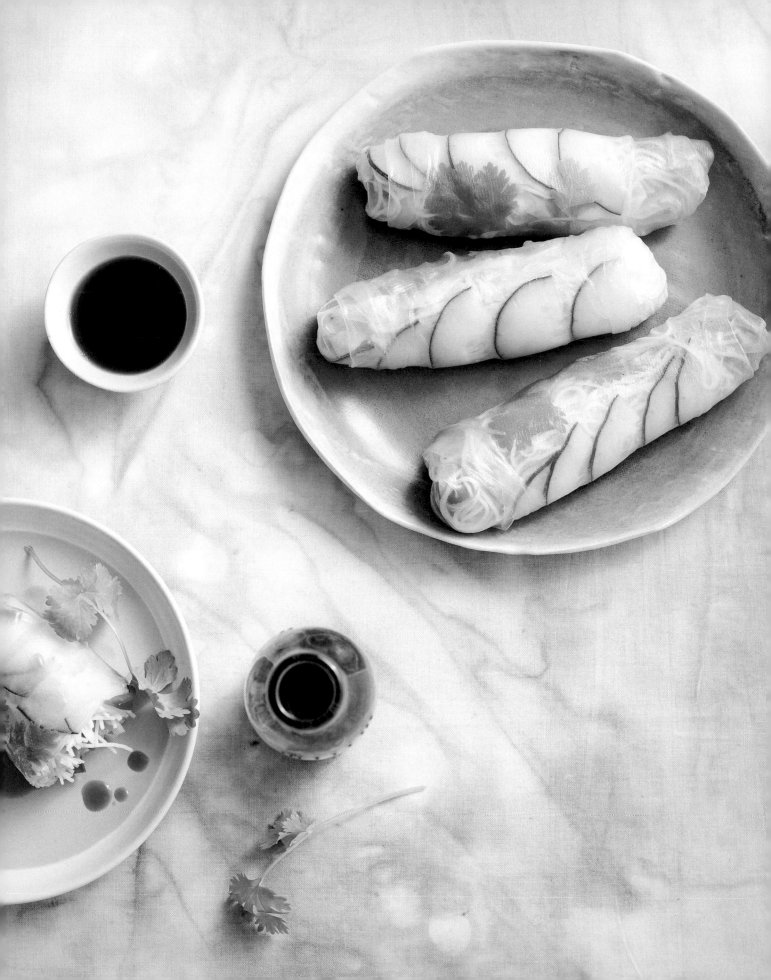

(A) VIETNAMESE ROLLS

SERVES 1
PREP TIME 15 MINUTES +
10 MINUTES SOAKING TIME
COOKING TIME 4 MINUTES
DIFFICULTY EASY

Vietnamese rolls (or "cold rolls" as we like to call them in South Australia) are one of my favourite meals because they are just full of mouth-watering flavours. Try making them the next time you are entertaining—they are so easy!

¼ oz rice vermicelli noodles

oil spray

2 large eggs, lightly whisked

4 small rice paper wrappers

½ Lebanese cucumber, thinly sliced

1 small handful bean sprouts

½ medium carrot, thinly sliced

¼ medium red bell pepper, seeds removed and thinly sliced

fresh cilantro leaves, to serve (optional)

salt-reduced tamari or soy sauce, to serve

Place the noodles in a heatproof bowl and cover with boiling water. Leave for 10 minutes, then loosen the noodles with a fork. Drain and refresh under cold water. Drain well and set aside to cool slightly. When cool enough to handle, cut into shorter lengths.

Meanwhile, heat a non-stick fry pan over medium heat and spray lightly with oil spray. Pour in the egg and swirl to cover the base of the pan. Cook for 1–2 minutes or until the egg is set. Place the omelette on a plate and set aside to cool. When cool enough to handle, slice into thin strips.

Place the rice paper wrappers, egg, noodles, and all the prepared vegetables on the clean workbench, ready to roll.

Fill a large bowl with warm water for the wrappers. Working with one wrapper at a time, dip into the water for 1 second to soften. Do not soak as the wrappers can become too soft and tear.

Place the wrapper on a chopping board and place one-quarter of the noodles, egg, and vegetables on the bottom third, adding a few cilantro leaves, if desired. Bring the bottom of the wrapper up and over the filling, fold in the sides and then roll up. Set the roll aside, seam-side down, while you prepare the remaining rolls. Repeat with the remaining ingredients to make four rolls in total.

Serve the rolls with a small dish of tamari or soy sauce for dipping.

LOADED SALAD SANDWICH with HUMMUS

SERVES 1
PREP TIME 10 MINUTES
DIFFICULTY EASY

This colourful sandwich contains a rainbow of vegetables. Amazing to look at and even better to eat!

5 oz hummus (see page 254)

2 slices whole wheat bread

1 small handful lettuce leaves

¼ medium tomato, thinly sliced

¼ medium carrot, coarsely grated

¼ Lebanese cucumber, thinly sliced

¼ small red onion, thinly sliced

1 small handful alfalfa sprouts

Spread the hummus over both slices of bread.

On one slice of bread, layer the lettuce, tomato, carrot, cucumber, red onion, and alfalfa sprouts.

Top with the other slice of bread.

To serve, place the sandwich on a serving plate and cut in half.

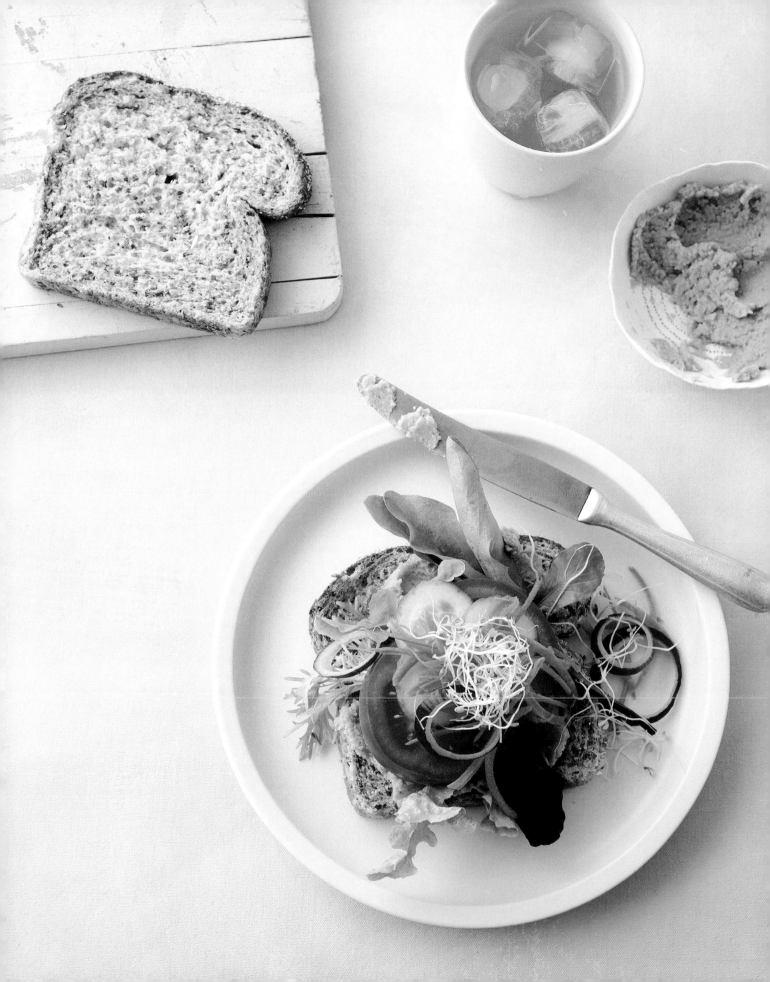

CRUNCHY GRAIN SALAD

SERVES 1
PREP TIME 10 MINUTES
COOKING TIME 35 MINUTES
DIFFICULTY EASY

Can't decide if you want rice or quinoa in your salad? Well, this recipe lets you have both! However, if you're short on time, then you can always leave one out: just remember to double the quantity of the one you're using.

2 tablespoons brown rice

1 oz quinoa

3 oz broccoli, cut into even-sized florets

3 semi-dried tomatoes, cut into slices

5 oz tinned chickpeas, drained and rinsed

1 tablespoon finely chopped fresh parsley

sea salt and ground black pepper, to taste

DRESSING

½ garlic clove, crushed

pinch of dried oregano

finely grated lemon zest and juice, to taste

Place the rice and ½ cup of water in a small saucepan over high heat and bring to a boil, stirring occasionally. Cover and reduce the heat to medium–low. Simmer for 20–25 minutes or until the liquid is absorbed and the rice is tender. Remove from the heat and let stand, covered, for 5 minutes. Set aside to cool.

Meanwhile, place the quinoa and ½ cup of water in a saucepan over high heat and bring to a boil, stirring occasionally. Cover and reduce the heat to low. Simmer for 10–12 minutes until the quinoa is tender. Drain off any excess liquid. Set aside to cool.

Fill a saucepan with water until 2 in deep and insert a steamer basket. Cover with a lid and bring the water to a boil over high heat, then reduce the heat to medium. Add the broccoli and steam for 2–3 minutes until tender-crisp. Place in a bowl of iced water to cool. Drain well and roughly chop.

To make the dressing, whisk the garlic, oregano, lemon zest and juice, and 2 teaspoons of water together in a small bowl.

To serve, place the rice, quinoa, broccoli, semi-dried tomatoes, chickpeas, and parsley in a serving bowl. Drizzle over the dressing and season with salt and pepper, if desired. Toss gently to combine.

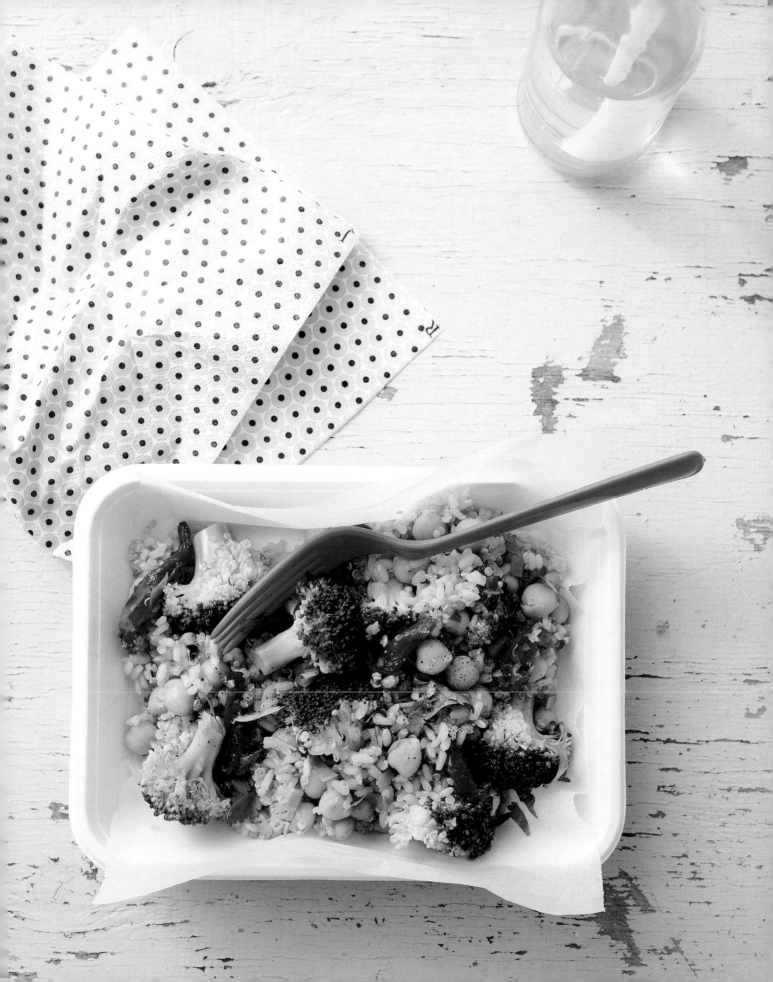

Ⓒ THAI BEEF NOODLE SALAD

SERVES 1

PREP TIME 15 MINUTES +
10 MINUTES SOAKING TIME

COOKING TIME 6 MINUTES

DIFFICULTY EASY

Fresh is the first word that comes to mind when I make this salad. Definitely a favourite of mine!

3½ oz rice vermicelli noodles

oil spray

3 oz lean beef steak

sea salt and ground black pepper, to taste

1 small handful mixed lettuce leaves

5 cherry tomatoes, halved

¼ small red onion, thinly sliced

¼ Lebanese cucumber, halved lengthways and thinly sliced

1 small handful bean sprouts

1 small handful fresh cilantro leaves

1 small handful fresh mint leaves

DRESSING

¼–½ teaspoon finely chopped fresh red chilli

1 garlic clove, crushed

2 teaspoons rinsed and finely chopped cilantro stalks

1 teaspoon honey, or to taste

1 tablespoon fish sauce, or to taste

1½ tablespoons lime juice, or to taste

To make the dressing, whisk the chilli, garlic, cilantro stalks, honey, fish sauce, and lime juice together in a small bowl. Adjust the balance with extra honey, fish sauce, and lime juice, if needed. Set aside.

Place the noodles in a heatproof bowl and cover with boiling water. Leave for 10 minutes, then loosen the noodles with a fork. Drain and refresh under cool running water. Drain well and set aside.

Heat a non-stick fry pan over high heat and spray lightly with oil spray. Season the steak with salt and pepper, if desired. Cook for 2–3 minutes on each side or continue to cook to your liking. Cover loosely with foil and set aside to rest. Slice the steak against the grain.

To serve, place the noodles, lettuce, tomato, onion, cucumber, bean sprouts, cilantro, and mint leaves into a serving bowl. Top with the sliced beef and drizzle over the dressing. Toss gently to combine.

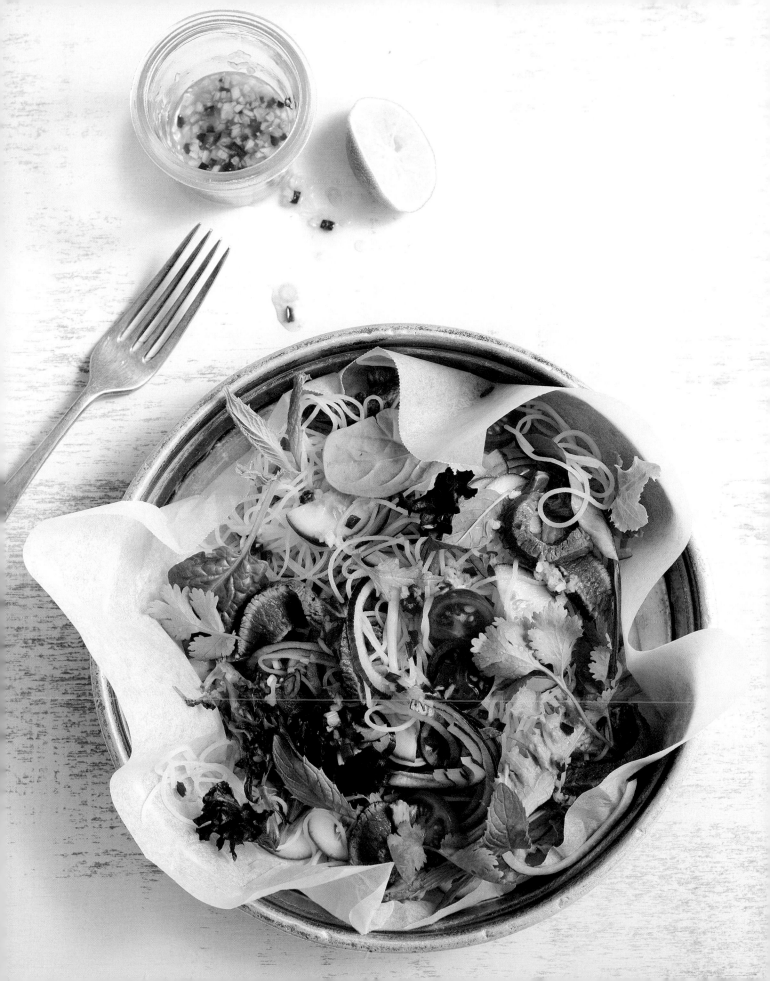

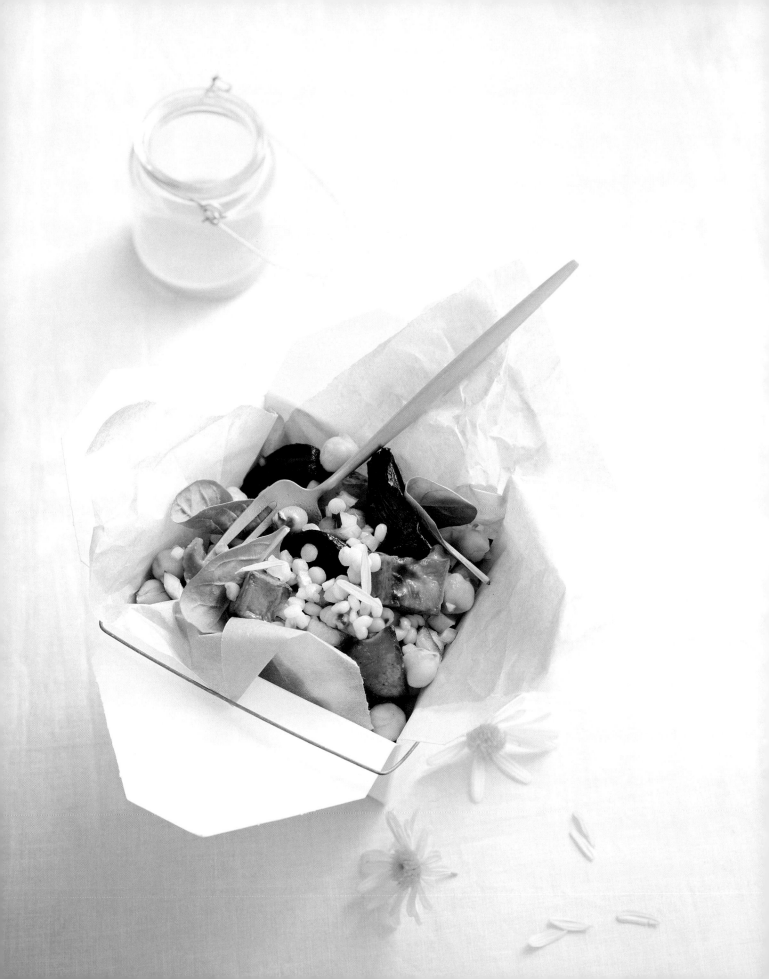

Ⓐ PEARL COUSCOUS, PUMPKIN & BEETROOT SALAD

SERVES 1
PREP TIME 15 MINUTES
COOKING TIME 35 MINUTES
DIFFICULTY EASY

Stuck for time? You can prepare the couscous, pumpkin and beetroot the night before and store them in separate airtight containers in the refrigerator. Just add the other salad ingredients and the dressing when you're ready to eat. Easy peasy, lemon squeezy ;)

1 small beetroot, cut into wedges
oil spray
sea salt and ground black pepper, to taste
2 oz pumpkin, cut into ½-in cubes
⅓ cup pearl couscous
1 small handful spinach leaves
¼ small red onion, thinly sliced

5 oz tinned chickpeas, drained and rinsed

DRESSING
juice of ½ lemon
1 teaspoon Dijon mustard
1 teaspoon honey
1 teaspoon red wine vinegar

Preheat the oven to 350°F (325°F convection) and line a baking sheet with parchment paper.

Place the beetroot wedges on the lined baking sheet and spray lightly with oil spray. Season with salt and pepper, if desired.

Bake in the oven for 10 minutes. Remove the sheet from the oven, add the pumpkin and spray lightly with oil spray. Season with salt and pepper, if desired. Bake in the oven for a further 15–20 minutes or until the beetroot is tender and the pumpkin is soft and lightly browned, turning the pumpkin with tongs every 10 minutes. Set aside to cool.

Fill a saucepan with water and bring to the boil. Stir in the pearl couscous and simmer over medium heat for 10–12 minutes until al dente. Drain and set aside to cool.

To make the dressing, whisk the lemon juice, mustard, honey, and vinegar together in a small bowl.

To serve, place the pumpkin, beetroot, couscous, spinach, onion, and chickpeas in a serving bowl. Drizzle over the dressing and toss gently to combine.

HUMMUS

MAKES 2¾ oz

PREP TIME 10 MINUTES

DIFFICULTY EASY

As you've probably noticed, this healthy oil-free hummus is one of my favourite staples! This recipe makes about 2¾ ounces—you can just multiply the ingredients to make larger quantities.

2¾ oz tinned chickpeas, drained and rinsed

¼ garlic clove, crushed

lemon juice, to taste

pinch of smoked paprika

sea salt, to taste

Place the chickpeas, garlic, lemon juice, paprika, salt, and 1½ tablespoons of water in a food processor. Pulse until smooth and creamy.

TZATZIKI

MAKES 1¾ oz

PREP TIME 10 MINUTES + OVERNIGHT STRAINING TIME

DIFFICULTY EASY

I love making a fresh batch of tzatziki and taking it to barbecues for my family and friends to enjoy! This recipe makes about 1¾ oz—you can just multiply the ingredients to make larger quantities.

1¾ oz low-fat plain yoghurt

¾-in piece Lebanese cucumber

lemon juice, to taste

¼ garlic clove, crushed

¼ teaspoon finely chopped fresh dill

sea salt and ground black pepper, to taste

Place the yoghurt in a strainer lined with cheesecloth over another bowl and leave in the fridge overnight. This will give the tzatziki a thicker consistency.

Peel and remove the seeds from the cucumber. Grate and squeeze out any excess water.

Place the yoghurt, cucumber, lemon juice, garlic, dill, salt, and pepper in a small bowl and mix until well combined.

⒟ GREEK SALAD PITA SANDWICH

SERVES 1
PREP TIME 10 MINUTES
DIFFICULTY EASY

One of the things I love about Greek cuisine is that it's often so light and fresh! Sometimes I'll make this with half a whole wheat wrap instead—just depends on what I have in my pantry at the time.

5 cherry tomatoes, quartered

¼ Lebanese cucumber, finely chopped

¼ small red onion, finely chopped

¼ medium green bell pepper, seeds removed and finely chopped

1 oz salt-reduced low-fat feta cheese, crumbled

1 tablespoon chopped fresh parsley

1 teaspoon red wine vinegar

sea salt and ground black pepper, to taste

2¾ oz hummus (see page 254)

½ whole wheat pita bread

Place the tomato, cucumber, onion, capsicum, feta, parsley, and vinegar in a bowl. Season with salt and pepper, if desired, and toss gently to combine.

To serve, spread the hummus on the inside of the pita half and fill with the Greek salad.

OPEN TUNA & SALAD SANDWICH

SERVES 1
PREP TIME 10 MINUTES
DIFFICULTY EASY

Tuna is one of my favourite sources of protein. I love adding a little extra lemon juice here for a bit more zing!

1½ oz tinned cannellini beans, drained and rinsed

1 small handful baby spinach leaves

½ Lebanese cucumber, cut into ribbons with a vegetable peeler

¼ small fennel bulb, thinly sliced

3½ oz tinned tuna in springwater, drained and flaked

¼ small red onion, finely chopped

2 teaspoons capers, rinsed and finely chopped

2 teaspoons finely chopped fresh parsley

ground black pepper, to taste

finely grated lemon zest and juice, to taste

1 slice whole wheat bread

Place the cannellini beans in a small bowl and roughly mash using a fork until a chunky paste has formed.

Place the spinach, cucumber, and fennel in another small bowl and toss gently to combine.

Place the tuna, onion, capers, parsley, pepper, lemon zest, and juice in a small bowl and mix until well combined.

To serve, place the slice of bread on a serving plate. Spread over the cannellini bean paste and top with cucumber mixture and tuna mixture. Squeeze over a little extra lemon juice, if desired.

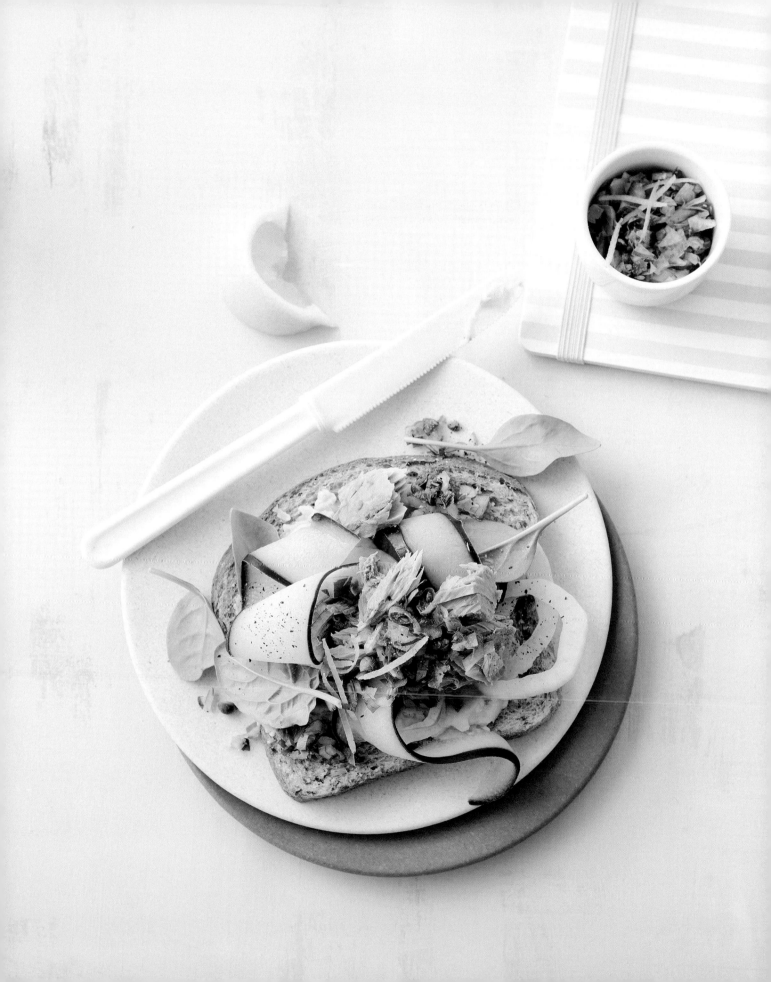

Ⓓ FATTOUSH SALAD

SERVES 1
PREP TIME 10 MINUTES
COOKING TIME 10 MINUTES
DIFFICULTY EASY

I love having toasted bread in my salads. It's super easy to make and gives your lunch an amazing texture boost.

½ whole wheat pita bread

oil spray

½ Lebanese cucumber, cut into ribbons with a vegetable peeler

5 cherry tomatoes, halved

1 radish, thinly sliced

¼ small red onion, thinly sliced

1 small handful fresh mint leaves

1 small handful fresh parsley leaves

1 oz salt-reduced low-fat feta cheese, crumbled

HUMMUS DRESSING

2¾ oz hummus (see page 254)

juice of ¼ lemon

Preheat the oven to 400°F (350°F convection) and line a baking sheet with parchment paper.

Lay the pita bread on the lined baking sheet and spray lightly with oil spray. Bake in the oven for 5 minutes until it begins to colour. Turn over and bake for a further 5–8 minutes or until both sides are lightly coloured and set aside to cool. When cool enough to handle, break into bite-sized pieces.

To make the hummus dressing, whisk the hummus, lemon juice, and 2 teaspoons of water together in a small bowl. If it is too thick, add ¼ teaspoon of water at a time until the desired consistency is reached.

To serve, place the pita pieces, cucumber, tomato, radish, onion, mint, and parsley in a serving bowl and toss gently to combine. Drizzle over the hummus dressing and top with the feta.

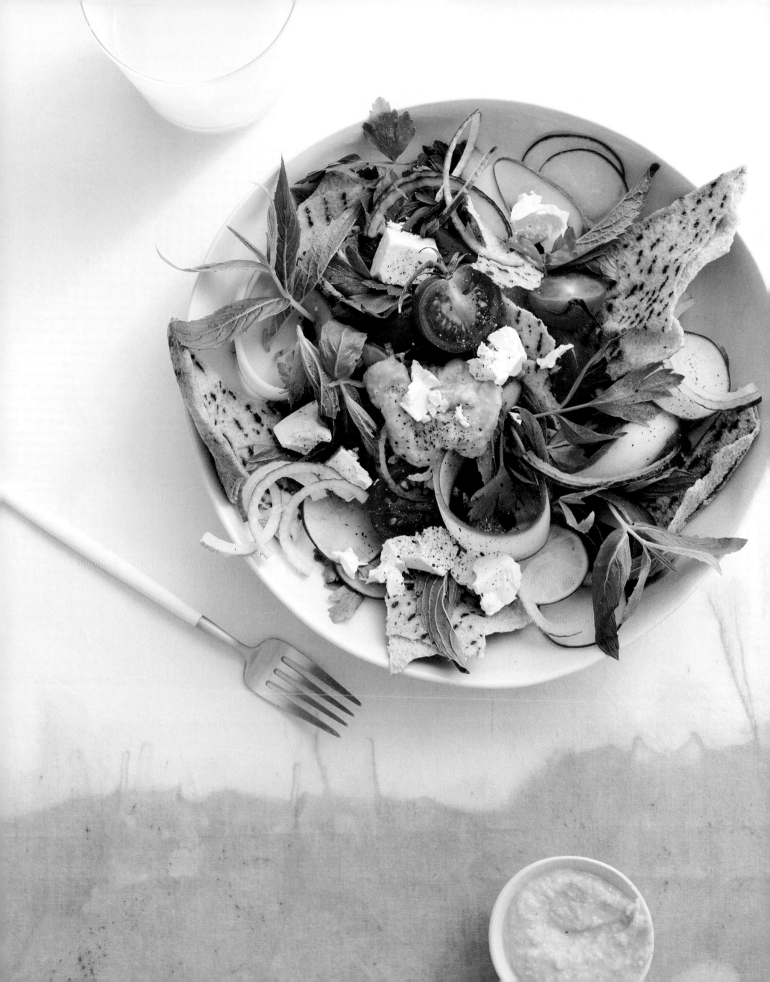

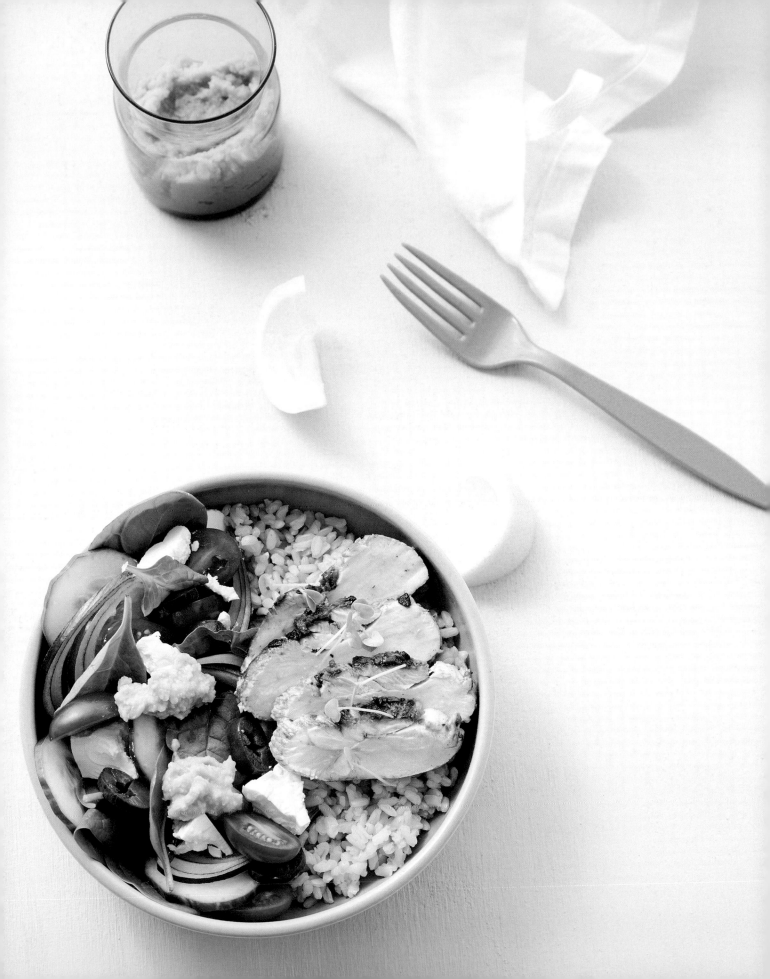

Ⓑ CHICKEN RICE BOWL

SERVES 1

PREP TIME 10 MINUTES +
30 MINUTES OR OVERNIGHT
MARINATING TIME

COOKING TIME 30 MINUTES

DIFFICULTY EASY

A hearty bowl packed with goodness and full of flavour. Prepare all the ingredients the night before and you'll be able to quickly throw this lunch together and head out the door. Easy!

lemon juice, to taste

2 teaspoons finely chopped fresh parsley

½ garlic clove, crushed

¼ teaspoon ground paprika

¼ teaspoon dried oregano

sea salt and ground black pepper, to taste

2¾ oz chicken breast fillet

2 oz brown rice

oil spray

1 small handful baby spinach leaves, chopped

5 cherry tomatoes, halved

¼ Lebanese cucumber, thinly sliced

¼ small red onion, thinly sliced

2 kalamata olives, pitted and sliced

1 oz salt-reduced low-fat feta cheese, crumbled

1½ oz hummus (see page 254)

lemon wedges, to serve

Whisk the lemon juice, parsley, garlic, paprika, oregano, salt, and pepper together in a medium bowl. Place the chicken in the bowl and rub with the spice mix. Ensure all the chicken is coated. Cover with plastic wrap and refrigerate for 30 minutes to marinate. Alternatively, leave to marinate overnight.

Place the rice and 1¼ cups of water in a small saucepan over high heat and bring to the boil, stirring occasionally. Cover and reduce the heat to medium–low. Simmer for 20–25 minutes or until the liquid is absorbed and the rice is tender. Remove from the heat and let stand, covered, for 5 minutes. Set aside to cool.

Heat a non-stick fry pan over medium heat and spray lightly with oil spray. Add the chicken and cook for 5–6 minutes on each side or until cooked through. Transfer to a plate and set aside to rest. Cut into thick slices.

Place the spinach, tomato, cucumber, onion, olives, and feta in a bowl and toss gently to combine.

To serve, place the rice into one half of a serving bowl. Place the salad into the other half and top with the chicken and hummus. Serve with lemon wedges on the side.

Ⓑ GRILLED VEGETABLE & SMASHED CHICKPEA TOASTIE

SERVES 1
PREP TIME 10 MINUTES
COOKING TIME 15 MINUTES
DIFFICULTY EASY

This Mediterranean-inspired toastie is super delicious. The chickpeas are a really nice addition! The vegetables can be grilled the night before and stored in an airtight container in the refrigerator.

¼ medium eggplant,
cut into ½-in thick slices

½ medium zucchini,
cut into ½-in thick slices

⅛ medium red bell pepper,
seeds removed and chopped

oil spray

2 slices whole wheat bread

1 small handful baby spinach leaves

1 oz salt-reduced low-fat feta cheese,
crumbled

SMASHED CHICKPEAS

5¼ oz tinned chickpeas,
drained and rinsed

½ garlic clove, crushed

pinch of sweet paprika

lemon juice, to taste

sea salt and ground black pepper,
to taste

Heat a barbecue grill-plate or chargrill pan over high heat.

Place the eggplant, zucchini, and bell pepper in a large bowl and spray with oil spray. Ensure that all the vegetables are lightly coated.

Working in batches if necessary, grill the eggplant, zucchini, and pepper for 4–6 minutes or until tender, turning occasionally. Set aside to cool.

Preheat a sandwich press.

To make the smashed chickpeas, place the chickpeas, garlic, paprika, lemon juice, salt, and pepper in a small bowl and roughly mash with a fork until a chunky paste has formed. If it is too thick, add a little cold water until the desired consistency is reached.

Place the slices of bread on a clean chopping board and spread over the smashed chickpeas. On one slice of bread, layer the spinach, grilled vegetables, and feta. Top with the other slice of bread.

Place the sandwich onto the sandwich press and gently press down the lid. Toast for 3–5 minutes or until the sandwich is golden.

To serve, place the toastie on a serving plate and cut in half.

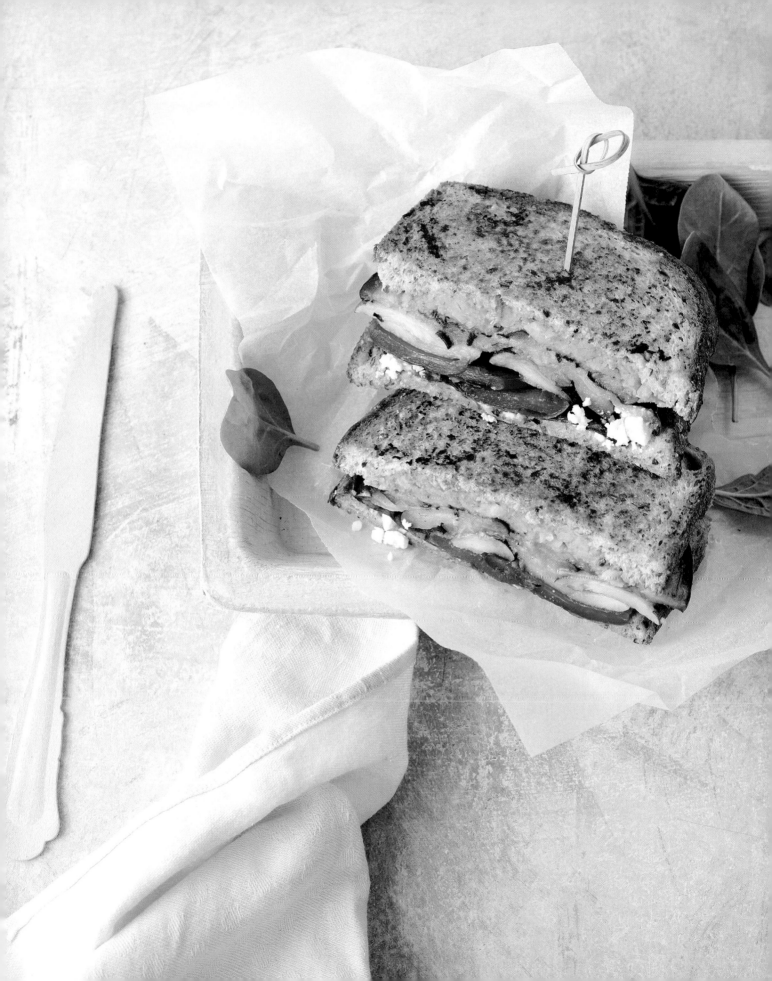

B BEEF & CARAMELISED ONION TOASTIE

SERVES 1
PREP TIME 10 MINUTES
COOKING TIME 35 MINUTES
DIFFICULTY EASY

This combination takes toasties to a whole new level! Beef not your thing? Replace it with chicken to still get that protein fix. The caramelised onion can be stored in an airtight container in the refrigerator for up to 5 days.

2 slices whole wheat bread

2⅓ oz cooked beef, sliced

½ medium tomato, sliced

1 oz salt-reduced low-fat feta cheese, crumbled

1 small handful arugula leaves

CARAMELISED ONION

oil spray

½ small brown onion, sliced

2 teaspoons pure maple syrup

2 teaspoons balsamic vinegar

To caramelise the onion, heat a small non-stick fry pan over low heat and spray lightly with oil spray. Add the onion and cook slowly for 15–20 minutes or until soft and golden, stirring occasionally. Don't be tempted to increase the heat as this can cause the onion to burn. Add the maple syrup and balsamic vinegar and cook for a further 5–10 minutes or until sticky and caramelised, stirring occasionally. Set aside to cool.

Preheat a sandwich press.

Place a slice of bread on a clean chopping board. Layer the caramelised onion, beef, tomato, feta, and arugula leaves. Top with the other slice of bread.

Place the sandwich on the sandwich press and gently press down the lid. Toast for 3–5 minutes or until the sandwich is golden.

To serve, place the toastie on a serving plate and cut in half.

Ⓑ CHICKEN & CHEESE TOASTIE

SERVES 1
PREP TIME 5 MINUTES
COOKING TIME 5 MINUTES
DIFFICULTY EASY

Sometimes a sandwich just doesn't cut it, which is why I LOVE making toasties! And what's a toastie without cheese?! I've used Jarlsberg in this one, but you could always use cheddar or mozzarella if you prefer.

2 slices whole wheat bread

1 large handful baby spinach leaves

3 oz cooked chicken, shredded

¼ small red onion, thinly sliced

3 semi-dried tomatoes, sliced

⅔ oz Jarlsberg cheese, sliced

Preheat a sandwich press.

Place a slice of bread on a clean chopping board. Layer the spinach, chicken, onion, tomato, and cheese. Top with the other slice of bread.

Place the sandwich on the sandwich press and gently press down the lid. Toast for 3–5 minutes or until the cheese is melted and the sandwich is golden.

To serve, place the toastie on a serving plate and cut in half.

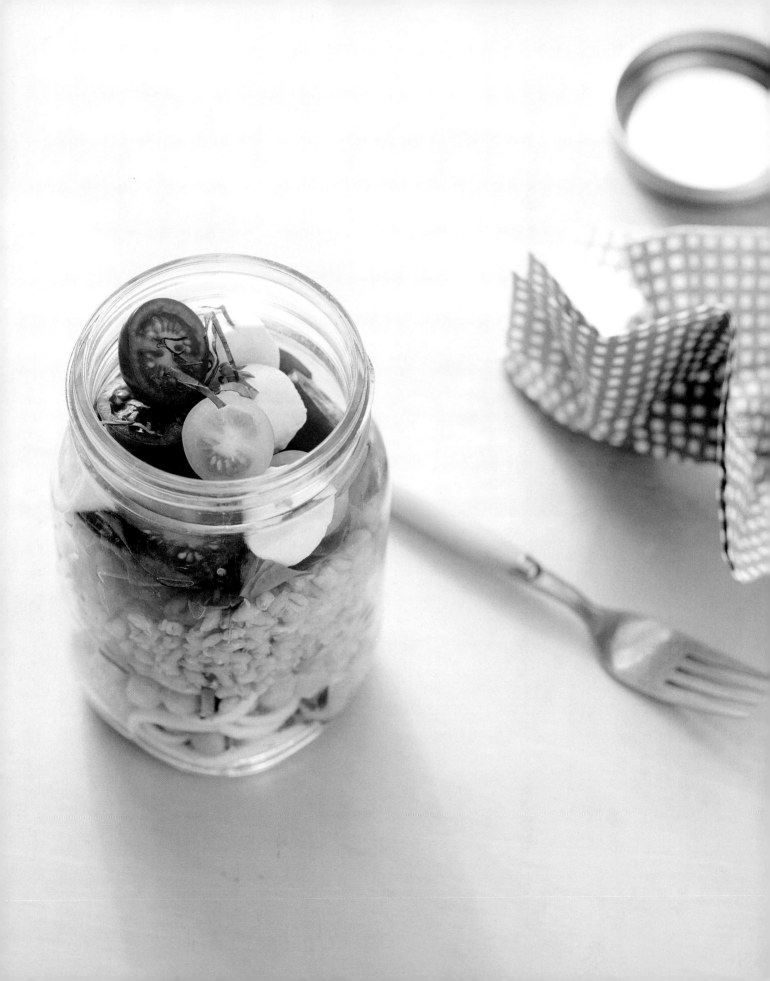

Ⓓ ZUCCHINI NOODLE & PEARL BARLEY MASON JAR SALAD

SERVES 1
PREP TIME 10 MINUTES
COOKING TIME 30 MINUTES
DIFFICULTY EASY

The trick to making the best mason-jar salad is the order! I suggest starting with the dressing and then adding the "harder" ingredients, such as vegetables, beans, grains, or pasta. Then add your cheese and protein, followed by your softer vegetables and then any nuts, seeds, or dried fruits. Finish it off with your leafy greens and you're good to go! The pearl barley can be cooked the night before and, when cool, stored in an airtight container in the refrigerator.

1½ oz pearl barley

1 teaspoon lemon juice

sea salt and ground black pepper, to taste

2 teaspoons finely chopped fresh basil

½ medium zucchini, spiralised

2¾ oz tinned chickpeas, drained and rinsed

⅔ oz baby bocconcini (mozzarella), halved

5 cherry tomatoes, halved

1 small handful baby spinach leaves, shredded

4 fresh basil leaves (extra), chopped

Place the pearl barley and ½ cup of water in a small saucepan over high heat and bring to the boil, stirring occasionally. Cover and reduce the heat to low. Simmer for 25–30 minutes or until the pearl barley is tender. Remove from the heat and let stand, covered, for 5 minutes. Drain off any excess liquid and set aside to cool.

Whisk the lemon juice, salt, pepper, basil, and 2 teaspoons of water together in a small bowl. Pour into the bottom of a mason jar.

Place the spiralised zucchini and chickpeas in a bowl and toss gently to combine. Transfer into the mason jar on top of the dressing.

Layer the pearl barley, bocconcini, tomato, spinach, and extra basil into the mason jar.

To serve, pour the contents of the mason jar into a serving bowl and toss gently to combine.

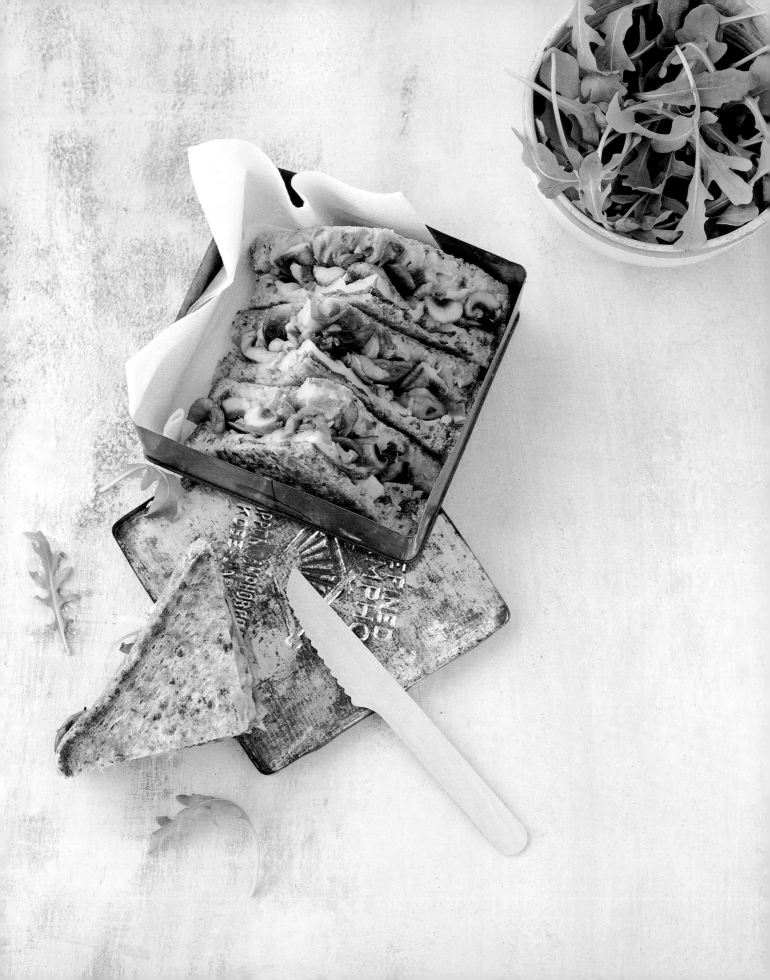

Ⓑ MUSHROOM MELT

SERVES 1
PREP TIME 10 MINUTES
COOKING TIME 20 MINUTES
DIFFICULTY EASY

This toastie recipe will seriously melt in your mouth ;)
I recommend using cremini or white button mushrooms.

oil spray
¼ small brown onion, thinly sliced
½ garlic clove, crushed
¼ teaspoon chopped fresh thyme
3½ oz mushrooms, sliced
2 teaspoons chopped fresh parsley
sea salt and ground black pepper, to taste

⅔ oz mozzarella cheese, grated
5¼ oz tinned cannellini beans, drained and rinsed
¼ teaspoon ground cumin
2 teaspoons lemon juice
2 slices whole wheat bread
1 small handful arugula leaves

Heat a non-stick fry pan over medium heat and spray with oil spray. Add the onion and cook for 5 minutes or until soft and translucent, stirring occasionally.

Add the garlic and thyme and cook for 1 minute or until fragrant, stirring constantly. Add the mushrooms and cook for 10 minutes or until soft. Remove from the heat and drain off any excess liquid.

Stir in the parsley and season with salt and pepper, if desired. Set aside to cool.

Once cooled, add the mozzarella and gently stir to combine.

Place the cannellini beans, cumin, and lemon juice in a small bowl and roughly mash with a fork until a chunky paste has formed. If it is too thick, add a little cold water until the desired consistency is reached.

Preheat a sandwich press.

Place a slice of bread on a clean chopping board and spread over the cannellini bean mixture. Layer the mushroom mixture and arugula. Top with the other slice of bread.

Place the sandwich on the sandwich press and gently press down the lid. Toast for 3–5 minutes or until the sandwich is golden.

To serve, place the toastie on a serving plate and cut in half or quarters.

(B) CHARGRILLED EGGPLANT & QUINOA SALAD

SERVES 1
PREP TIME 10 MINUTES
COOKING TIME 15 MINUTES
DIFFICULTY EASY

Move over boring salad—this one wins the day! If you're not super keen on eggplant, chargrilled zucchini also works really well.

2 oz quinoa

¼ medium eggplant, cut into ½-in thick slices

oil spray

4 kalamata olives, pitted and sliced

1 small handful arugula leaves

5¼ oz tinned chickpeas, drained and rinsed

1 tablespoon fresh basil leaves

freshly ground black pepper (optional)

1 oz salt-reduced low-fat feta cheese, crumbled

Place the quinoa and ⅔ cup of water in a saucepan over high heat and bring to the boil, stirring occasionally. Cover and reduce the heat to low. Simmer for 10–12 minutes until the liquid is absorbed and quinoa is tender.

Heat a barbecue grill-plate or chargrill pan over high heat.

Lightly spray the eggplant slices with oil spray. Grill for 4–6 minutes or until tender, turning occasionally. Set aside to cool.

To serve, place the quinoa, olives, arugula, chickpeas, basil, and eggplant in a serving bowl. Season with pepper if desired, and toss gently to combine. Sprinkle over the feta.

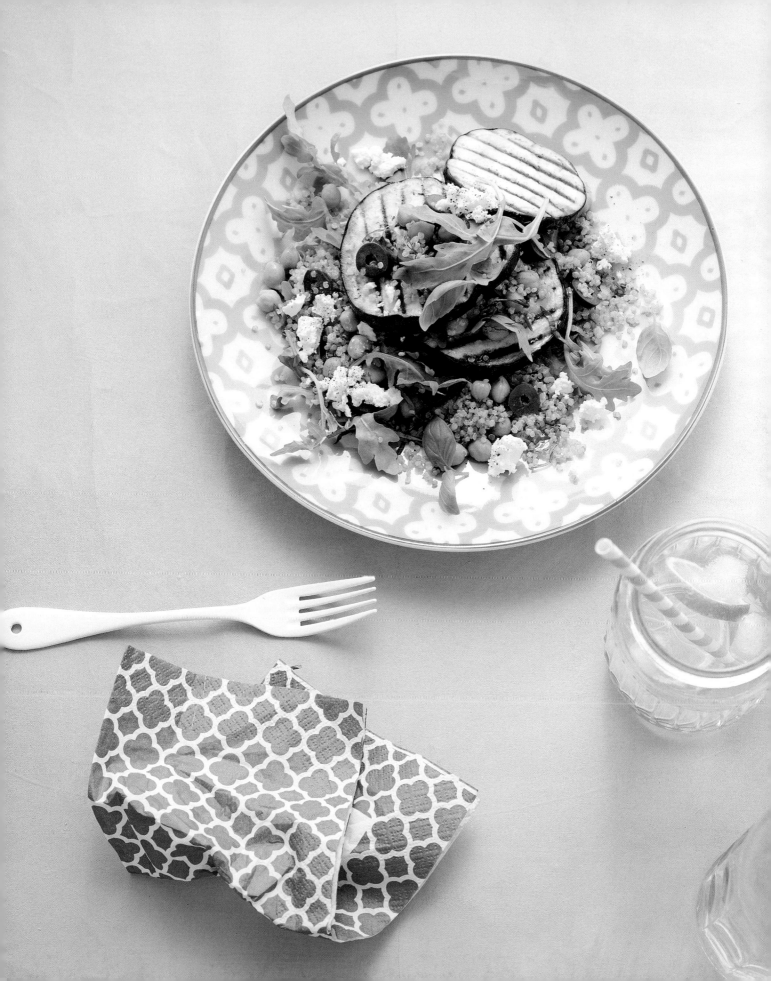

Ⓑ MEDITERRANEAN TACOS

SERVES 1
PREP TIME 10 MINUTES
COOKING TIME 12 MINUTES
DIFFICULTY EASY

Sink your teeth into this delicious lunch! It's such an easy meal that is full of vegetables—and lots of flavour. It is also a perfect way to use up any leftover chicken breast.

2 cups salt-reduced vegetable stock

3 oz boneless, skinless chicken breast

5 cherry tomatoes, quartered

¼ Lebanese cucumber, diced

¼ small red onion, diced

1 teaspoon red wine vinegar

sea salt and ground black pepper, to taste

1 whole wheat pita bread

1½ oz hummus (see page 254)

1 small handful lettuce leaves, shredded

2 kalamata olives, pitted and sliced

1 oz salt-reduced low-fat feta cheese, crumbled

Heat the stock in a small saucepan over medium heat. Add the chicken and reduce the heat to medium–low. Cook for 10–12 minutes until the chicken is cooked through. Drain off excess liquid. Coarsely shred the chicken using two forks and set aside to cool completely. To save time, the chicken can be cooked the night before and stored in an airtight container in the refrigerator.

Place the tomato, cucumber, onion, vinegar, salt, and pepper in a small bowl and toss gently to combine.

Warm the pita bread in a large dry pan over medium–high heat for 30 seconds on each side. Remove from the heat.

To serve, spread the hummus over the pita and layer the chicken, lettuce, tomato mixture, olives, and feta. Fold in half.

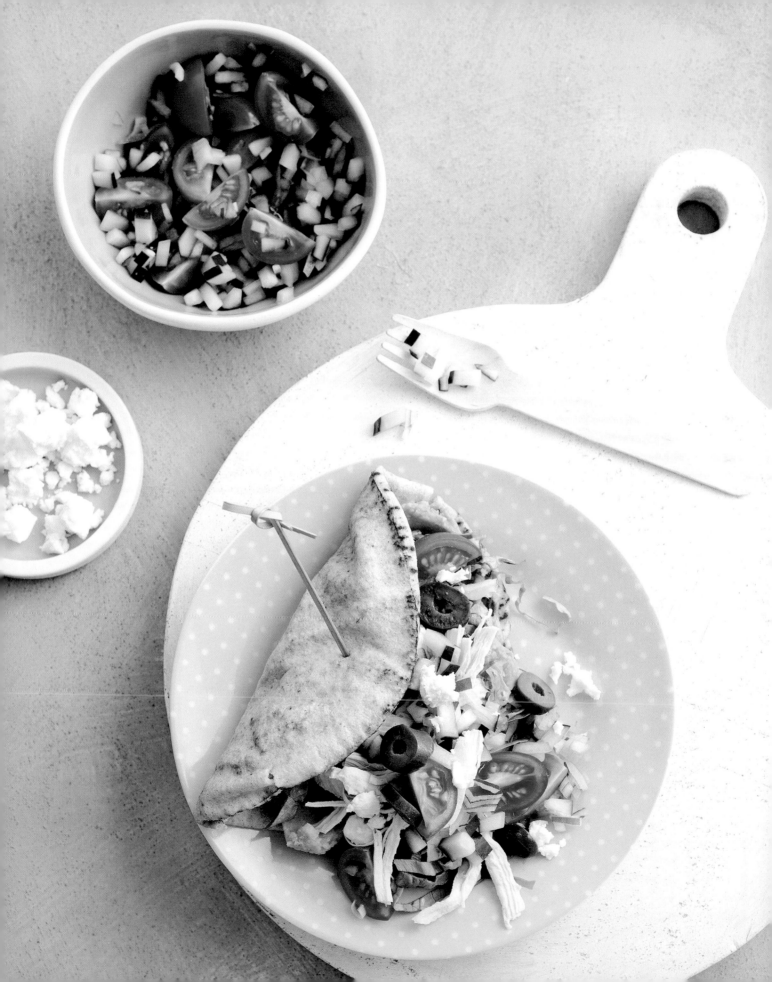

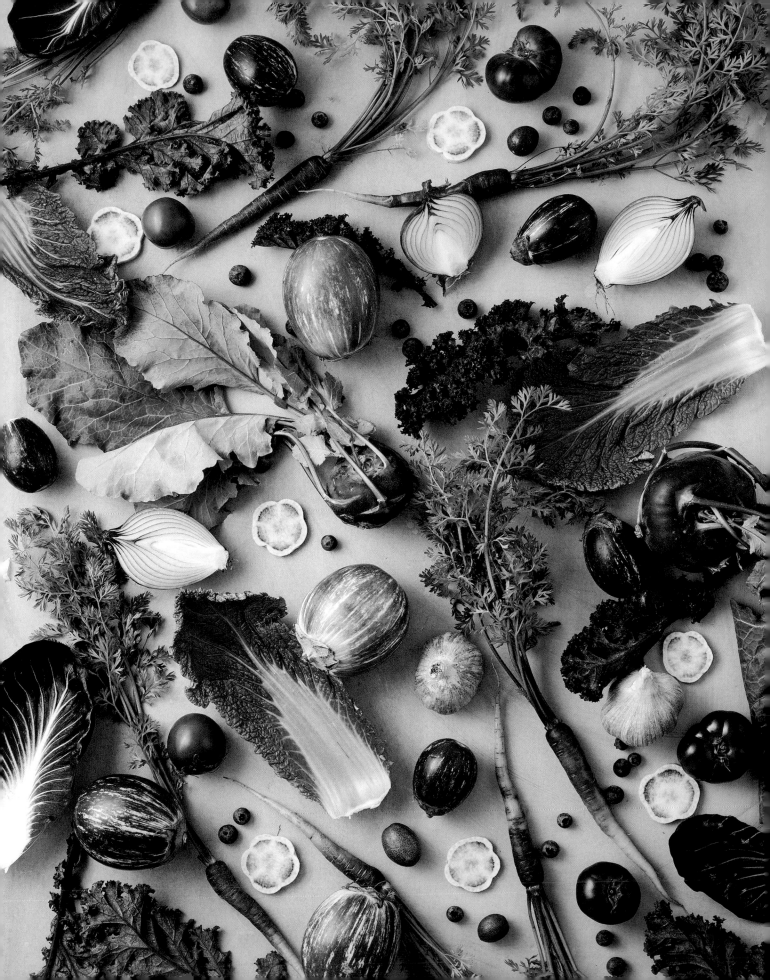

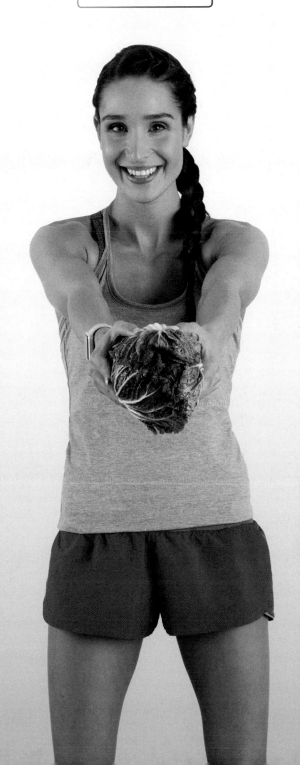

Ⓑ CAJUN CHICKEN BURGER

SERVES 2

PREP TIME 15 MINUTES +
30 MINUTES MARINATING TIME

COOKING TIME 10 MINUTES

DIFFICULTY EASY

Chicken, spice, and all things nice—this recipe is such a great change from your standard beef burger.

7 oz boneless, skinless chicken breast, cut into 4 even pieces

oil spray

3½ oz low-fat plain yoghurt

lime juice, to taste

2 whole wheat bread rolls

1 large handful lettuce leaves

1 small handful baby spinach leaves

1 medium tomato, sliced

1 Lebanese cucumber, sliced

½ small red onion, thinly sliced

⅔ oz reduced-fat cheddar cheese, sliced

CAJUN SPICE MIX

2 teaspoons ground cumin

2 teaspoons ground coriander

2 teaspoons sweet paprika

1 teaspoon cayenne pepper

Place the chicken pieces on a clean chopping board between two pieces of plastic film and lightly pound with a rolling pin to flatten slightly. Try to keep the pieces at an even thickness.

To make the Cajun spice mix, place the cumin, coriander, paprika, and cayenne in a small bowl and stir to combine.

Place the chicken pieces in the bowl and rub with the Cajun spice mix. Ensure that all the chicken is coated. Cover with plastic wrap and refrigerate for 30 minutes.

Heat a large non-stick fry pan over medium–high heat and spray lightly with oil spray. Add the chicken and cook for 2–3 minutes on each side or until cooked through. Transfer to a plate and set aside to rest.

Meanwhile, whisk the yoghurt and lime juice together in a small bowl.

To serve, cut the bread rolls in half and toast lightly in a toaster or under a hot oven broiler. On one half of each roll, layer half of the yoghurt dressing, lettuce, spinach, chicken, tomato, cucumber, onion, and cheese. Top with the other half of the roll.

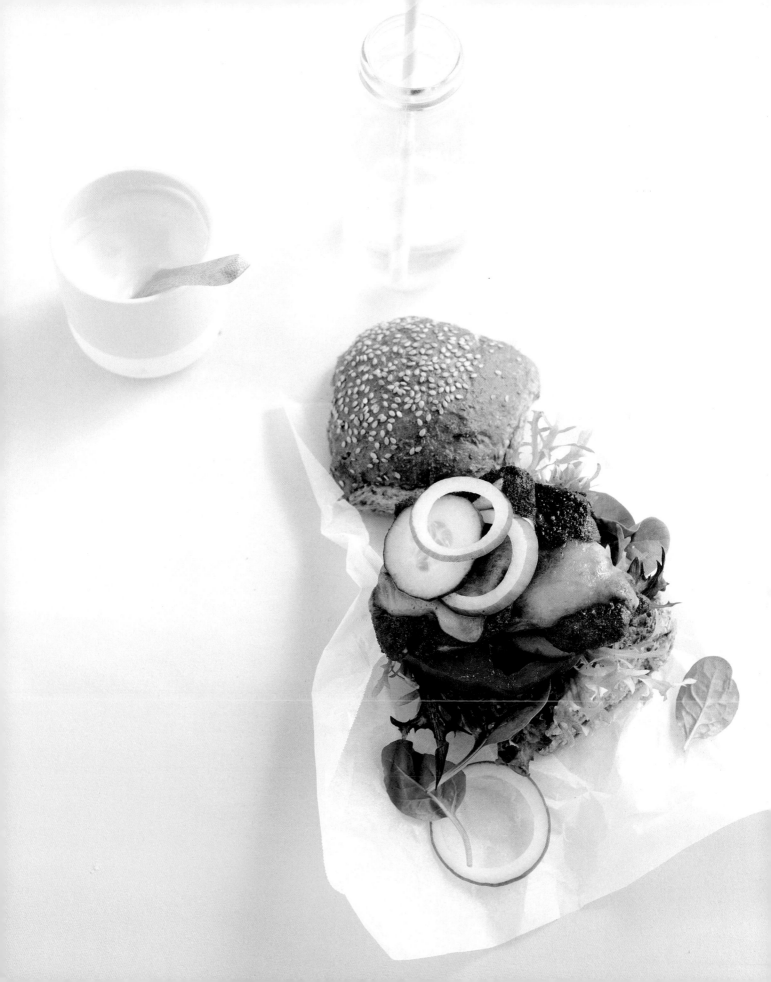

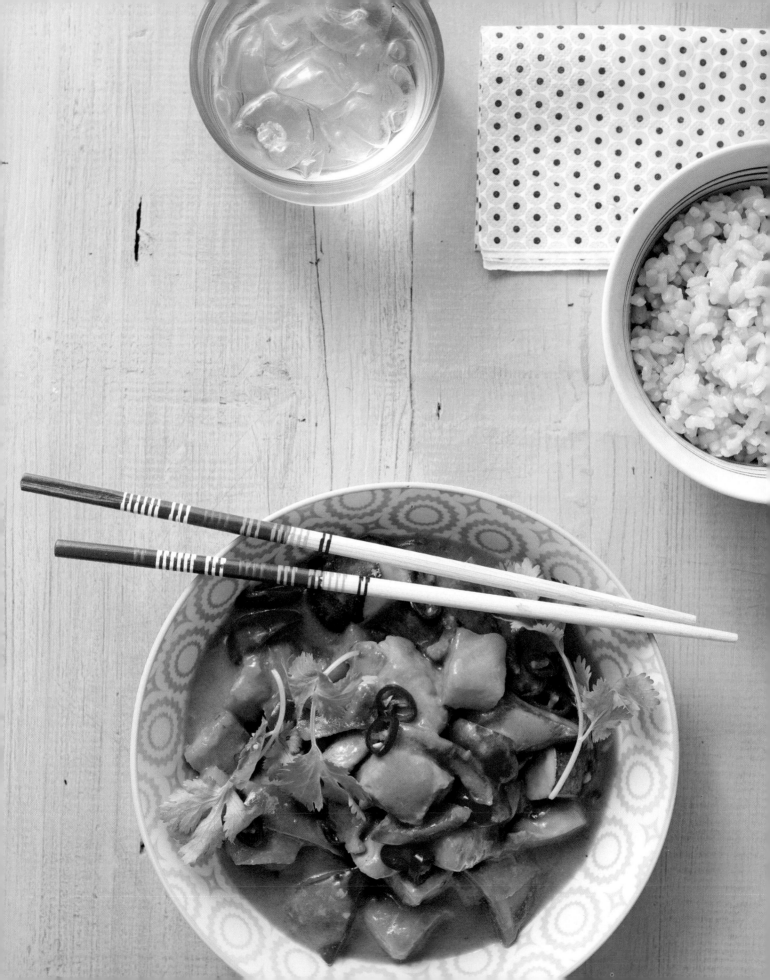

Ⓓ SWEET & SOUR CHICKEN with RICE

SERVES 2
PREP TIME 15 MINUTES
COOKING TIME 45 MINUTES
DIFFICULTY MEDIUM

This recipe is way better than the takeaway version—and healthier too!

2 oz brown rice

3 teaspoons sunflower oil

½ small red onion, roughly chopped

½ medium carrot, roughly chopped

1 garlic clove, crushed

½ teaspoon finely grated fresh ginger

7 oz boneless, skinless chicken breast, cut into 1-in pieces

½ medium green bell pepper, seeds removed and roughly chopped

½ medium red bell pepper, seeds removed and roughly chopped

1 medium zucchini, chopped

9 oz pineapple, cut into chunks

1 cup low-fat milk

3 teaspoons cornstarch

1 tablespoon fresh cilantro leaves

sliced fresh red chilli, to garnish

SWEET & SOUR SAUCE

3 oz cored pineapple flesh

2 tablespoons salt-reduced tamari or soy sauce

1 tablespoon honey

2 teaspoons white vinegar

¼ teaspoon dried chilli flakes (optional)

To make the sauce, place the pineapple in a high-powered blender or food processor and blend to a juice. Pour into a small bowl. Add the tamari or soy sauce, honey, vinegar, and chilli flakes (if using) and whisk until well combined.

Place the rice and 1 cup of water in a small saucepan over high heat and bring to a boil, stirring occasionally. Cover and reduce the heat to medium–low. Simmer for 20–25 minutes or until the liquid is absorbed and the rice is tender. Remove from the heat and let stand, covered, for 5 minutes.

Meanwhile, heat the oil in a large non-stick fry pan over medium–high heat. Add the onion and carrot and cook for 2–3 minutes, stirring occasionally. Add the garlic, ginger, and chicken and cook for 5–7 minutes or until the chicken is cooked through, stirring frequently.

Reduce the heat to medium and add the green and red bell peppers and zucchini. Cook for 4–5 minutes or until tender-crisp. Add the pineapple and cook for a further 2 minutes.

Add the sauce mixture to the chicken and vegetables and bring to a boil, stirring occasionally.

Whisk the milk and cornstarch together in a small bowl, then gradually stir into the chicken and vegetable mixture. Cook for 2–3 minutes or until the sauce has thickened, stirring constantly.

To serve, place the rice in two serving bowls and top with the sweet and sour chicken. Sprinkle over the cilantro and chilli.

SALMON with SUMMER SALSA

SERVES 2
PREP TIME 10 MINUTES
COOKING TIME 30 MINUTES
DIFFICULTY EASY

Give this recipe a try and it will soon become your go-to summer salad! Packed with fresh and nutritious ingredients like avocado, tomato, lime, and salmon, this is the perfect dish to share with friends on a warm evening.

4¼ oz brown rice
1½ medium tomatoes, finely diced
1½ Lebanese cucumbers, finely diced
½ small red onion, finely diced
3½ oz avocado, finely diced
finely chopped fresh chives, to taste

finely chopped fresh dill, to taste
juice of 1 lime
2 tablespoons capers, rinsed (optional)
oil spray
6 oz salmon fillet, deboned
1 small handful baby spinach leaves

Place the rice and 1¼ cups of water in a small saucepan over high heat and bring to a boil, stirring occasionally. Cover and reduce the heat to medium–low. Simmer for 20–25 minutes or until the liquid is absorbed and the rice is tender. Remove from the heat and let stand, covered, for 5 minutes. Set aside to cool.

Meanwhile, place the tomato, cucumber, onion, and avocado in a medium bowl. Add the chives, dill, lime juice, and capers (if using) and gently toss to combine.

Heat a medium non-stick fry pan over medium heat and spray lightly with oil spray. Add the salmon and cook for 7–10 minutes or until cooked to your liking, turning occasionally. Transfer to a plate and set aside to rest for 2 minutes. Cut into thick slices.

To serve, place the spinach on two serving plates. Top with the rice, salsa, and salmon.

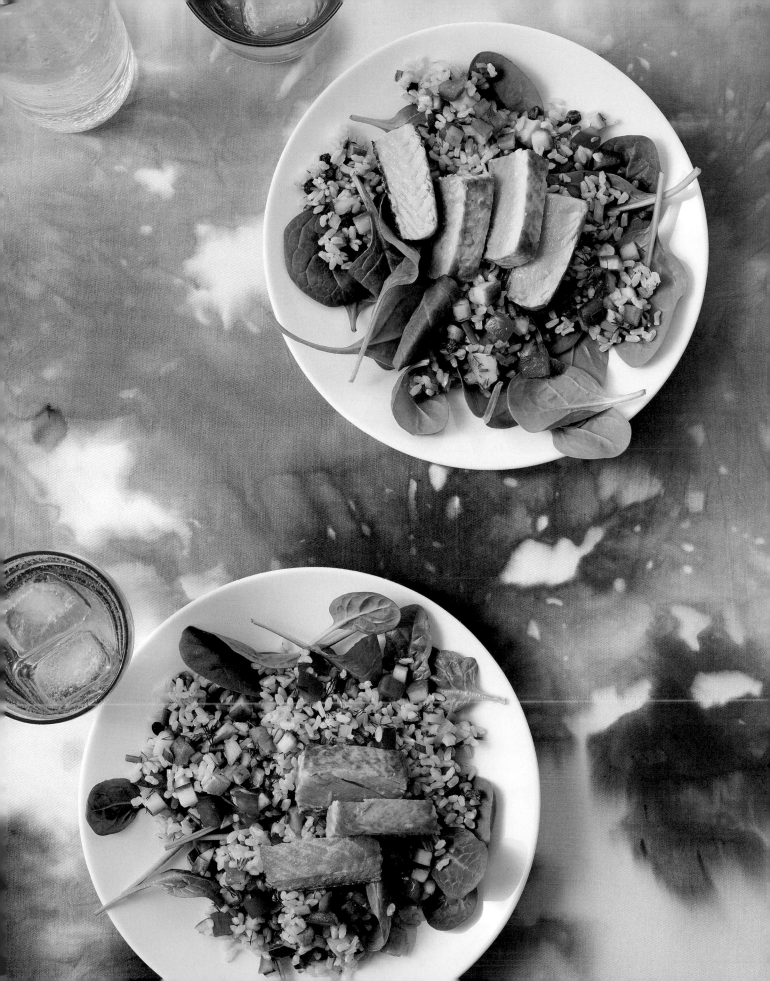

(D) SWEET POTATO & BLACK BEAN ENCHILADAS with GUACAMOLE

SERVES 4
PREP TIME 15 MINUTES
COOKING TIME 45 MINUTES
DIFFICULTY MEDIUM

Don't get me wrong, I love regular guacamole, but the addition of the pomegranate seeds here is amazing! They bring such a vibrant colour, flavour, and texture. Best!

oil spray

½ small red onion, finely chopped

2 garlic cloves, crushed

2 teaspoons chilli powder

½ teaspoon ground cumin

½ teaspoon sweet paprika

pinch of dried oregano

sea salt and ground black pepper, to taste

16 oz tinned crushed tomatoes

½ cup salt-reduced vegetable stock

2 medium sweet potatoes, peeled and cut into ¾ in cubes

21 oz tinned black beans, drained and rinsed

8 dried apricots, finely diced

2 whole wheat wraps

3 oz reduced-fat cheddar cheese, coarsely grated

GUACAMOLE

3½ oz avocado

2 pomegranates

lime juice, to taste

finely chopped fresh green chilli, to taste

½ small red onion, finely chopped

2 tablespoons fresh cilantro leaves

sea salt and ground black pepper, to taste

Preheat the oven to 400°F (350°F convection).

Heat a large saucepan over medium heat and spray lightly with oil spray. Add the onion and cook for 5–7 minutes or until soft and translucent, stirring frequently. Add the garlic, chilli powder, cumin, paprika, oregano, salt, and pepper and cook for 1 minute or until fragrant, stirring constantly.

Remove the pan from the heat and stir in the tomatoes. Using a stick blender, carefully blend until smooth. Transfer half the mixture to a bowl.

Return the pan to the heat and bring to a simmer over medium–low heat. Add the sweet potato and cook, covered, for 10–15 minutes or until the sweet potato is tender, stirring occasionally. Remove from the heat and stir through the black beans and dried apricots.

Place the wraps on a clean chopping board and cut in half. Top each wrap half with one-quarter of the sweet potato and tomato mixture. Roll up each wrap to enclose the filling. Place in the baking dish seam-side down.

Spoon over the reserved tomato mixture and sprinkle over the cheese. Bake in the oven for 20 minutes or until the cheese has melted and the filling is heated through.

Meanwhile, to make the guacamole, scoop the avocado out into a small bowl and roughly mash with a fork. Cut the pomegranates in half and gently tap into the bowl to remove the seeds. Add the lime juice, chilli, onion, and cilantro and gently mix to combine. Season with salt and pepper, if desired.

To serve, place the enchiladas on four serving plates and top with the guacamole.

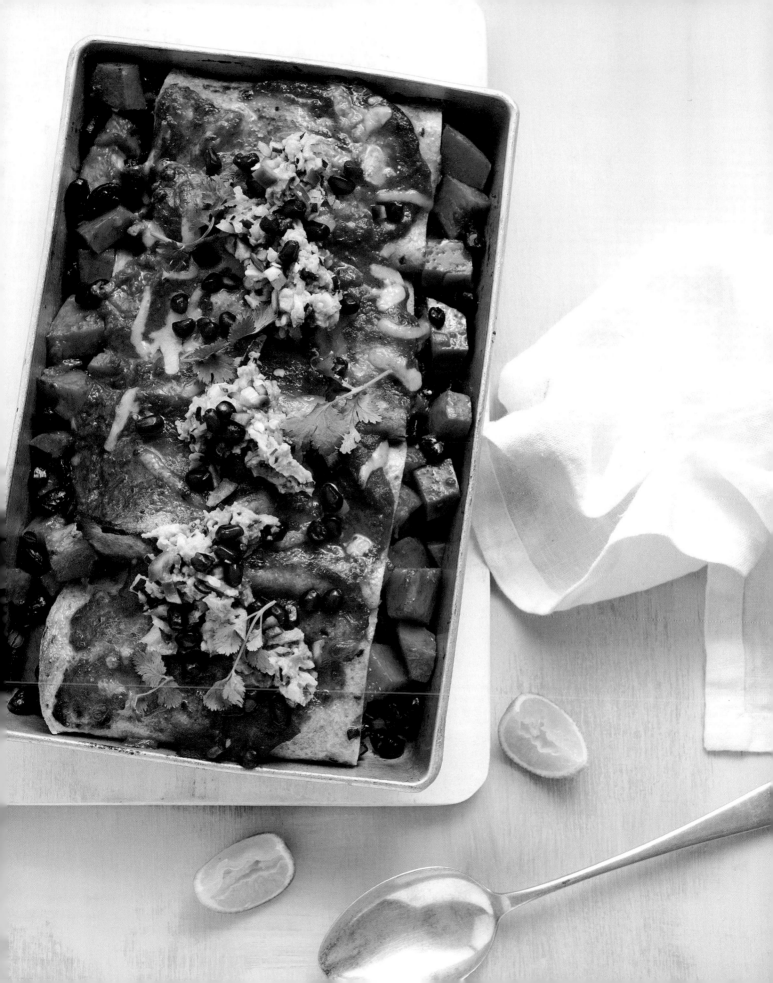

Ⓐ FISH CURRY

SERVES 2
PREP TIME 10 MINUTES
COOKING TIME 30 MINUTES
DIFFICULTY EASY

Not sure what fish you should use in this curry? Snapper, mahi mahi, ling, or trevalla all work really well.

4¼ oz brown rice

3 teaspoons olive oil

½ small brown onion, finely diced

1 tablespoon yellow curry paste

½ medium green bell pepper, seeds removed and sliced

15 green beans, trimmed and sliced

1½ cups salt-reduced vegetable stock

½ cup light coconut milk

1 teaspoon fish sauce

lime juice, to taste

9 oz white fish fillet, cut into 1½-in cubes

1 large handful baby spinach leaves

sea salt and ground black pepper, to taste

1 scallion, sliced

Place the rice and 1¼ cups of water in a small saucepan over high heat and bring to the boil, stirring occasionally. Cover and reduce the heat to medium–low. Simmer for 20–25 minutes or until the liquid is absorbed and the rice is tender. Remove from the heat and leave to stand, covered, for 5 minutes.

Meanwhile, heat the oil in a saucepan over medium heat. Add the onion and cook for 2–3 minutes or until soft, stirring occasionally.

Add the curry paste and cook for 1–2 minutes or until fragrant, stirring occasionally.

Add the bell pepper and beans and stir to coat in the paste. Cook for 2–3 minutes, stirring occasionally.

Stir in the vegetable stock and bring to a boil. Reduce the heat to medium–low then stir in the coconut milk, fish sauce, and lime juice.

Add the fish and stir gently to combine. Simmer for 10–15 minutes or until the fish is cooked through. In the last 5 minutes, add the spinach and stir gently to combine. Season with salt and pepper, if desired.

To serve, place the rice in two bowls and top with the fish curry. Sprinkle over the scallion.

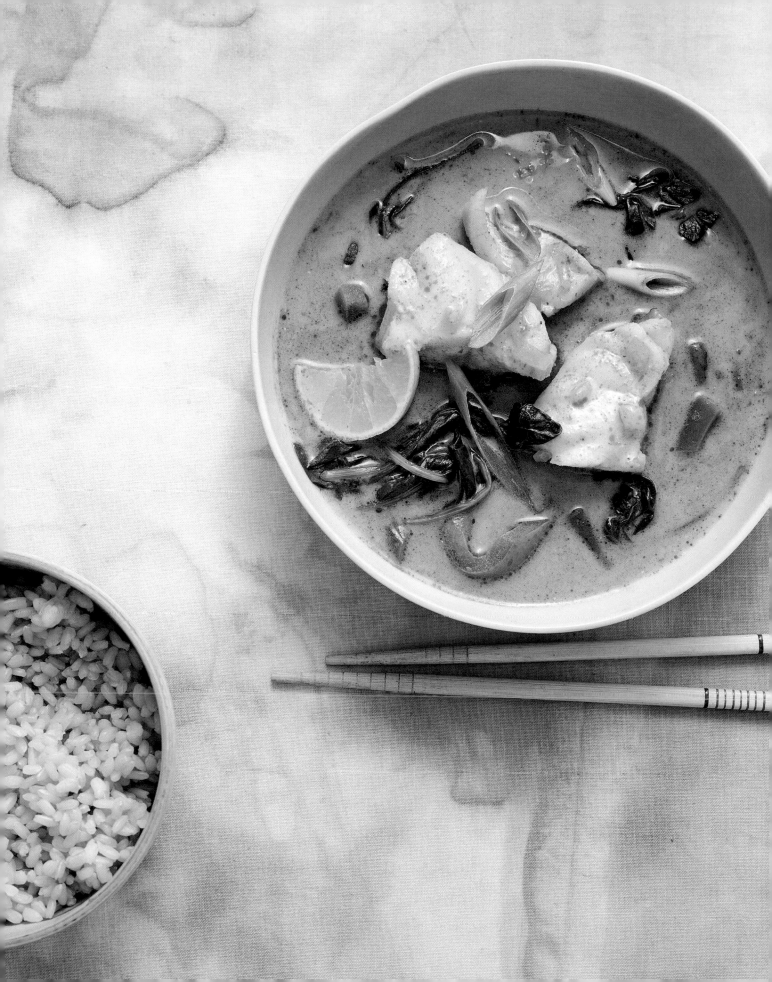

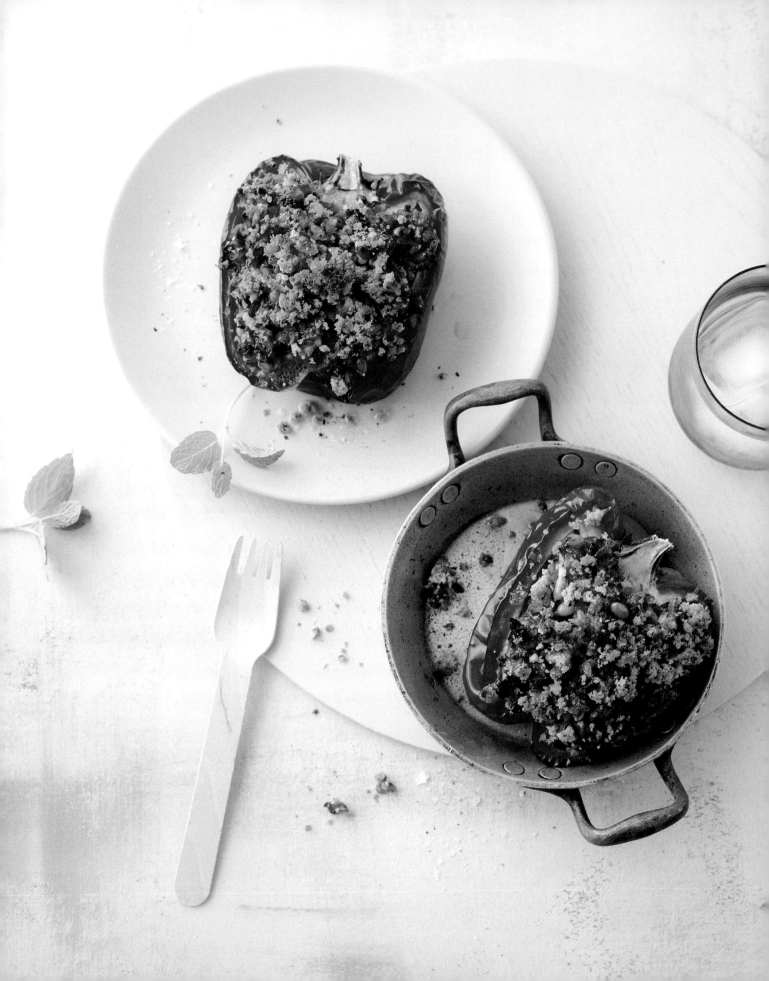

YEMISTA (STUFFED PEPPER with RICE)

SERVES 2

PREP TIME 10 MINUTES

COOKING TIME 1 HOUR 20 MINUTES

DIFFICULTY MEDIUM

When I was growing up, every time I visited my yiayia, she'd ask what I would like for dinner. My answer was always, "Yemista!" I still love this dish and I'm sure you will too!

3 oz brown rice

1 slice whole wheat bread

3 teaspoons olive oil

½ small brown onion, finely chopped

1 garlic clove, crushed

7¾ oz turkey or ground chicken

5¼ oz tinned crushed tomatoes

1 tablespoon tomato paste

2 tablespoons pine nuts

1 tablespoon finely chopped fresh parsley

2 teaspoons finely chopped fresh mint

finely grated zest and juice of 1 lemon

sea salt and ground black pepper, to taste

1 medium red bell pepper, halved lengthways and seeds removed

Place the rice and 1 cup of water in a small saucepan over high heat and bring to a boil, stirring occasionally. Cover and reduce the heat to medium–low. Simmer for 20–25 minutes or until the liquid is absorbed and the rice is tender. Remove from the heat and let stand, covered, for 5 minutes.

Tear the bread into small pieces. Place in a food processor and process until coarse crumbs form.

Preheat the oven to 350°F (325°F convection) and line a baking sheet with parchment paper.

Heat 2 teaspoons of oil in a large non-stick fry pan over medium heat. Add the onion, garlic, and ground chicken and cook for 10 minutes or until the chicken is browned, stirring frequently with a wooden spoon to break the meat up. Remove from the heat.

Add the rice, tomatoes, tomato paste, pine nuts, parsley, mint, lemon zest and juice, salt, and pepper and stir gently to combine.

Fill each bell pepper half with half of the stuffing.

Place the stuffed pepper halves on the lined baking sheet. Sprinkle over the breadcrumbs and drizzle over the remaining oil.

Bake in the oven for 40–45 minutes or until the pepper is tender. Serve.

Ⓑ VEGETARIAN PIZZA

SERVES 2
PREP TIME 10 MINUTES
COOKING TIME 10 MINUTES
DIFFICULTY EASY

No meat? No problem! By adding lentils to the passata, you can create a healthy veggie pizza that still packs a protein punch.

10¾ oz tinned brown lentils, drained and rinsed

2¾ oz tomato passata (tomato puree)

2 whole wheat pita breads

½ medium eggplant, thinly sliced

3½ oz mushrooms, thinly sliced

1 medium tomato, sliced

1½ oz mozzarella cheese, coarsely grated

sea salt and ground black pepper, to taste

1 small handful arugula leaves

Preheat the oven to 350°F (325°F convection) and line a baking sheet with parchment paper.

Place the lentils and passata in a bowl and mix until well combined.

Lay the pita breads on a clean work surface and spread over the lentil and passata mixture. Scatter over the eggplant, mushrooms, and tomato. Sprinkle over the cheese and season with salt and pepper, if desired.

Place the pizzas on the lined baking sheet and bake for 8–10 minutes or until the toppings are hot, the cheese has melted, and the edges are golden brown.

To serve, top the pizzas with the arugula.

Ⓒ BEEF & LENTIL SOUP

SERVES 4
PREP TIME 20 MINUTES
COOKING TIME 1 HOUR 40 MINUTES
DIFFICULTY EASY

This is the perfect go-to soup for winter when it's cold and raining outside. It's also a great way to use up any leftover vegetables in your fridge.

3 teaspoons olive oil

¾ lb lean beef chuck, cut into ¾-in cubes

1 small brown onion, diced

2 medium carrots, diced

2 celery stalks, diced

2 garlic cloves, crushed

2 teaspoons chopped fresh rosemary

2 cups salt-reduced vegetable stock

1 bay leaf

2 medium sweet potatoes, peeled and cut into ¼-in cubes

3 medium tomatoes, diced

15 green beans, trimmed and chopped

2 oz frozen peas

10¾ oz tinned brown lentils, drained and rinsed

1 small handful chopped fresh parsley

ground black pepper, to taste

3 oz reduced-fat cheddar cheese, grated

Heat half of the oil in a large saucepan over medium–high heat. Cook the beef for 2–3 minutes or until browned, stirring frequently. Transfer to a plate.

Heat the remaining oil in the pan over medium heat. Add the onion, carrot, and celery and cook for 5–7 minutes or until the vegetables start to soften, stirring occasionally. Add the garlic and rosemary and cook for 1 minute or until fragrant, stirring frequently. Return the beef to the pan.

Add the stock, bay leaf, and 1 cup of water and bring to the boil over high heat. Reduce the heat to medium–low and simmer, covered, for 1 hour, stirring occasionally. Carefully skim off and discard any foam that rises to the surface.

Add the sweet potato, tomato, beans, peas, and lentils and simmer, covered, for 20–30 minutes or until the beef is tender. Stir through the parsley and season with pepper, if desired.

To serve, ladle the soup into bowls and sprinkle over the cheese.

Ⓑ LAMB KOFTAS with QUINOA TABOULI & TZATZIKI

SERVES 2

PREP TIME 20 MINUTES +
30 MINUTES CHILLING TIME

COOKING TIME 25 MINUTES

DIFFICULTY EASY

I love tzatziki! My best tip is to leave the yoghurt in a strainer lined with muslin cloth over another bowl overnight. You'll wake up to deliciously thick yoghurt that will seriously take your tzatziki to the next level!

6 oz lean ground lamb
½ small brown onion, finely chopped
½ teaspoon sweet paprika
½ teaspoon ground cumin
pinch of ground cinnamon
1 tablespoon finely chopped fresh cilantro
1 tablespoon finely chopped fresh mint
finely grated lemon zest, to taste
sea salt and ground black pepper, to taste
oil spray
7 oz tzatziki (see page 254)

QUINOA TABOULI

4¼ oz quinoa
1 garlic clove, crushed
1 large handful fresh parsley, chopped
1 medium tomato, finely chopped
1 Lebanese cucumber, finely chopped
½ small red onion, finely chopped
1 large handful baby spinach leaves, chopped
lemon juice, to taste
sea salt and ground black pepper, to taste

Place the ground lamb, onion, paprika, cumin, cinnamon, cilantro, mint, and lemon zest in a medium bowl. Season with salt and pepper and stir until well combined.

Form the mixture into eight small sausage shapes. Place on a plate, cover with plastic wrap, and refrigerate for 30 minutes.

Preheat the oven to 350°F (325°F convection) and line a baking sheet with parchment paper.

Heat a large non-stick fry pan over medium–high heat and spray lightly with oil spray. Add the koftas and cook for 2 minutes on each side until lightly browned. Transfer to the lined baking sheet and bake in the oven for a further 10 minutes or until cooked through.

To make the quinoa tabouli, place the quinoa and 1¼ cups of water in a saucepan over high heat and bring to the boil, stirring occasionally. Cover and reduce the heat to low. Simmer for 10–12 minutes until the liquid is absorbed and quinoa is tender. Set aside to cool.

Place the quinoa, garlic, parsley, tomato, cucumber, onion, spinach, and lemon juice in a mixing bowl. Season with salt and pepper, if desired, and toss gently to combine.

To serve, place the quinoa tabouli on two serving plates. Top with the lamb koftas and drizzle over the tzatziki.

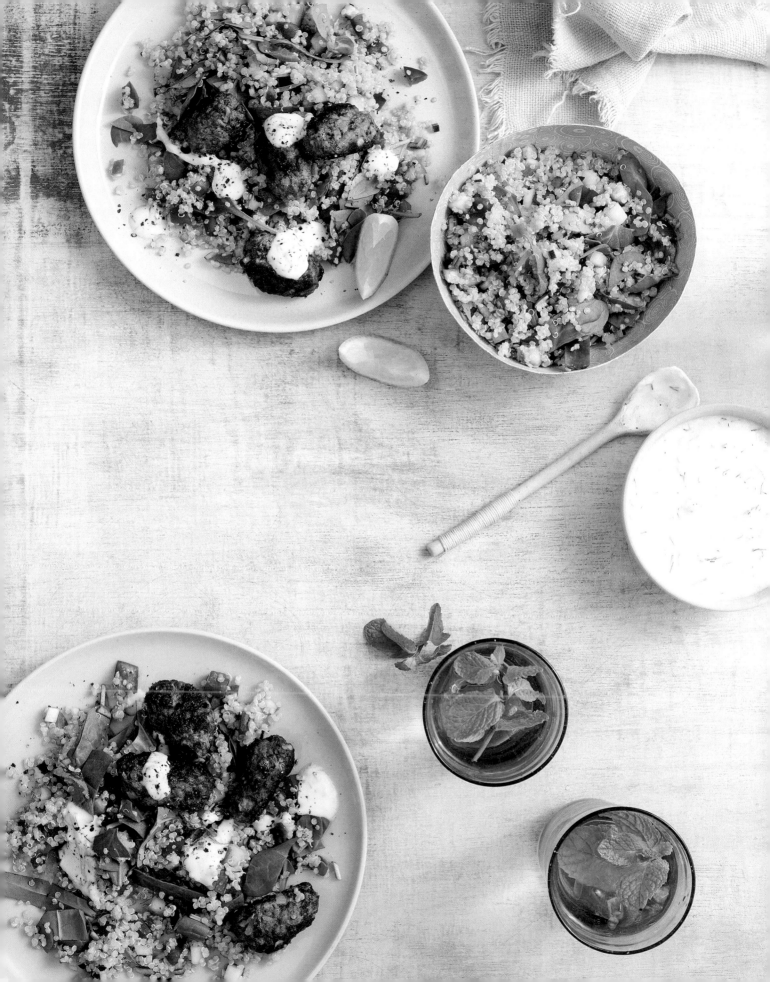

Ⓒ CHICKEN, POTATO & SWEETCORN CHOWDER

SERVES 4
PREP TIME 15 MINUTES
COOKING TIME 40 MINUTES
DIFFICULTY EASY

Feeling sick and under the weather? Then this chowder is exactly what the doctor ordered!

3 teaspoons olive oil

1 small brown onion, finely chopped

2 celery stalks, diced

1 medium carrot, diced

1 bay leaf

2 garlic cloves, crushed

2 medium potatoes, cut into ½-in cubes

21 oz boneless skinless chicken breast, cut into 1-in pieces

3 cups salt-reduced vegetable stock

8½ oz tinned corn kernels, drained and rinsed

5¼ oz tinned cannellini beans, drained and rinsed

2 cups low-fat milk

2 scallions, sliced

sea salt and ground black pepper, to taste

2 teaspoons cornstarch

Heat the oil in a large saucepan over medium heat. Add the onion, celery, carrot, and bay leaf and cook for 5–7 minutes or until the vegetables start to soften, stirring occasionally. Add the garlic and cook for 1 minute or until fragrant, stirring frequently.

Add the potato, chicken, and stock and bring to a simmer over medium heat. Reduce the heat to medium–low and cook for 20–25 minutes or until the potato and chicken are tender, stirring occasionally.

Stir through the corn, cannellini beans, milk, and half of the scallions. Cook for 5 minutes or until heated through, stirring occasionally. Season with salt and pepper, if desired.

To thicken the soup, mix the cornstarch with 2 tablespoons of the soup liquid in a small bowl. Pour back into the soup and cook for a further 2–3 minutes or until thickened, stirring gently.

To serve, ladle the soup into bowls and sprinkle over the remaining scallions.

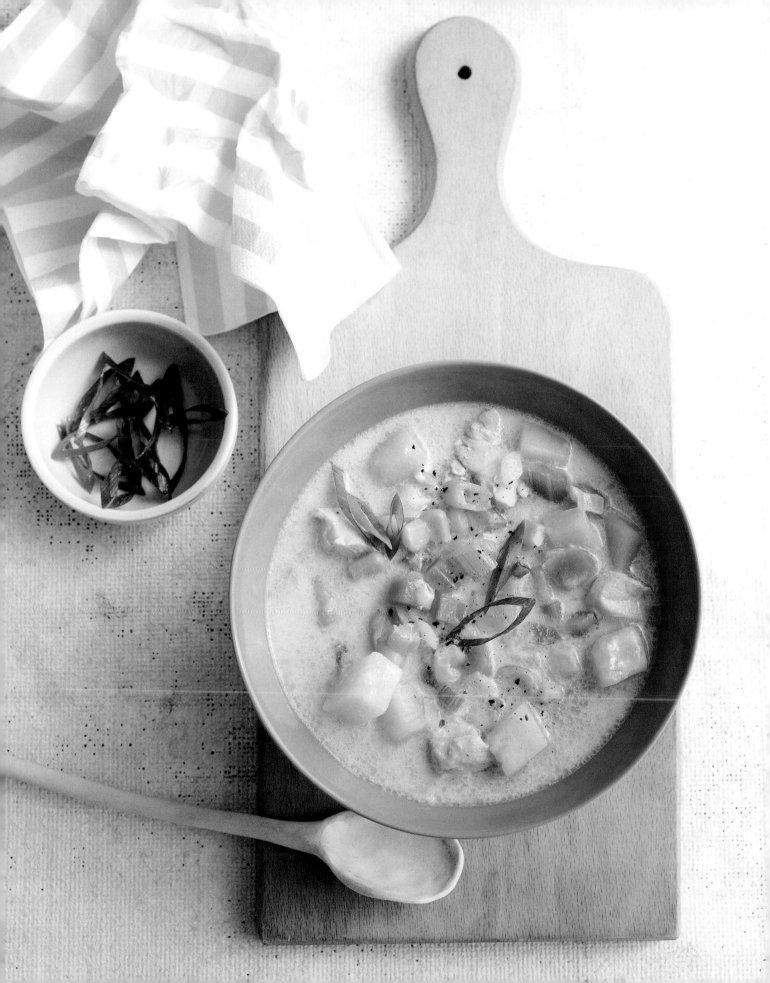

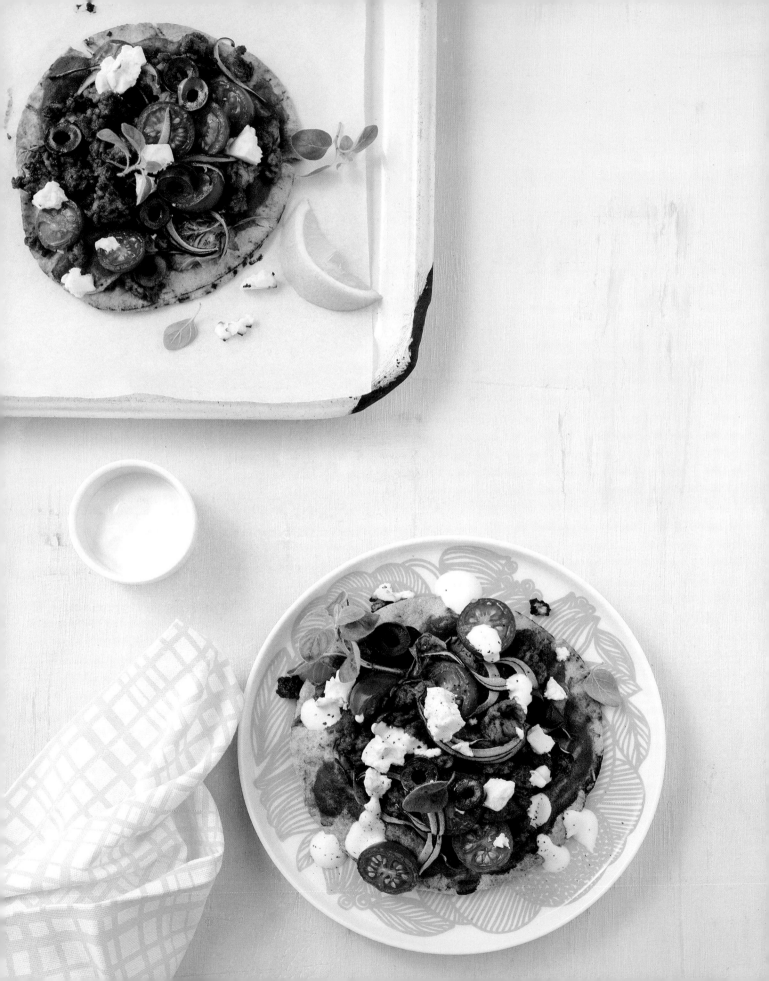

Ⓑ GREEK LAMB PIZZA

SERVES 2
PREP TIME 10 MINUTES
COOKING TIME 20 MINUTES
DIFFICULTY EASY

Love a good gyro or lamb on the spit? Then you are definitely going to love this pizza! It has all of the same Greek flavours and is super easy to put together. Perfect for a Friday night in.

oil spray
1 garlic clove, crushed
4¼ oz lean ground lamb
sea salt and ground black pepper, to taste
2 whole wheat pita breads
2¾ oz tomato passata (tomato puree)
1 large handful baby spinach leaves
½ small red onion, thinly sliced

10 cherry tomatoes, halved
8 kalamata olives, pitted and sliced
1 oz salt-reduced low-fat feta cheese, crumbled

YOGHURT SAUCE
3½ oz low-fat plain yoghurt
½ garlic clove, crushed
lemon juice, to taste

Preheat the oven to 350°F (325°F convection) and line a baking sheet with parchment paper.

Heat a large non-stick fry pan over medium heat and spray lightly with oil spray. Add the garlic and ground lamb and cook for 5–7 minutes or until browned, stirring frequently with a wooden spoon to break the meat up. Season with salt and pepper, if desired. Drain off any excess liquid.

Lay the pita breads on a clean work surface and spread over the passata. Sprinkle over the spinach, lamb, onion, tomato, olives, and feta.

Place the pizzas on the lined baking sheet and bake for 8–10 minutes or until the toppings are hot and the edges are golden brown.

Meanwhile, to make the yoghurt sauce, whisk the yoghurt, garlic, and lemon juice together in a small bowl.

To serve, top the pizzas with the yoghurt sauce.

SHRIMP STIR-FRY

SERVES 2

PREP TIME 10 MINUTES +
10 MINUTES SOAKING TIME

COOKING TIME 10 MINUTES

DIFFICULTY EASY

This stir-fry is one of my favourite mid-week dinners. It's so easy
to prepare and so quick to put together, which is great when you've
had a long day at work!

7 oz hokkien noodles

3 teaspoons sesame oil

20 medium raw king prawns,
peeled and deveined, tails intact

½ small red onion, thinly sliced

½ medium green bell pepper,
seeds removed and thinly sliced

1 medium carrot, thinly sliced

4¼ oz snow peas, trimmed and halved

2 tablespoons unsalted cashew nuts,
roughly chopped

HONEY LEMON SAUCE

1 cup salt-reduced vegetable stock

1 teaspoon honey

¾ in fresh ginger, peeled
and finely chopped

lemon juice, to taste

½ teaspoon salt-reduced tamari
or soy sauce

Place the noodles in a heatproof bowl and cover with boiling water.
Leave for 10 minutes, then loosen the noodles with a fork. Drain and
refresh under cool running water. Drain well and set aside.

Meanwhile, to make the sauce, whisk the stock, honey, ginger, lemon juice,
and tamari or soy sauce together in a small bowl.

Heat a wok over high heat until hot. Add half of the oil and carefully swirl
it around to coat the sides of the wok. Heat until very hot.

Add the prawns and stir-fry for 2–3 minutes or until they change colour.
Transfer to a plate and set aside to rest.

Heat the remaining oil in the wok over high heat. Add the onion, bell
pepper, and carrot and stir-fry for 3–4 minutes until tender-crisp. Add the
snow peas and stir-fry for 1 minute.

Pour in the sauce and toss gently to coat. Add the prawns and cook for
1–2 minutes or until the prawns are just cooked through. Add the noodles
and toss gently to combine.

To serve, place the stir-fry in two serving bowls and sprinkle over
the cashews.

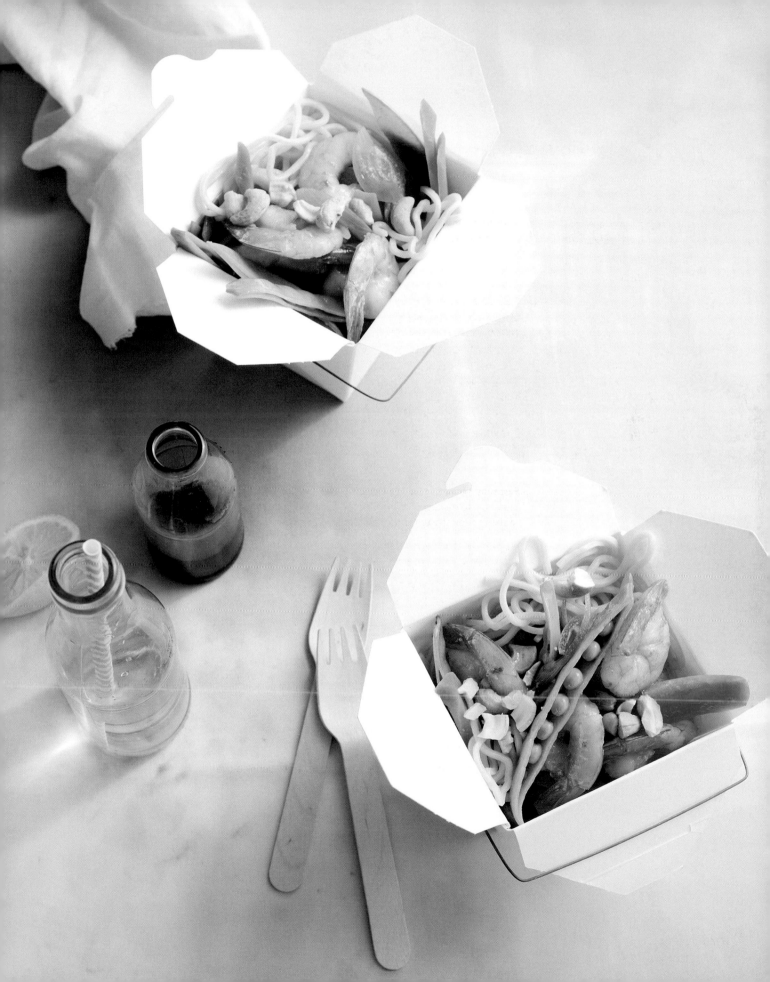

⒟ QUINOA PILAF with CHICKEN

SERVES 2
PREP TIME 10 MINUTES
COOKING TIME 35 MINUTES
DIFFICULTY EASY

Quinoa is all the rage at the moment, so I thought I'd give this pilaf dish a modern spin by using it instead of rice. And the results are incredible! The quinoa adds a delicious texture, which I know you'll love. However, if you prefer your pilaf the traditional way, just replace the quinoa with an equal amount of brown rice.

oil spray

7 oz boneless, skinless chicken breast, cut into ¾-in pieces

½ small brown onion, finely chopped

1 garlic clove, crushed

½ teaspoon garam masala

¼ teaspoon ground turmeric

2 oz quinoa

⅔ cup salt-reduced vegetable stock

5 oz broccoli, cut into florets

2 oz frozen peas

2 oz dried cranberries

2 tablespoons unsalted cashew nuts

2 tablespoons fresh cilantro leaves

7 oz low-fat plain yoghurt

Heat a large saucepan over medium–high heat and spray with oil spray. Add half the chicken and cook for 5 minutes or until browned, stirring occasionally. Set aside on a plate. Repeat with the remaining chicken and set aside.

Reheat the saucepan over medium heat and spray lightly with oil spray. Add the onion and cook for 5 minutes or until soft and translucent, stirring occasionally. Add the garlic, garam masala, and turmeric and cook for 1 minute or until fragrant, stirring constantly.

Add the quinoa, stock, and chicken and bring to a boil over high heat. Reduce the heat to low and simmer, covered, for 15–20 minutes or until the liquid is absorbed and the quinoa is tender.

Fill a saucepan with water until 2 in deep and insert a steamer basket. Cover with a lid and bring the water to the boil over high heat, then reduce the heat to medium.

Add the broccoli florets and steam, covered, for 3 minutes. Add the peas and steam for a further 2–3 minutes or until both the broccoli and peas are tender.

Add the broccoli and peas to the chicken and quinoa mixture and stir gently to combine.

To serve, place the pilaf in two serving bowls. Sprinkle over the cranberries, cashews, and cilantro and drizzle over the yoghurt.

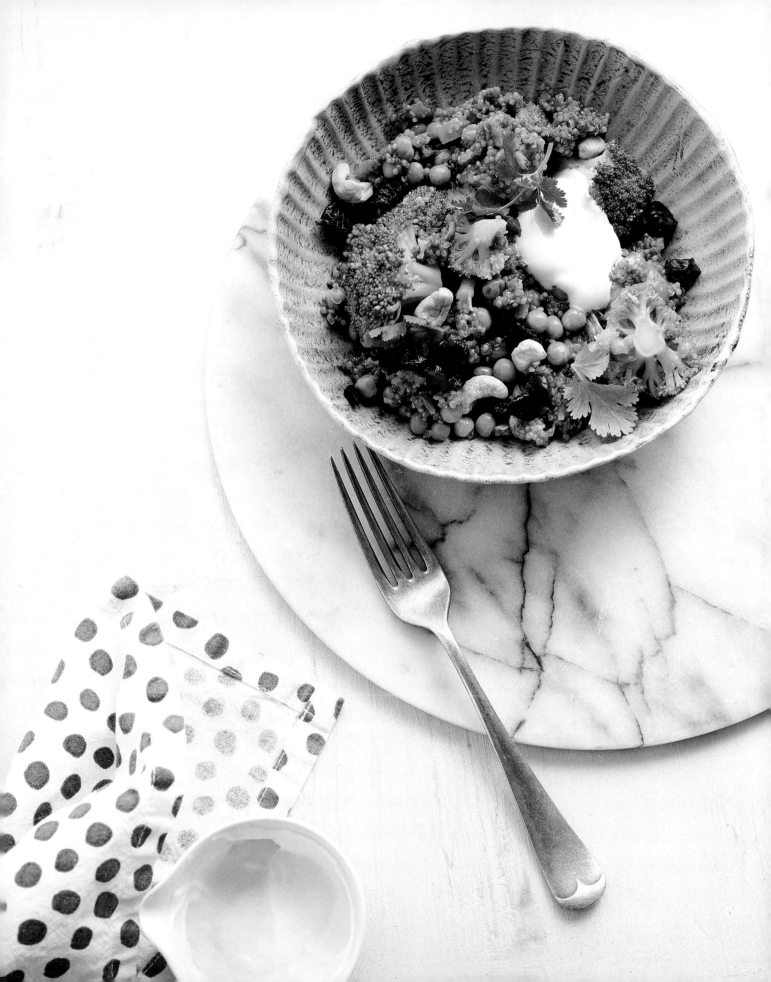

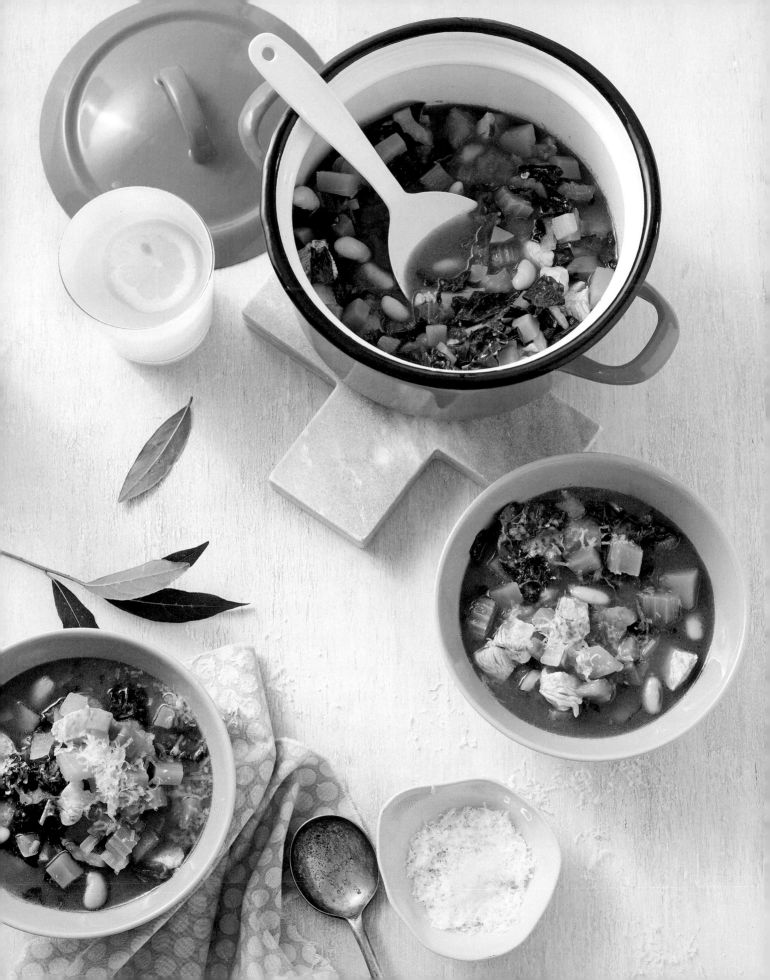

Ⓒ TUSCAN BEAN & CHICKEN SOUP

SERVES 4
PREP TIME 15 MINUTES
COOKING TIME 40 MINUTES
DIFFICULTY EASY

This Italian-inspired soup is so hearty! I recommend making a big batch and then freezing extra portions to enjoy later.

3 teaspoons olive oil

1 small brown onion, finely chopped

2 medium carrots, chopped

4 celery stalks, chopped

2 garlic cloves, crushed

½ teaspoon chopped fresh thyme

½ teaspoon chopped fresh rosemary

1 bay leaf

14 oz boneless skinless chicken breast, cut into bite-sized pieces

3 cups salt-reduced vegetable stock

14 oz pumpkin, cut into ¾-in cubes

10¾ oz tinned crushed tomatoes

3 large handfuls kale, chopped

10¾ oz tinned cannellini beans, drained and rinsed

sea salt and ground black pepper, to taste

3 oz parmesan cheese, grated

Heat the oil in a large saucepan over medium heat. Add the onion, carrot, and celery and cook for 8–10 minutes or until soft, stirring occasionally.

Add the garlic, thyme, rosemary, and bay leaf and cook for 1 minute or until fragrant, stirring occasionally.

Add the chicken and cook for 5 minutes or until lightly browned, stirring frequently.

Stir in the stock, pumpkin, tomatoes, and kale and bring to a boil over high heat. Reduce the heat to low and simmer for 10 minutes. Add the cannellini beans and simmer for a further 10–15 minutes. Season with salt and pepper, if desired.

To serve, ladle the soup into serving bowls and sprinkle over the grated parmesan.

Ⓑ CHICKPEA & BEETROOT BURGER

SERVES 2

PREP TIME 10 MINUTES +
30 MINUTES CHILLING TIME

COOKING TIME 45 MINUTES

DIFFICULTY EASY

You'll be seeing red with this burger patty . . . but in a good way!
I absolutely love the bright, vibrant colour. It's almost too pretty to eat!

10¾ oz tinned chickpeas,
drained and rinsed

oil spray

½ small brown onion, finely chopped

1 garlic clove, crushed

2 small beetroots, peeled and grated

2 teaspoons balsamic vinegar

2 teaspoons chopped fresh parsley

sea salt and ground black pepper,
to taste

2 whole wheat bread rolls

⅔ oz reduced-fat cheddar cheese

1 Lebanese cucumber, sliced

1 small handful alfalfa sprouts

3½ oz low-fat plain yoghurt

Place the chickpeas in a mixing bowl and mash with a potato masher.
Don't mash the chickpeas completely as the mixture should be chunky.
Set aside.

Heat a non-stick fry pan over medium heat and spray lightly with oil spray.
Add the onion and cook for 5 minutes or until soft and translucent, stirring
occasionally. Add the garlic and cook for 1 minute, stirring occasionally.

Add the beetroot to the pan and cook for 5–6 minutes or until the beetroot
is cooked. Stir through the vinegar, then remove from the heat. Add the
beetroot mixture and parsley to the chickpeas and mix until well combined.
Season with salt and pepper, if desired, and set aside to cool.

Shape the beetroot chickpea mixture into two even patties. Place on
a plate, cover with plastic wrap and refrigerate for 30 minutes.

Preheat the oven to 350°F (325°F convection) and line a baking sheet with
parchment paper.

Place the patties on the lined baking sheet and spray lightly with oil spray.
Bake for 15 minutes, then turn carefully and cook for a further 15 minutes.
Remove from the oven and set aside to rest for 5 minutes.

To serve, cut the bread rolls in half and toast lightly in a toaster or under
a hot oven broiler. On one half of each roll, layer half of the cheese,
cucumber, and alfalfa, a patty. Drizzle over the yoghurt and top with the
other half of each roll.

Ⓓ VEGETABLE PILAF

SERVES 2
PREP TIME 15 MINUTES
COOKING TIME 30 MINUTES
DIFFICULTY EASY

The creaminess of the goat's cheese and the crunch of the pistachios bring amazing texture to this dish. You'll see once you try it!

oil spray

½ small brown onion, diced

1 garlic clove, crushed

1 teaspoon ground turmeric

1 teaspoon ground cumin

1 teaspoon ground coriander

½ teaspoon ground cinnamon

1 teaspoon chilli powder

2 oz brown rice

1 oz cremin mushrooms, sliced

½ medium carrot, coarsely grated

15 green beans, trimmed and sliced

1 cup salt-reduced vegetable stock

10¾ oz tinned chickpeas, drained and rinsed

1¾ oz sultanas

sea salt and ground black pepper, to taste

1 tablespoon chopped fresh parsley

⅔ oz unsalted pistachio kernels, chopped

1¾ oz soft goat's cheese, crumbled

Heat a large saucepan over medium heat and spray with oil spray. Add the onion and cook for 5 minutes or until soft and translucent, stirring occasionally.

Add the garlic, turmeric, cumin, coriander, cinnamon, and chilli powder and cook for 1 minute or until fragrant, stirring constantly.

Add the rice, mushrooms, carrot, and beans and cook for 3 minutes, stirring constantly.

Stir in the stock and bring to a boil over high heat. Reduce the heat to low and simmer, covered, for 15–20 minutes or until the liquid is absorbed and the rice is tender. Remove from the heat and stir in the chickpeas and sultanas. Let stand, covered, for 5 minutes before fluffing with a fork to separate the grains. Season with salt and pepper, if desired.

To serve, place the pilaf in two serving bowls and sprinkle over the parsley, pistachios, and goat's cheese.

YELLOW CURRY with TOFU

SERVES 2
PREP TIME 15 MINUTES
COOKING TIME 30 MINUTES
DIFFICULTY EASY

Like the look of this curry, but not a fan of tofu? Just replace it with a serve of your favourite protein instead.

4¼ oz brown rice

3 teaspoons olive oil

1 tablespoon yellow curry paste

1 medium carrot, chopped

1 fresh red chilli, seeds removed and thinly sliced

3 oz broccoli, cut into florets

1 oz frozen peas

3½ oz mushrooms, sliced

1 cup salt-reduced vegetable stock

5¼ oz tinned chickpeas, drained and rinsed

6 oz firm tofu, cut into 3-in cubes

2 teaspoons salt-reduced tamari or soy sauce

½ cup light coconut milk

1 teaspoon cornstarch (optional)

lime wedges, to serve

Place the rice and 1¼ cups of water in a small saucepan over high heat. Bring to a boil, then cover with a lid and reduce the heat to low. Simmer for 20–25 minutes or until the liquid is absorbed and the rice is tender. Remove from the heat and let stand, covered, for 5 minutes.

Meanwhile, heat the oil in a medium saucepan over medium heat. Add the curry paste and cook for 2–3 minutes until fragrant, stirring occasionally.

Add the carrot, chilli, broccoli, peas, and mushrooms and cook for 5 minutes, stirring occasionally.

Add the stock, chickpeas, and tofu and cook for 1 minute, stirring occasionally. Reduce the heat to medium–low and simmer, covered, for 10–15 minutes or until the vegetables are tender.

Stir in the tamari or soy sauce and coconut milk and cook, uncovered, for 2–3 minutes.

If the curry looks too thin, mix the cornstarch and 2 tablespoons of curry liquid together in a small bowl. Pour back into the curry and cook for a further 2–3 minutes or until thickened, stirring gently.

To serve, place the rice in two serving bowls and top with the yellow curry. Serve with lime wedges on the side.

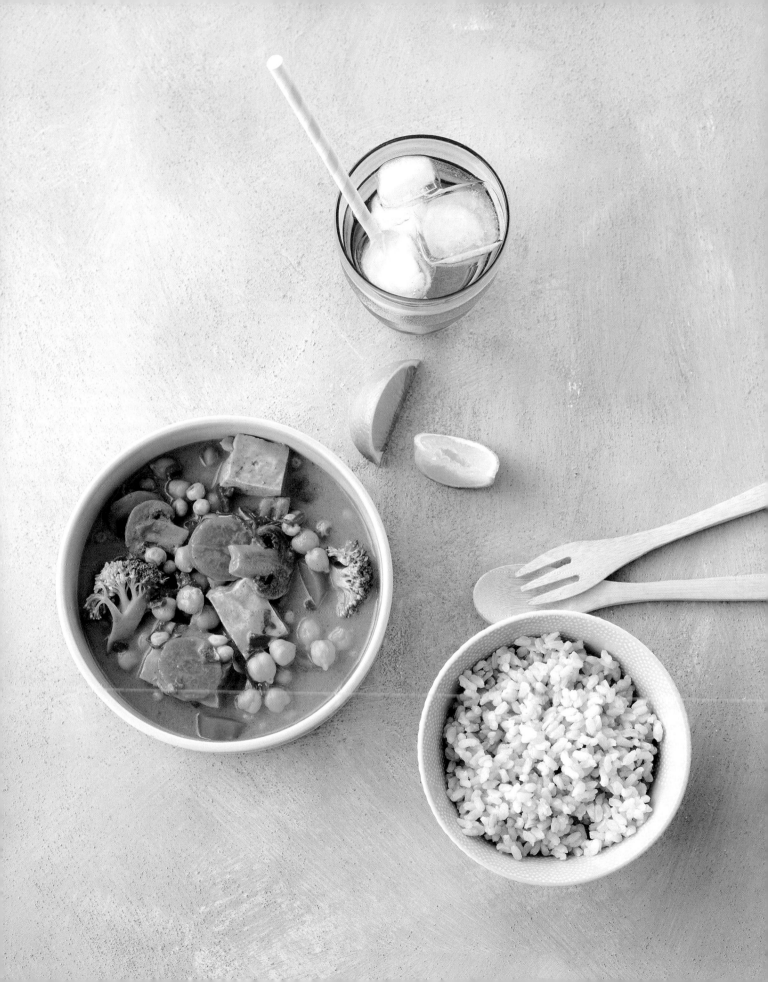

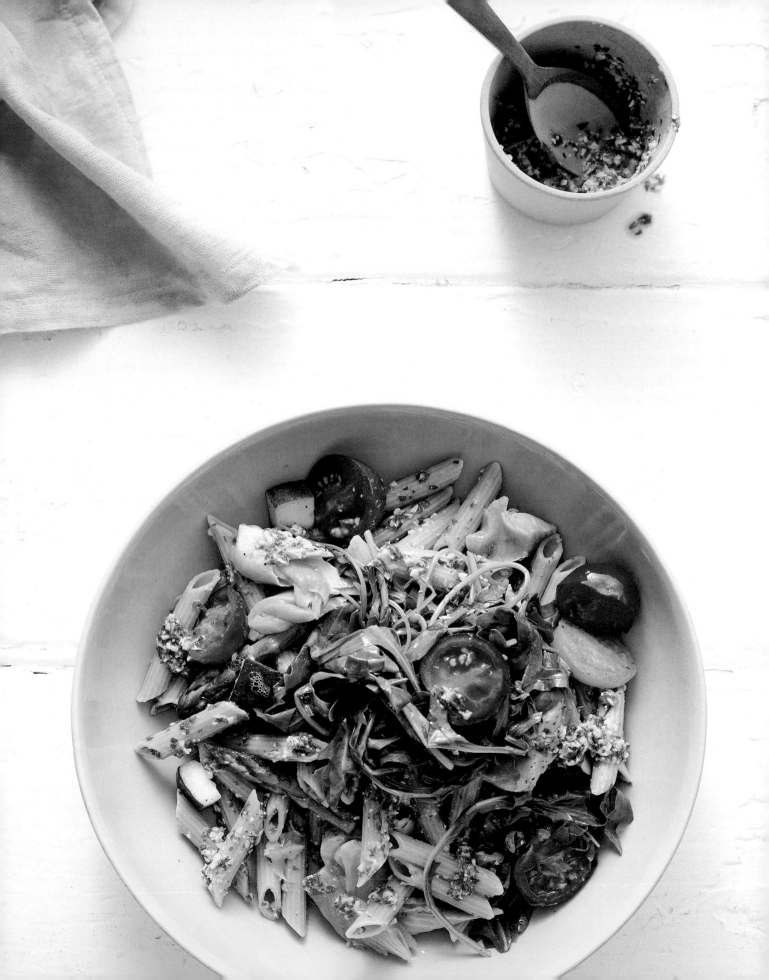

SALMON PESTO PASTA

SERVES 2
PREP TIME 15 MINUTES
COOKING TIME 20 MINUTES
DIFFICULTY MEDIUM

I've used basil in this pesto recipe, but you could also use coriander or parsley for something a little different. You could also try almonds or cashews instead of pine nuts. So many options!

5¾ oz whole wheat pasta

oil spray

6 oz salmon fillet, skin removed and deboned

¼ small brown onion, diced

1 medium zucchini, chopped

6 asparagus spears, trimmed and sliced

8 cherry tomatoes, halved

1 large handful arugula leaves

sea salt and ground black pepper, to taste

PESTO

2 large handfuls fresh basil leaves

1 garlic clove, crushed

2 tablespoons pine nuts

½ teaspoon finely grated lemon zest

2 tablespoons lemon juice

3 teaspoons olive oil

sea salt and ground black pepper, to taste

To make the pesto, place the basil leaves, garlic, pine nuts, lemon zest, and juice together in a food processor until finely chopped. Add the oil and 3 tablespoons of water and process until smooth. If the mixture is too thick, add 1 tablespoon of water at a time until the desired consistency is reached. Season with salt and pepper, if desired.

Fill a large saucepan with water, add a pinch of salt and bring to a boil. Add the pasta and cook until al dente (see the pasta packet for the recommended cooking time). Drain and set aside.

Meanwhile, heat a non-stick fry pan over medium heat and spray lightly with oil spray. Add the salmon and cook for 5–6 minutes or until cooked to your liking, turning occasionally. Transfer to a plate and set aside to rest for 2 minutes. Coarsely flake the salmon using two forks.

Wipe the fry pan clean, heat over medium heat and spray lightly with oil spray. Add the onion and cook for 3 minutes or until soft but not coloured, stirring occasionally.

Add the zucchini, asparagus, and tomato and cook for 5 minutes or until the vegetables start to soften.

Add the arugula and cook for 1 minute or until it starts to wilt. Remove from the heat and stir through the pesto. Add the pasta and toss gently to combine. Season with salt and pepper, if desired.

To serve, place the pesto pasta and salmon in two serving bowls.

(D) STUFFED TOMATOES with QUINOA & LENTILS

SERVES 2
PREP TIME 15 MINUTES
COOKING TIME 40 MINUTES
DIFFICULTY EASY

Rice is almost always used when stuffing capsicum or tomatoes in Greek cooking. But with this recipe, I decided to experiment a little bit by using quinoa and a touch of dried fruit—and I really liked how it turned out :)

2 oz quinoa (about ⅓ cup)

4 small tomatoes

oil spray

½ small brown onion, finely chopped

½ garlic clove, crushed

½ teaspoon dried basil

½ medium zucchini, coarsely grated

1 large handful baby spinach leaves, finely chopped

10¾ oz tinned brown lentils, drained and rinsed

1¾ oz dried currants

2 tablespoons pine nuts, roughly chopped

2 oz salt-reduced low-fat feta cheese, crumbled

sea salt and ground black pepper, to taste

Preheat the oven to 350°F (325°F convection) and line a baking sheet with parchment paper.

Place the quinoa and ⅔ cup of water in a saucepan over high heat and bring to the boil, stirring occasionally. Cover and reduce the heat to low. Simmer for 10–12 minutes until the liquid is absorbed and the quinoa is tender. Set aside to cool slightly.

Cut the tops off the tomatoes and set aside for later use. Without breaking the skin, carefully scoop out the tomato flesh and roughly chop it into small pieces.

Heat a non-stick fry pan over medium heat and spray lightly with oil spray. Add the onion, garlic, and basil and cook for 5 minutes or until the onion is soft and translucent, stirring frequently. Add the chopped tomato flesh, zucchini, and spinach and cook for a further 2–3 minutes or until the zucchini is soft and the spinach has wilted, stirring occasionally.

Place the quinoa, zucchini and spinach mixture, lentils, currants, pine nuts, feta, salt, and pepper in a bowl and toss gently to combine.

Fill the tomatoes evenly with the quinoa mixture, sit the tomato lids on top and place on the lined baking sheet.

Bake for 20–25 minutes or until the tomatoes are tender and the filling is heated through. Serve.

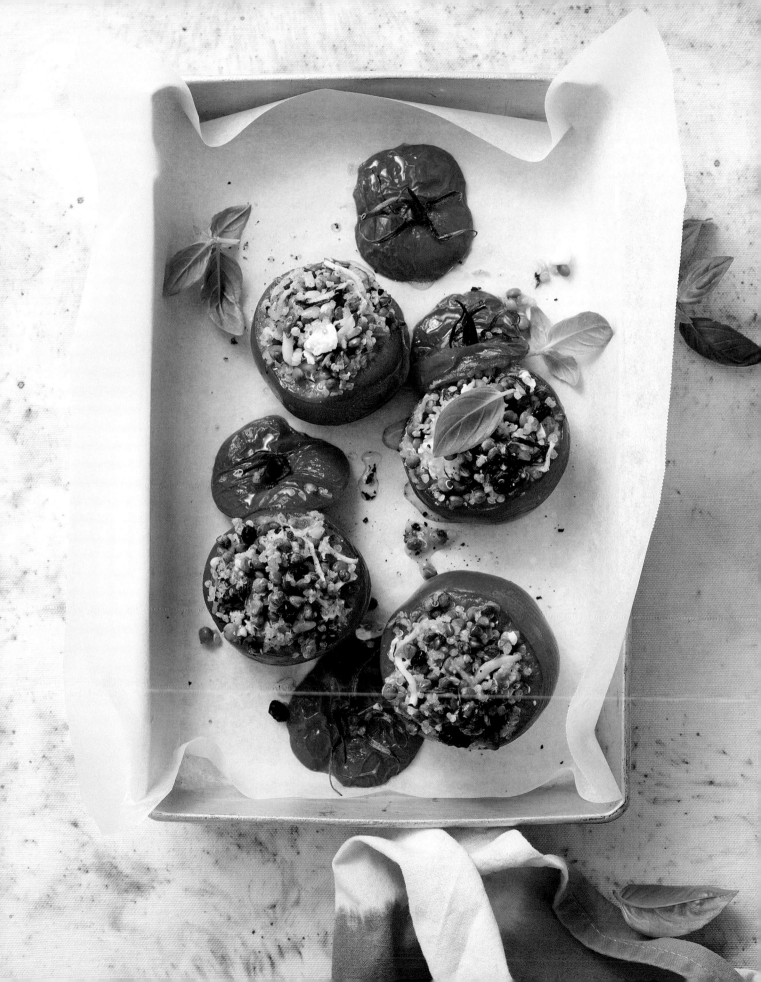

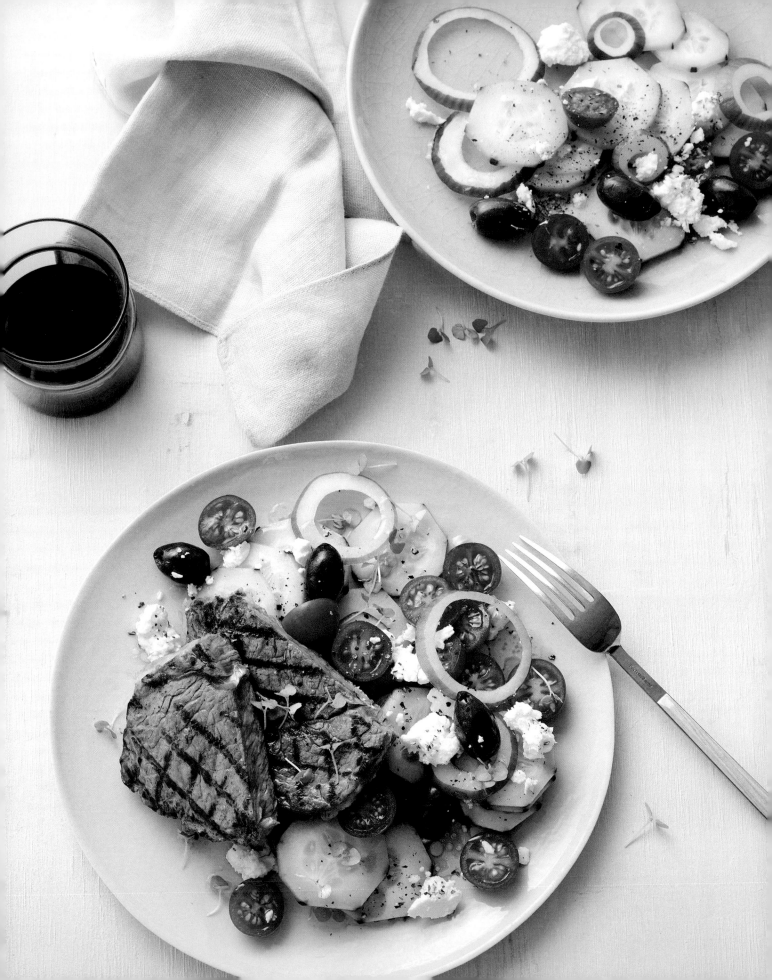

Ⓒ GRILLED STEAK with *HORIATIKI* (GREEK SALAD)

SERVES 2
PREP TIME 10 MINUTES
COOKING TIME 12 MINUTES
DIFFICULTY EASY

So simple and so delicious. My mum makes this dinner for Tobi all the time—it's one of his favourites!

Two 4½-oz steaks (porterhouse or rib eye)

oil spray

sea salt and ground black pepper, to taste

20 cherry tomatoes, halved

2 Lebanese cucumbers, peeled and sliced

1 small red onion, thinly sliced

16 kalamata olives, pitted

2 oz salt-reduced low-fat feta cheese, crumbled

DRESSING

1½ teaspoons extra virgin olive oil

1 teaspoon red wine vinegar

½ teaspoon dried oregano

Heat a barbecue grill-plate or chargrill pan over medium–high heat.

Place the steaks on a plate and lightly spray both sides with oil spray. Season with salt and pepper, if desired.

Grill the steaks for 4–5 minutes or until slightly charred. Turn the steaks over and cook for a further 5 minutes for medium or continue until cooked to your liking. Loosely cover with foil and set aside to rest for 2 minutes.

To make the dressing, whisk the oil, vinegar, and oregano together in a small bowl.

Place the tomatoes, cucumber, onion, olives, and feta in a large bowl. Drizzle over the dressing and toss gently to combine.

To serve, place the steaks on two serving plates with the Greek salad on the side.

ⓒ CHARGRILLED BEEF with CHIMICHURRI SAUCE

SERVES 2
PREP TIME 20 MINUTES
COOKING TIME 25 MINUTES
DIFFICULTY MEDIUM

Chimi-what?! Chimichurri is a bright green sauce, a bit similar to pesto. And it tastes amazing with grilled meat!

oil spray

1 medium sweet potato, peeled and diced

1 medium zucchini, diced

1 medium red bell pepper, seeds removed and diced

2 oz frozen corn kernels, thawed

5¼ oz tinned cannellini beans, drained and rinsed

1 small handful arugula leaves

6 oz lean beef steak

CHIMICHURRI SAUCE

1 large handful fresh parsley

2 teaspoons oregano leaves

1 garlic clove, crushed

1 scallion, chopped

½ teaspoon dried chilli flakes

2 teaspoons lemon juice

¾ teaspoon olive oil

2 teaspoons white wine vinegar

sea salt and ground black pepper, to taste

TAHINI YOGHURT DRESSING

7 oz low-fat plain yoghurt

1 teaspoon tahini

½ garlic clove, crushed

lemon juice, to taste

sea salt and ground black pepper, to taste

To make the chimichurri sauce, place the parsley, oregano, garlic, scallion, chilli flakes, lemon juice, oil, vinegar, salt, and pepper in a food processor and pulse until well combined. Set aside.

Heat a large non-stick fry pan over medium heat and spray lightly with oil spray. Add the sweet potato and cook for 5 minutes, stirring occasionally. Add the zucchini, bell pepper, and corn and cook for a further 5 minutes or until the sweet potato is tender (you should be able to easily push a fork into it). Add the cannellini beans and cook for a further minute or until warmed through.

Place the arugula and cooked vegetables in a large bowl and toss gently to combine.

To make the tahini yoghurt dressing, whisk the yoghurt, tahini, garlic, lemon juice, salt, and pepper together in a small bowl.

Heat a barbecue grill-plate or chargrill pan over high heat. Grill the steak for 4–5 minutes or until slightly charred. Turn the steak over and cook for a further 5–7 minutes for medium or continue until cooked to your liking. Cover loosely with foil and set aside to rest for 2 minutes. Slice the steak into bite-sized pieces.

To serve, place the vegetable and arugula salad on two serving plates and top with the sliced steak. Drizzle over the chimichurri sauce and tahini yoghurt dressing.

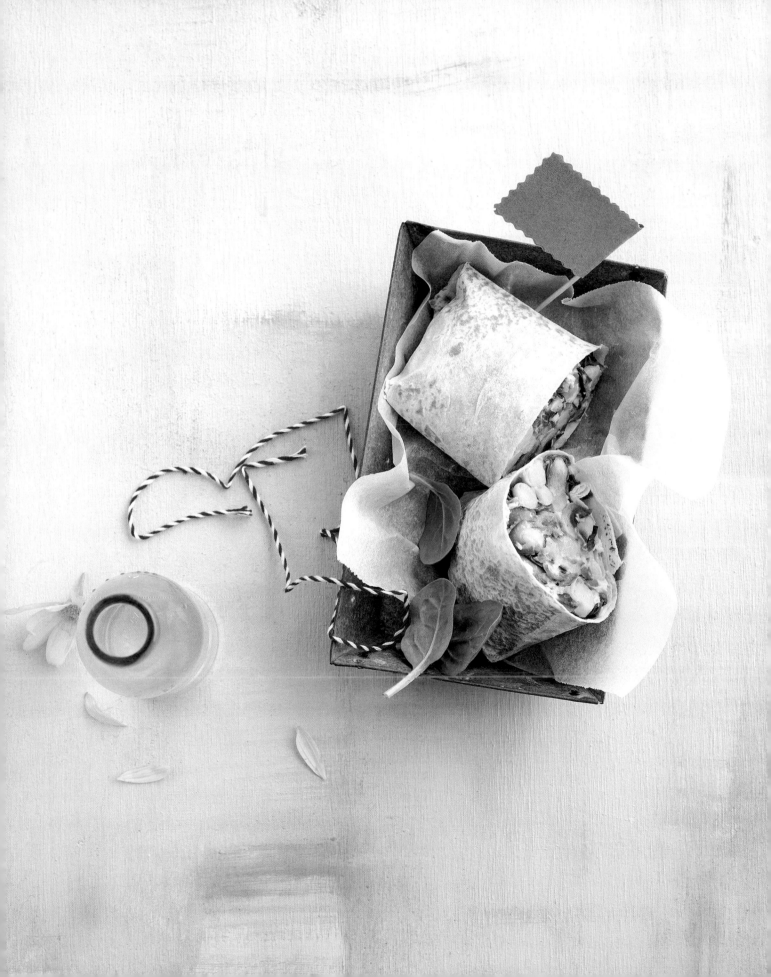

Ⓑ CHOC PEANUT BUTTER SMOOTHIE BOWL

SERVES 1

PREP TIME 5 MINUTES +
30 MINUTES SOAKING TIME

DIFFICULTY EASY

This recipe is like a healthy Snickers in a bowl! If you're not a fan of peanut butter, you can replace with another nut butter of your choice. I like almond butter and cashew butter.

3 medjool dates, pitted

2 teaspoons 100% natural peanut butter

1¼ oz tinned chickpeas, drained and rinsed

1 tablespoon raw cacao powder (see page 49)

3½ oz low-fat plain yoghurt

1 cup low-fat milk

TOPPINGS

1 oz natural muesli

½ medium banana, peeled and sliced

1 tablespoon raw cacao nibs

In a heatproof bowl, cover the dates with boiling water and let soak for 30 minutes to soften. Drain.

Place the dates, peanut butter, chickpeas, cacao powder, yoghurt, and milk in a high-powered blender and blend until smooth.

To serve, pour the smoothie mixture into a bowl and top with the muesli, banana, and cacao nibs.

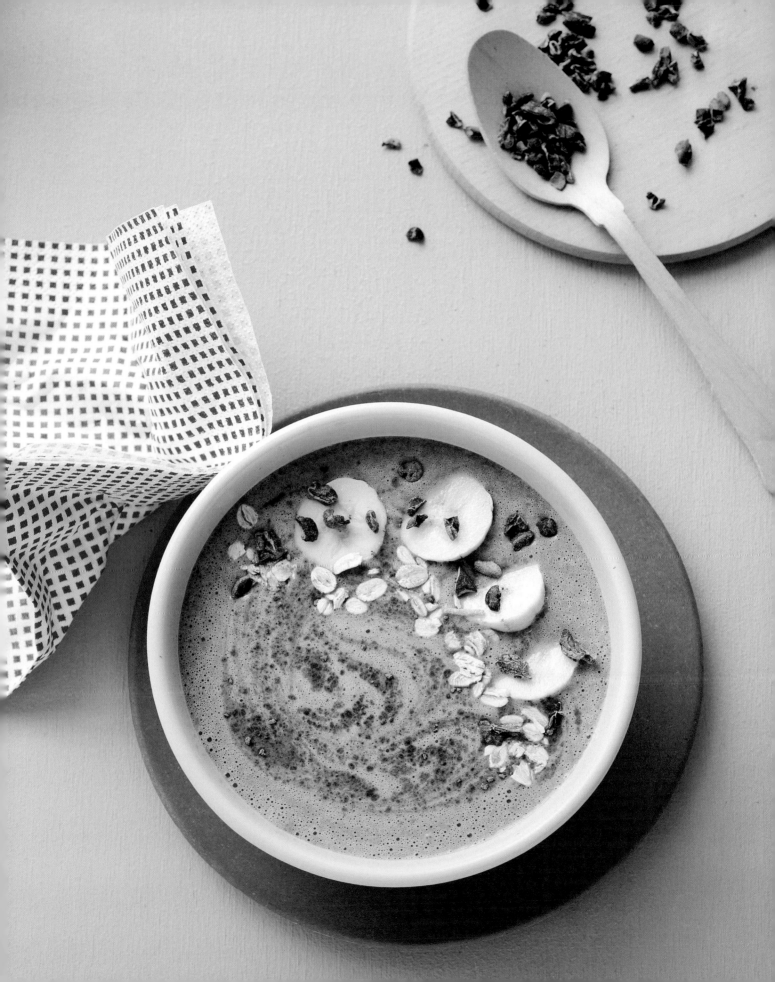

ⓓ BIG BREAKFAST

SERVES 1
PREP TIME 10 MINUTES
COOKING TIME 30 MINUTES
DIFFICULTY EASY

This is the ultimate big breakfast recipe to keep you energised all morning! If you're not a fan of goat's cheese, you can always substitute 1 oz of feta instead.

1 teaspoon white vinegar

2 large eggs

¼ medium sweet potato, peeled and grated

½ tablespoon whole wheat flour

sea salt and ground black pepper, to taste

1½ teaspoons olive oil

1¾ oz button mushrooms, thinly sliced

2 slices whole wheat bread

1 oz soft goat's cheese

Fill a saucepan with water until 3 in deep. Add the vinegar and bring to a boil over medium heat, then reduce the heat to medium–low. Break the eggs into the water and cook for 2–3 minutes for a semi-soft yolk or 3–4 minutes for a firm yolk. Remove the eggs with a slotted spoon and allow to drain on paper towel.

Using your hands, squeeze out as much liquid from the grated sweet potato as possible. Transfer the sweet potato to a mixing bowl. Add the flour, salt, and pepper and mix to combine.

Heat half the oil in a small non-stick fry pan over medium heat. Add the sweet potato mixture and flatten out with the back of a metal spoon. Cook for 2–3 minutes or until the bottom of the rosti is golden and crisp. Carefully flip over and cook further for 2–3 minutes. Transfer to a plate, cover with foil, and set aside.

Heat the remaining oil in the fry pan over medium heat. Add the mushrooms and cook for 7–10 minutes or until soft, stirring occasionally.

Meanwhile, toast the bread to your liking.

To serve, place the toast, sweet potato rosti, and mushrooms on a serving plate. Top with the poached eggs and sprinkle over the goat's cheese.

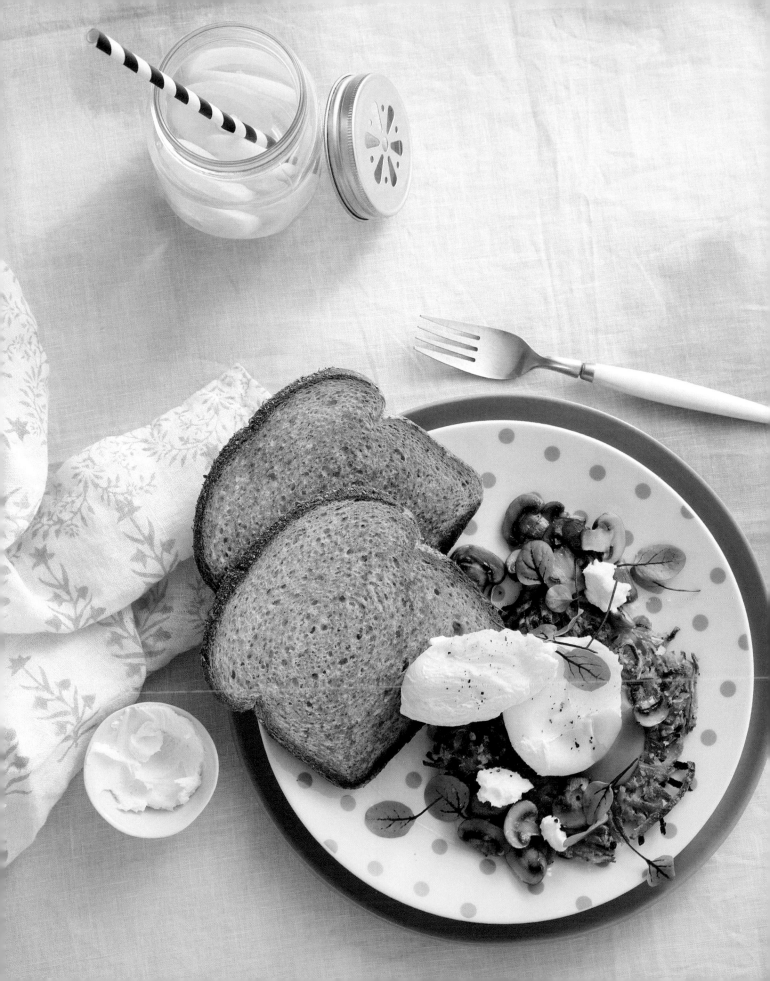

BANANA & STRAWBERRY BRUSCHETTA

SERVES 1
PREP TIME 5 MINUTES
COOKING TIME 2 MINUTES
DIFFICULTY EASY

I love the combination of banana and strawberry, and the drizzle of maple syrup takes this bruschetta to the next level! If you want to play around with different fruit combinations, feel free—use what's in season for the freshest flavours.

2 slices raisin bread
3½ oz low-fat ricotta cheese
4½ oz strawberries, hulled and sliced

½ medium banana, peeled and sliced
2 teaspoons pure maple syrup

Toast the bread to your liking.

To serve, place the toast on a serving plate and spread over the ricotta. Top with the strawberries and banana and drizzle with maple syrup.

Ⓑ CHOC BANANA SMOOTHIE BOWL

SERVES 1
PREP TIME 5 MINUTES
DIFFICULTY EASY

Treat yourself with my decadent (but healthy) creation that features one of my favourite flavour combos: chocolate and banana!

1 medium banana, peeled
and chopped

½ medium zucchini, chopped

1 tablespoon raw cacao powder

7 oz low-fat plain yoghurt

½ cup low-fat milk

TOPPINGS

1 oz natural muesli

½ medium banana, peeled and sliced

1 heaping tablespoon hazelnuts,
roughly chopped

Place the banana, zucchini, cacao powder, yoghurt, and milk in a high-powered blender and blend until smooth.

To serve, pour the smoothie mixture into a serving bowl and top with the muesli, banana, and hazelnuts.

Ⓓ ZUCCHINI, TOMATO & RICE FRITTATA

SERVES 1
PREP TIME 10 MINUTES
COOKING TIME 35 MINUTES
DIFFICULTY EASY

I have cooked the rice fresh here, but this recipe is a great way to use up any rice leftover from another meal. To save time, the frittata can also be cooked the night before and stored in an airtight container in the refrigerator.

2 tablespoons brown rice

oil spray

1½ teaspoons olive oil

½ medium zucchini, coarsely grated

½ medium tomato, diced

1 oz salt-reduced low-fat feta cheese, crumbled

2 teaspoons chopped fresh parsley

2 large eggs

1 slice whole wheat bread

Place the rice and ½ cup of water in a small saucepan over high heat and bring to a boil, stirring occasionally. Cover and reduce the heat to medium–low. Simmer for 20–25 minutes or until the liquid is absorbed and the rice is tender. Remove from the heat and let stand, covered, for 5 minutes. Set aside to cool.

Preheat the oven to 350°F (325°F convection) and grease a 3-in ramekin with oil spray.

Heat the oil in a small non-stick fry pan over medium heat. Add the zucchini and tomato and cook for 3–4 minutes or until soft, stirring occasionally. Set aside to cool slightly.

Place the rice, zucchini and tomato mixture, feta, and parsley in a mixing bowl and stir until well combined. Transfer to the prepared ramekin.

Whisk the eggs and 2 tablespoons of water together in a small bowl. Pour the egg mixture into the prepared ramekin.

Bake in the oven for 15–20 minutes or until golden and set.

Meanwhile, toast the bread to your liking.

Serve the frittata with the toast on the side.

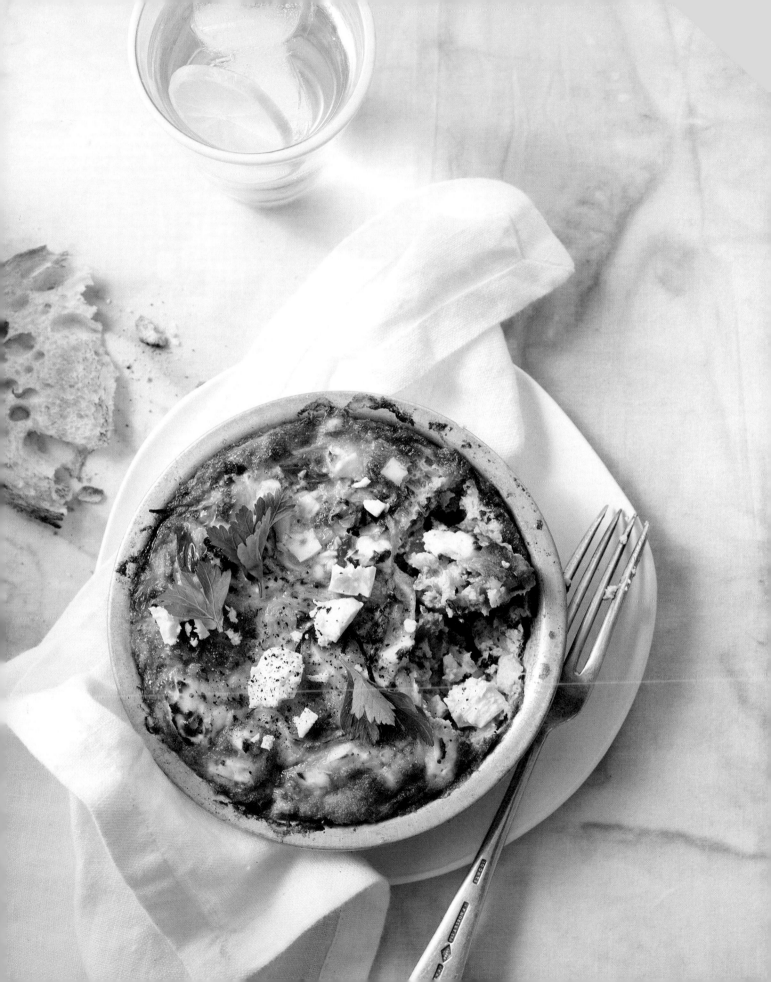

BUCKWHEAT & BANANA PARFAIT

SERVES 1

PREP TIME 8 HOURS OR
OVERNIGHT SOAKING TIME +
10 MINUTES CHILLING TIME

DIFFICULTY EASY

This brilliant breakfast will have your tastebuds buzzing!

3¼ buckwheat kernels

7 oz low-fat plain yoghurt

1 teaspoon honey

1 medium banana, peeled and sliced

Soak the buckwheat in a bowl of cold water for 8 hours or overnight. Drain and rinse.

Place the yoghurt and honey in a small bowl and mix until well combined.

Layer the buckwheat, honey, yoghurt, and banana in a glass.

Place in the refrigerator to chill for 10 minutes. Serve.

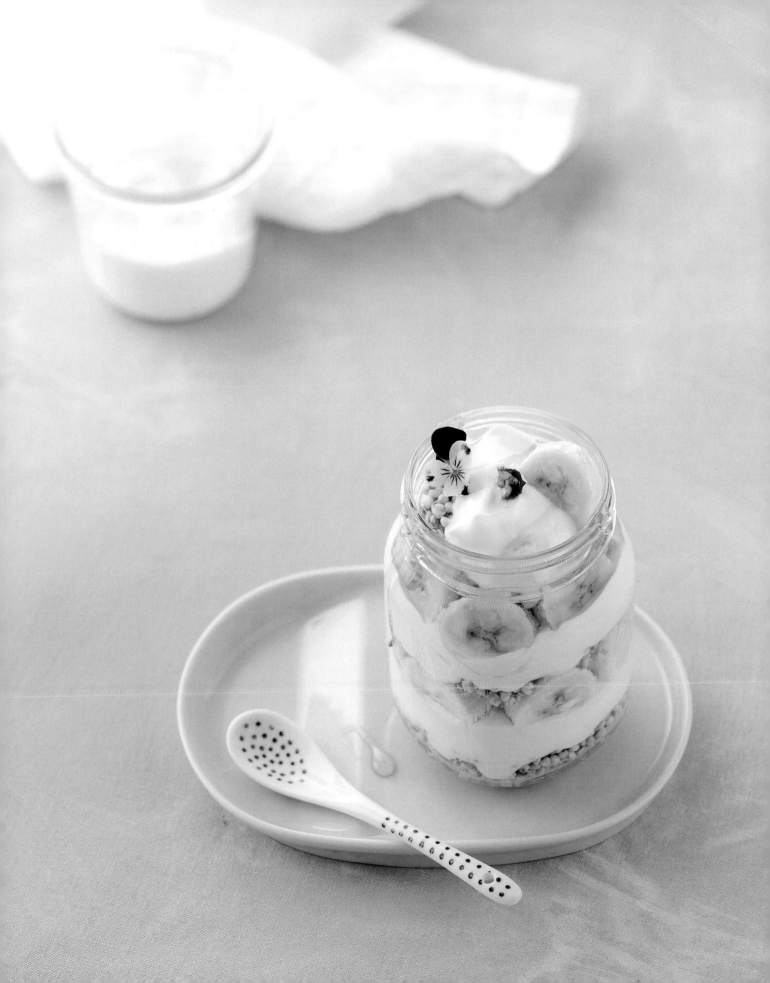

PEACH PARFAIT

SERVES 1

PREP TIME 5 MINUTES +
10 MINUTES CHILLING TIME

DIFFICULTY EASY

Only four ingredients needed to make this refreshing parfait.
Simple and delicious!

7 oz low-fat plain yoghurt

1 teaspoon honey

2 oz natural muesli

5¼ oz tinned diced peaches
in fruit juice, drained

Place the yoghurt and honey in a small bowl and mix until well combined.

Layer the honey yoghurt, muesli, and peaches in a glass.

Place in the refrigerator to chill for 10 minutes. Serve.

Ⓓ POACHED EGGS with ASPARAGUS

SERVES 1
PREP TIME 5 MINUTES
COOKING TIME 10 MINUTES
DIFFICULTY EASY

Who can resist a poached egg for breakfast? The toasted pumpkin seeds add a really nice texture . . . you'll see!

1 teaspoon white vinegar

2 large eggs

⅓ oz pumpkin seeds (pepitas)

6 asparagus spears, trimmed

2 slices whole wheat bread

⅔ oz parmesan cheese, shaved

Fill a saucepan with water until 3 in deep. Add the vinegar and bring to a boil over medium heat, then reduce the heat to medium–low. The water should just be simmering. Break the eggs into the water and cook for 2–3 minutes for a semi-soft yolk or 3–4 minutes for a firm yolk. Remove the eggs with a slotted spoon and allow to drain on paper towel.

Heat a non-stick fry pan over medium heat. Add the pumpkin seeds and cook for 4–5 minutes or until a pale gold colour, stirring constantly. Remove from the pan and set aside to cool.

Heat the fry pan over medium–high heat. Add the asparagus spears and cook for 3–5 minutes or until they start to change colour and are the desired tenderness.

Meanwhile, toast the bread to your liking.

To serve, place the toast on a serving plate and top with the asparagus spears and poached eggs. Sprinkle over the parmesan and pumpkin seeds.

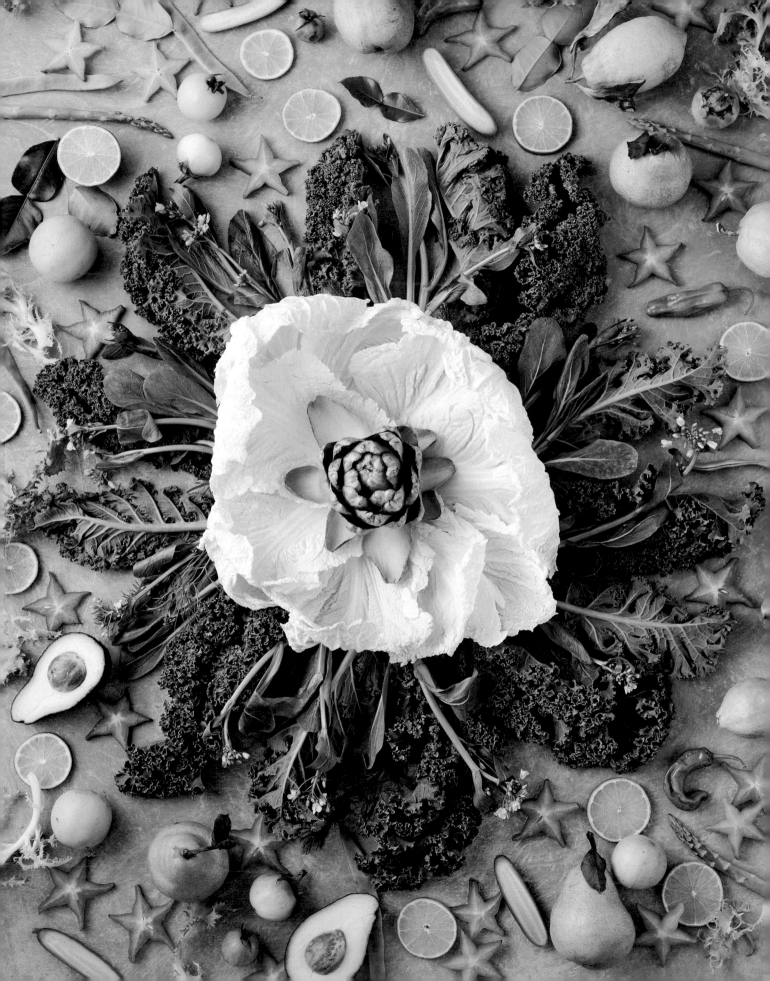

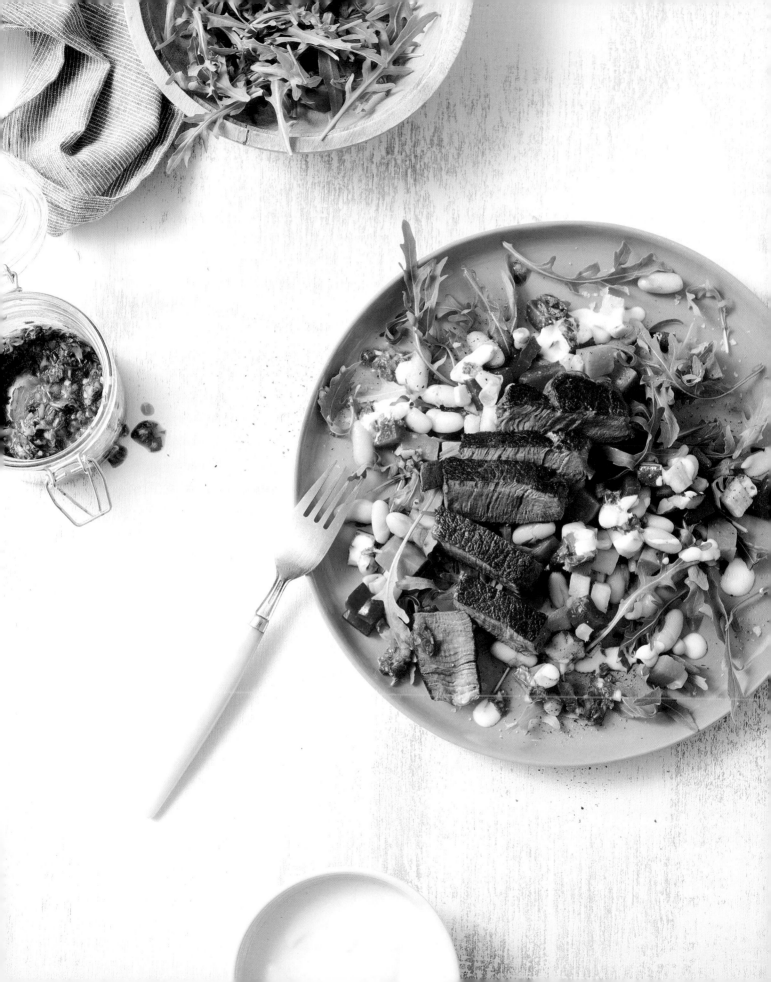

⒟ GRILLED BABY OCTOPUS with FENNEL, ROCKET & APPLE SALAD

SERVES 2

PREP TIME 15 MINUTES + 2 HOURS OR OVERNIGHT MARINATING TIME

COOKING TIME 15 MINUTES

DIFFICULTY MEDIUM

This salad makes a regular appearance at our family barbecues. It's so light and fresh!

10½ oz baby octopus, cleaned

3 teaspoons olive oil

1 teaspoon red wine vinegar

finely grated lemon zest and juice, to taste

1 garlic clove, crushed

sea salt and ground black pepper, to taste

2 oz salt-reduced low-fat feta cheese, crumbled

1 tablespoon finely chopped fresh parsley

FENNEL, ROCKET & APPLE SALAD

2 small fennel bulbs, thinly sliced

1 large handful arugula leaves

2½ oz tinned chickpeas, drained and rinsed

2 medium green apples, cored and thinly sliced

juice of ½ lemon

CROUTONS

2 slices sourdough bread

oil spray

½ garlic clove

Place the baby octopus in a steamer basket over a saucepan of boiling water. Cover and steam for 5–6 minutes or until the octopus has curled slightly and is cooked through. Transfer to a bowl and set aside.

Whisk the oil, vinegar, lemon zest and juice, garlic, salt, and pepper together in a medium bowl.

Place the octopus in the bowl containing the marinade. Cover with plastic wrap and refrigerate for 2 hours or overnight to marinate.

Preheat a barbecue grill-plate or chargrill pan over medium–high heat.

To make the salad, place the fennel, arugula, chickpeas, and apple in a bowl. Drizzle over the lemon juice and toss gently to combine.

To make the croutons, spray both sides of the sourdough bread slices with oil spray. Place on the barbecue grill-plate or chargrill pan and grill for 1–2 minutes on each side or until toasted. Rub the cut garlic clove over the charred bread for flavour.

Drain the octopus and grill on the barbecue grill-plate or chargrill pan for 4–5 minutes or until the edges are slightly charred and the flesh is warmed through, turning frequently.

To serve, place the fennel, arugula, and apple salad on two serving plates and top with the grilled octopus. Sprinkle over the feta and parsley. Serve the croutons on the side.

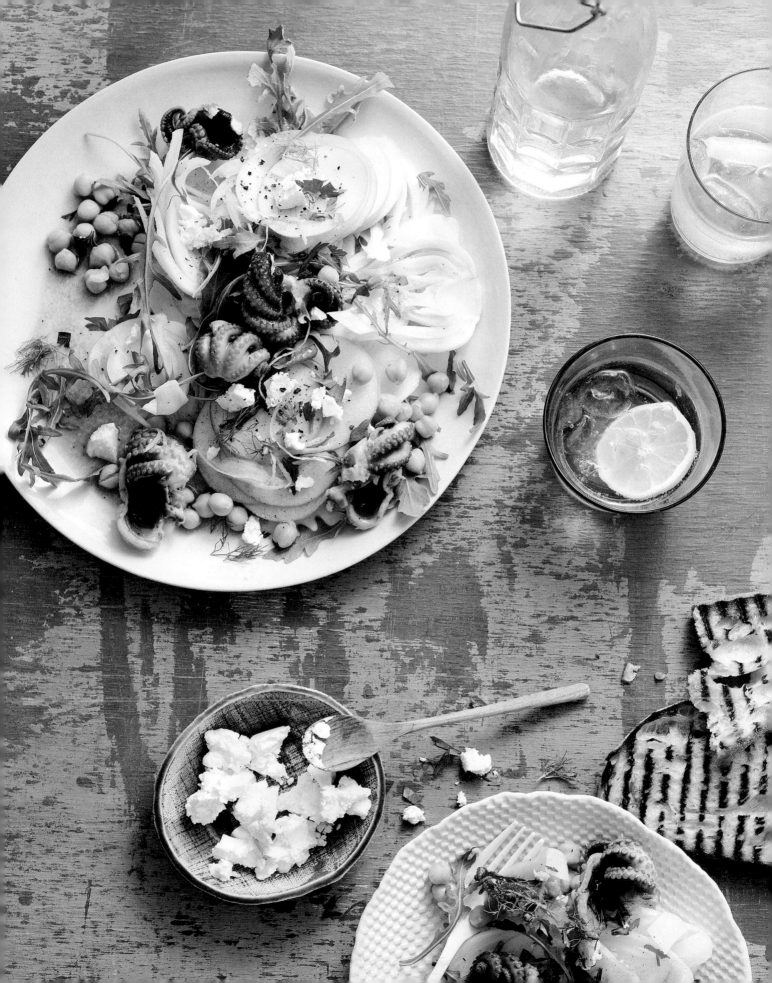

Ⓑ CHICKEN TACOS

SERVES 2
PREP TIME 15 MINUTES +
30 MINUTES MARINATING TIME
COOKING TIME 15 MINUTES
DIFFICULTY EASY

I like mixing things up every now and again, but for this one I've stuck with traditional Mexican flavours. You just can't go wrong!

1 teaspoon ground cumin
½ teaspoon sweet paprika
pinch of chilli powder
½ garlic clove, crushed
juice of 1 lime
7 oz boneless skinless chicken breast
oil spray
1 medium tomato, diced
½ small red onion, diced
2 oz frozen corn kernels, thawed
¼ medium bell pepper, seeds removed and diced

2 whole wheat wraps
1 large handful lettuce leaves, shredded
⅔ oz reduced-fat cheddar cheese, grated

DRESSING
3½ oz low-fat plain yoghurt
lime juice, to taste
1 tablespoon chopped fresh parsley

Whisk the cumin, paprika, chilli powder, garlic, and lime juice together in a medium bowl. Place the chicken in the bowl and rub with the spice mix. Cover with plastic wrap and refrigerate for 30 minutes to marinate.

Heat a non-stick fry pan over medium heat and spray lightly with oil spray. Add the chicken and cook for 4–6 minutes on each side or until cooked through. Transfer to a plate and set aside to rest.

To make the dressing, whisk the yoghurt, lime juice, and parsley together in a small bowl.

Place the tomato, onion, corn, and bell pepper in a small bowl and toss gently to combine.

Warm the wraps in a large dry fry pan over medium–high heat for 30 seconds on each side. Remove from the heat and cut in half.

To serve, place the wrap halves on two serving plates. Top with the lettuce, cheese, chicken, and tomato mixture. Drizzle over the dressing and fold in half.

Ⓐ SPICED CAULIFLOWER & CHICKPEA CURRY

SERVES 2
PREP TIME 10 MINUTES
COOKING TIME 30 MINUTES
DIFFICULTY EASY

Feeling hot, hot, hot? Feel free to add some extra chilli to this veggie curry if you like a little more heat!

4¼ oz brown rice

3 teaspoons olive oil

½ small brown onion, finely chopped

2 garlic cloves, crushed

¾ in fresh ginger, peeled and grated

½ teaspoon ground coriander

1 teaspoon ground cumin

1 teaspoon garam masala

2 teaspoons ground turmeric

pinch of dried chilli flakes

5¼ oz tinned crushed tomatoes

1 cup salt-reduced vegetable stock

5¼ oz cauliflower, cut into florets

10¾ oz tinned chickpeas, drained and rinsed

½ cup light coconut milk

1 oz frozen peas

sea salt and ground black pepper, to taste

2 tablespoons chopped fresh cilantro

Place the rice and 1¼ cups of water in a small saucepan over high heat and bring to a boil, stirring occasionally. Cover and reduce the heat to medium–low. Simmer for 20–25 minutes or until the liquid is absorbed and the rice is tender. Remove from the heat and let stand, covered, for 5 minutes.

Meanwhile, heat the oil in a large saucepan over medium heat. Add the onion, garlic, and ginger and cook for 5 minutes or until the onion is soft and translucent, stirring occasionally. Add the ground coriander, cumin, garam masala, turmeric, and chilli flakes. Cook for a further 2–3 minutes or until fragrant, stirring constantly.

Stir in the tomatoes, stock, cauliflower, chickpeas, coconut milk, and peas and bring to a boil over high heat. Reduce the heat to medium–low and simmer, covered, for 15 minutes, stirring occasionally.

Remove the lid and cook for a further 5 minutes or until the sauce has thickened a little, stirring occasionally. Season with salt and pepper, if desired.

To serve, place the rice in two serving bowls and top with the cauliflower and chickpea curry. Sprinkle over the cilantro.

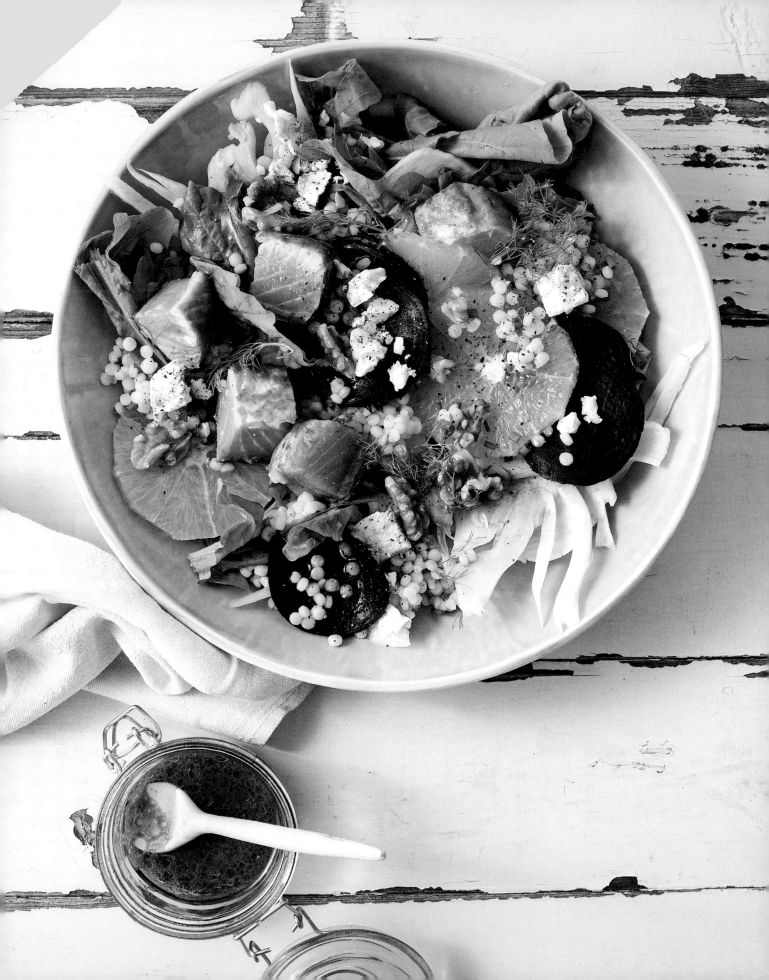

D SALMON with BEETROOT, FENNEL & ORANGE SALAD & PEARL COUSCOUS

SERVES 2
PREP TIME 15 MINUTES
COOKING TIME 45 MINUTES
DIFFICULTY EASY

This salad looks just as good as it tastes! The beetroot can be cooked the night before and stored in an airtight container in the refrigerator until needed.

2 oz pearl couscous

oil spray

6 oz salmon fillet, skin removed and deboned

1 tablespoon walnuts

2 oz salt-reduced low-fat feta cheese, crumbled

2 teaspoons chopped fresh dill

2 teaspoons chopped fresh chives

BEETROOT, FENNEL & ORANGE SALAD

2 small beetroots

2 medium oranges

1 small fennel bulb, thinly sliced

1 large handful arugula leaves

DRESSING

1½ teaspoons olive oil

1 teaspoon red wine vinegar

½ teaspoon Dijon mustard

sea salt and ground black pepper, to taste

Preheat the oven to 350°F (325°F convection).

Wrap the beetroot in foil with 1 tablespoon of water (this helps the beetroot to steam). Place in a small roasting pan and bake in the oven for 30–40 minutes or until tender. Test the beetroot with a skewer—it is cooked if a skewer pierces the flesh easily. Set aside to cool. When cool enough to handle, peel and slice the beetroot.

Fill a saucepan with water and bring to a boil. Stir in the pearl couscous and simmer over medium heat for 10–12 minutes until al dente. Drain and set aside to cool.

Meanwhile, peel the oranges over a medium bowl to catch the juice. Slice the oranges or cut into segments. Squeeze the remaining orange membrane to extract any extra juice into the bowl and set aside.

To make the dressing, whisk the oil, vinegar, mustard, and reserved orange juice together in a small bowl. Season with salt and pepper, if desired.

Heat a non-stick fry pan over medium heat and spray lightly with oil spray. Add the salmon and cook for 5–6 minutes or until cooked to your liking, turning occasionally. Transfer to a plate and set aside to rest for 2 minutes. Slice the salmon into bite-sized pieces.

Place the beetroot, orange segments, fennel, and arugula in a mixing bowl. Drizzle over the dressing and toss gently to combine.

To serve, place the pearl couscous on two serving plates. Top with the beetroot, fennel, and orange salad, and salmon. Sprinkle over the walnuts, feta, dill, and chives.

Ⓑ PUMPKIN "CHILLI CON CARNE"

SERVES 2
PREP TIME 10 MINUTES
COOKING TIME 45 MINUTES
DIFFICULTY EASY

This recipe puts a veggie spin on a Mexican classic, but you don't have to be a vegetarian to enjoy it!

4¼ oz brown rice

8½ oz pumpkin,
cut into ¾-in cubes

oil spray

½ small brown onion,
finely chopped

1 garlic clove, crushed

1 fresh green chilli, chopped,
plus extra to garnish
(optional)

7¾ oz tinned crushed
tomatoes

½ cup salt-reduced vegetable
stock

5¼ oz tinned black beans,
drained and rinsed

5¼ oz tinned chickpeas,
drained and rinsed

1–2 teaspoons chilli powder

½ teaspoon ground cumin

½ teaspoon sweet paprika

¼ teaspoon dried oregano

sea salt and ground black
pepper, to taste

7 oz low-fat plain yoghurt

Place the rice and 1¼ cups of water in a small saucepan over high heat and bring to a boil, stirring occasionally. Cover and reduce the heat to medium–low. Simmer for 20–25 minutes or until the liquid is absorbed and the rice is tender. Remove from the heat and let stand, covered, for 5 minutes.

Fill a saucepan with water until 2 in deep and insert a steamer basket. Cover with a lid and bring the water to the boil over high heat, then reduce the heat to medium. Add the pumpkin and steam, covered, for 10–12 minutes or until tender. There should be a little resistance when a knife is inserted—the pumpkin will finish cooking in later steps.

Roughly mash half of the pumpkin.

Heat a saucepan over medium heat and spray lightly with oil spray. Add the onion and cook for 3 minutes, stirring occasionally. Add the garlic and green chilli (if using) and cook for a further 2 minutes or until soft and fragrant, stirring occasionally.

Add the mashed pumpkin, pumpkin pieces, tomatoes, stock, black beans, and chickpeas. Stir in the chilli powder, cumin, paprika, and oregano. Taste to check the seasoning and add additional cumin and chilli powder, if desired.

Bring the chilli con carne to a boil over high heat, stirring occasionally to ensure the ingredients are well mixed. Reduce the heat to low and simmer for 20 minutes, stirring occasionally. If the sauce is too thick towards the end of cooking time, stir in a small amount of water. Season with salt and pepper, if desired.

To serve, place the pumpkin chilli con carne in two serving bowls and top with the yoghurt. Sprinkle over the extra green chilli (if using) and serve the rice on the side.

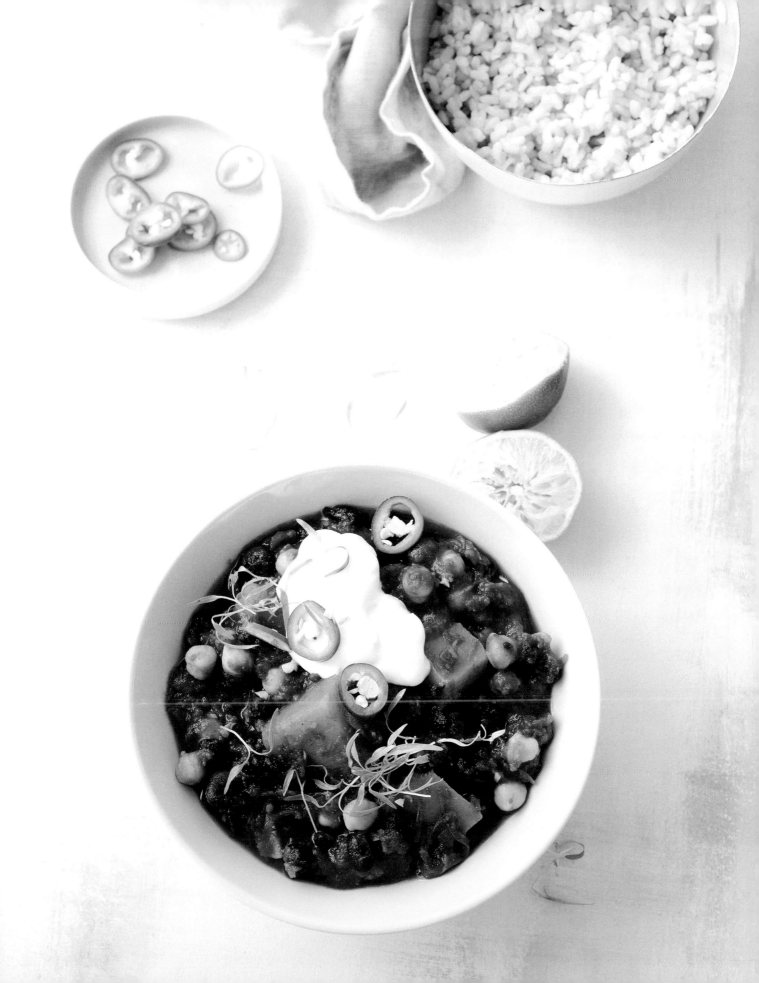

COCONUT-INFUSED SALMON
with ASIAN GREENS

SERVES 2
PREP TIME 10 MINUTES
COOKING TIME 30 MINUTES
DIFFICULTY EASY

I absolutely love the flavour of coconut. This is such a fragrant dish, complemented by the fresh Asian greens. Yum!

4¼ oz brown rice

¾ cup light coconut milk

½ lemongrass stalk, inner core of the white part only, finely chopped

¾ in fresh ginger, peeled and thinly sliced

finely grated zest and juice of 1 lime

2 teaspoons fish sauce

2 teaspoons honey

1 scallion, thinly sliced

Two 3-oz salmon fillets, skin removed and deboned

6⅓ oz bok choy, roughly chopped

15 green beans, trimmed and halved

3 oz snow peas, trimmed and halved

2 teaspoons sesame seeds

Place the rice and 1¼ cups of water in a small saucepan over high heat. Bring to a boil, then cover with a lid and reduce the heat to low. Simmer for 20–25 minutes or until the liquid is absorbed and the rice is tender. Remove from the heat and let stand, covered, for 5 minutes.

Meanwhile, place the coconut milk, lemongrass, ginger, lime zest and juice, fish sauce, honey, and scallion in a saucepan and bring to a simmer over medium heat.

Add the salmon and simmer for 8–10 minutes or until cooked to your liking and the coconut sauce has thickened.

Fill a saucepan with water until 2 in deep and insert a steamer basket. Cover with a lid and bring the water to the boil over high heat, then reduce the heat to medium. Add the bok choy and green beans and steam, covered, for 3 minutes. Add the snow peas and steam for a further 2–3 minutes or until the vegetables are tender-crisp.

To serve, place the rice in two bowls and top with the salmon fillet and steamed greens. Spoon over the coconut sauce and sprinkle over the sesame seeds.

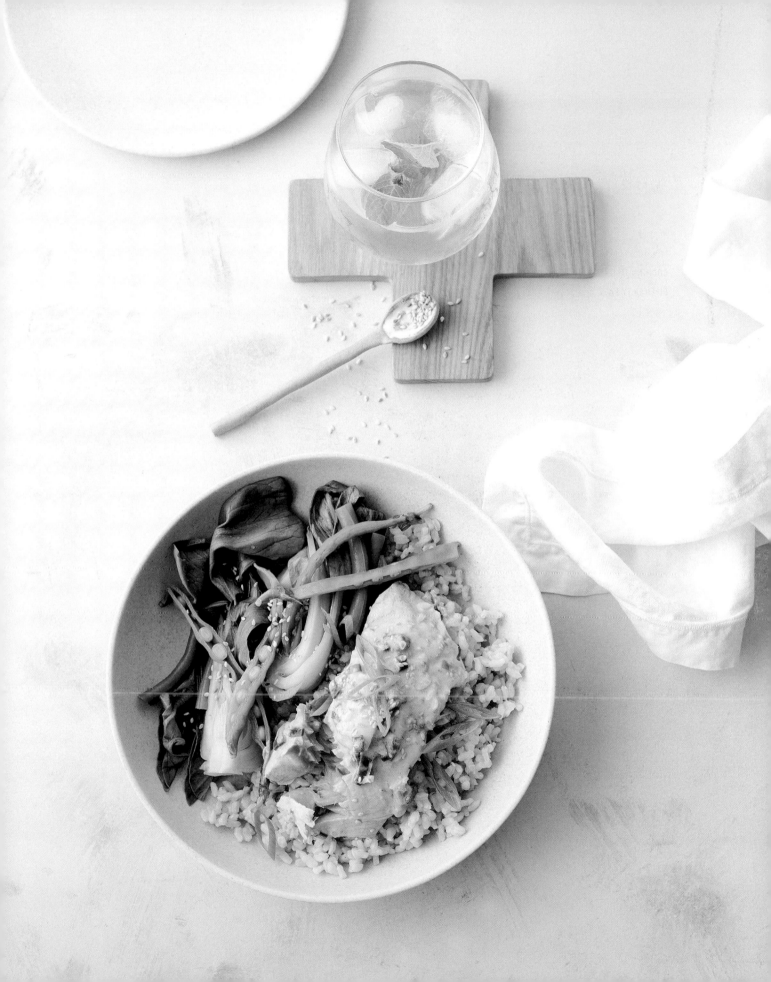

Ⓒ VEAL OSSO BUCCO

SERVES 2
PREP TIME 15 MINUTES
COOKING TIME 2 HOURS
DIFFICULTY EASY

I'm one of those people that really enjoys cleaning in my spare time (I just can't deal with a messy house, haha)! Because this is a slow-cook recipe, I'll sometimes put this in the oven while I'm cleaning. It's soooo comforting in the middle of winter—I love it!

2 small pieces veal osso bucco

1 tablespoon whole wheat flour

sea salt and ground black pepper, to taste

1½ teaspoons olive oil

1 small brown onion, diced

3 garlic cloves, crushed

1 medium carrot, diced

2 celery stalks, diced

2 bay leaves

10¾ oz tinned crushed tomatoes

1 cup salt-reduced vegetable stock

1 teaspoon dried thyme

1 teaspoon dried oregano

chopped fresh parsley, to garnish

SWEET POTATO MASH

1 medium sweet potato, peeled and cut into ¾-in cubes

¼ cup low-fat milk

1 oz parmesan cheese, grated

sea salt and ground black pepper, to taste

Preheat the oven to 300°F (275°F convection).

Place the osso bucco, flour, salt, and pepper in an oven bag (or zip-top bag) and shake to lightly coat each piece of osso bucco. Remove from the bag and shake off any excess flour.

Heat the oil in a saucepan over medium heat. Add the osso bucco and cook for 4–5 minutes or until lightly browned, turning occasionally. Remove the osso bucco from the saucepan and set aside.

Add the onion, garlic, carrot, celery, and bay leaves to the pan and cook for 3–4 minutes or until soft, stirring occasionally. Add the tomatoes, stock, thyme, oregano, salt, and pepper and bring to the boil.

Transfer the osso bucco and vegetable mixture to a casserole dish and cover with a lid or foil. Cook in the oven for 1½ hours.

Remove the lid or foil and cook for a further 15 minutes to allow the sauce to thicken.

Meanwhile, to make the mash, bring a saucepan of water to a boil over medium–high heat. Add the sweet potato and cook for 10 minutes or until tender. Drain and return the sweet potato to the warm saucepan. Shake over low heat for 30 seconds or until the excess moisture evaporates. Remove from the heat.

Using a potato masher, roughly mash the sweet potato. Gradually add the milk and mash until smooth. Add the parmesan, salt, and pepper and stir until combined.

To serve, place the mashed potato on two serving plates and top with the osso bucco. Sprinkle over the parsley.

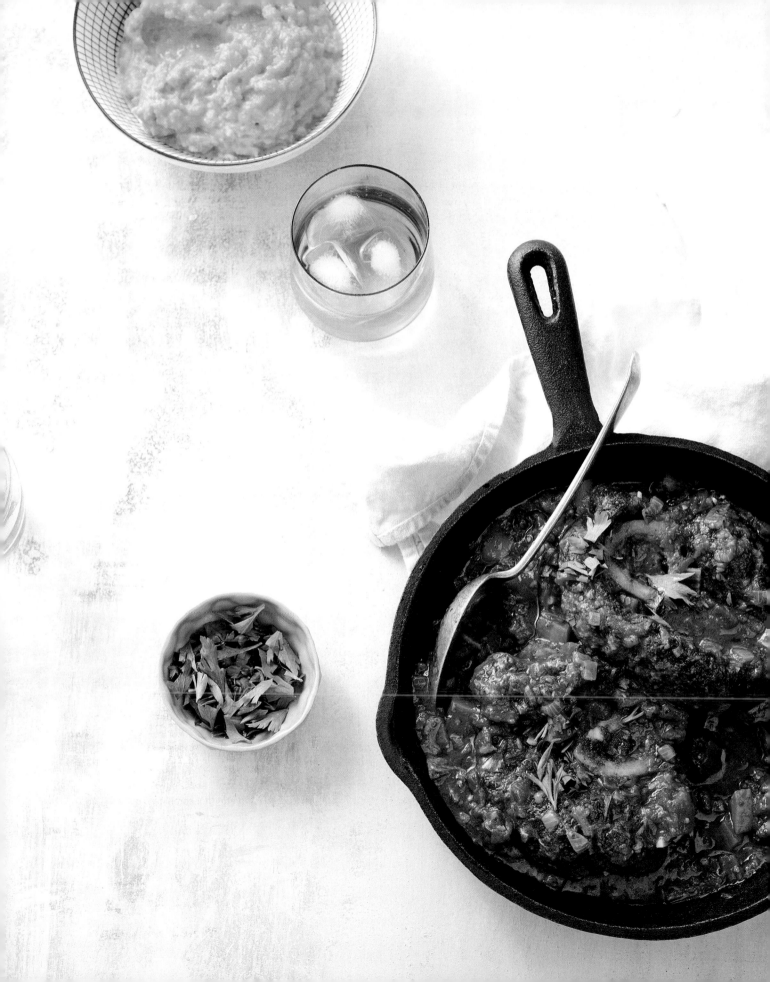

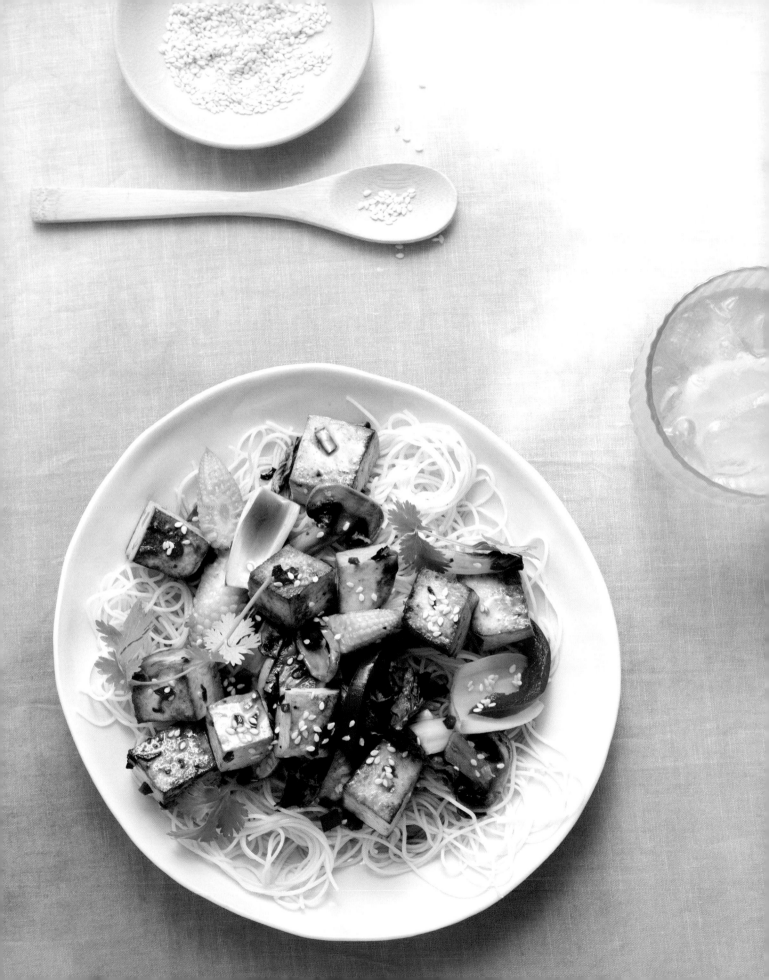

CHILLI TOFU STIR-FRY

SERVES 2

PREP TIME 20 MINUTES +
10 MINUTES SOAKING TIME +
15 MINUTES MARINATING TIME

COOKING TIME 15 MINUTES

DIFFICULTY EASY

This delicious stir-fry is jam-packed with fresh and satisfying ingredients. The combination of chilli and tofu will excite your tastebuds and leave you wanting more! But if you don't like spicy food, then just reduce the amount of chilli to your liking.

7 oz rice vermicelli noodles

1 fresh long red chilli, seeds removed and finely diced

1 garlic clove, crushed

¾ in fresh ginger, finely grated

⅓ cup salt-reduced tamari or soy sauce

12 oz firm tofu, cut into ¾-in cubes

3 teaspoons sesame oil

½ medium red bell pepper, seeds removed and thinly sliced

3½ oz mushrooms, sliced

2 oz baby corn, sliced

4¼ oz bok choy, roughly chopped

1 tablespoon sesame seeds

fresh cilantro leaves, to garnish

Place the noodles in a heatproof bowl and cover with boiling water. Leave for 10 minutes, then loosen the noodles with a fork. Drain and refresh under cool running water. Drain well and set aside.

Whisk the chilli, garlic, ginger, and tamari or soy sauce together in a shallow bowl. Add the tofu and turn gently to coat. Cover with plastic wrap and place in the refrigerator for 15 minutes to marinate.

Remove the tofu and reserve the marinade. Heat a wok over high heat. Add half the oil and carefully swirl it around to coat the sides of the wok. Heat until very hot. Add half of the tofu and cook for 3 minutes or until golden, stirring gently. Transfer to a plate. Reheat the wok and repeat with the remaining tofu.

Heat the remaining oil in the wok over high heat. Add the bell pepper, mushrooms, baby corn, and bok choy and stir-fry for 3–4 minutes or until tender-crisp.

Add the tofu and reserved marinade and stir-fry for 1 minute. Add the noodles and toss gently until heated through, taking care not to break up the tofu.

To serve, place the stir-fry in two serving bowls and sprinkle over the sesame seeds and cilantro.

Ⓒ VEGETARIAN MOUSSAKA

SERVES 2
PREP TIME 15 MINUTES
COOKING TIME 1 HOUR
DIFFICULTY MEDIUM

Moussaka is one of my favourite Greek dishes. Traditionally it is made with meat, but I have created this version so that my vegetarian friends don't miss out!

1 medium eggplant, thinly sliced

oil spray

1½ teaspoons olive oil

½ small brown onion, finely diced

1 garlic clove, crushed

1 medium carrot, coarsely grated

1 teaspoon dried oregano

7¾ oz tinned crushed tomatoes

½ cup salt-reduced vegetable stock

16 oz tinned brown lentils, drained and rinsed

1 medium potato, peeled

1½ oz reduced-fat cheddar cheese, grated

Preheat the oven to 350°F (325°F convection) and line a baking sheet with parchment paper.

Lay the eggplant on the lined baking sheet in a single layer and spray lightly with oil spray. Bake for 15–20 minutes or until tender. Set aside.

Meanwhile, heat the oil in a large saucepan over medium heat. Add the onion, garlic, and carrot and cook for 5 minutes or until soft, stirring occasionally. Add the oregano and cook for 1 minute or until fragrant, stirring constantly.

Stir in the tomatoes, stock, and lentils. Reduce the heat to medium–low and simmer, covered, for 15 minutes, stirring occasionally.

Place the potato in a saucepan and pour in enough cold water to almost cover it. Bring to a boil over high heat and boil for 15 minutes or until the potato is tender, then drain and set aside to cool. When cool enough to handle, cut into ¼-in thick slices.

Spread a small ladle of lentil mixture over the base of a 2-quart capacity baking dish. Layer half of the eggplant slices over the top, followed by half of the remaining lentil mixture. Repeat the layers again, finishing with the lentil mixture on top.

Arrange the potato slices over the lentil mixture and sprinkle over the grated cheese.

Bake in the oven for 30 minutes or until the potato is golden. Let stand for 5 minutes and serve.

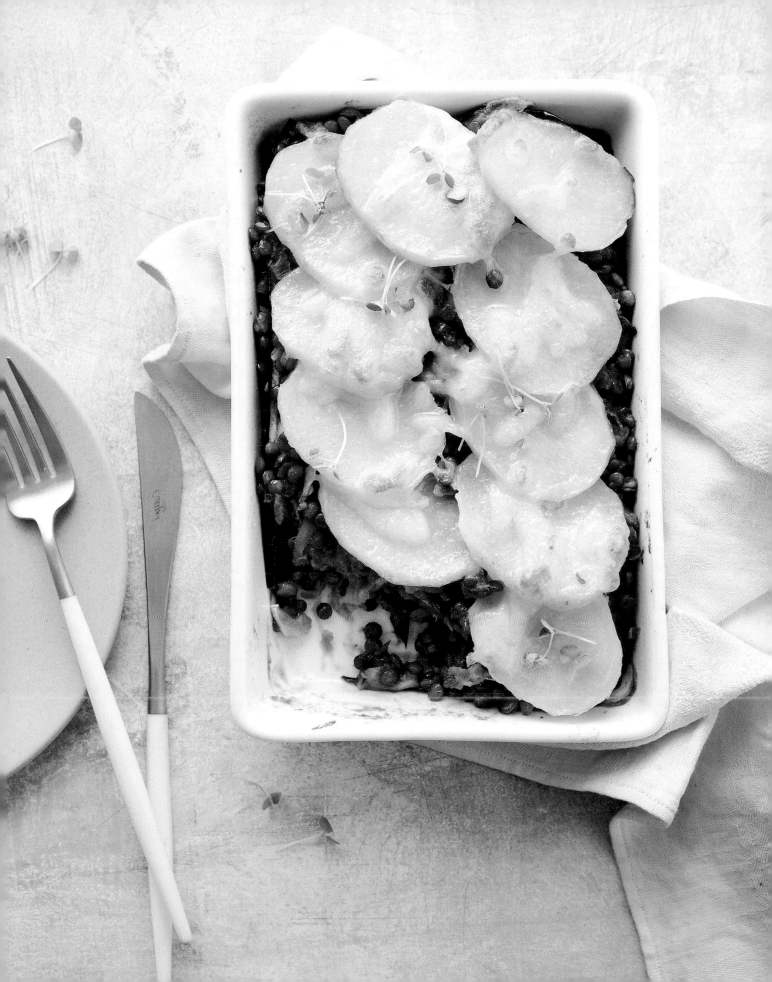

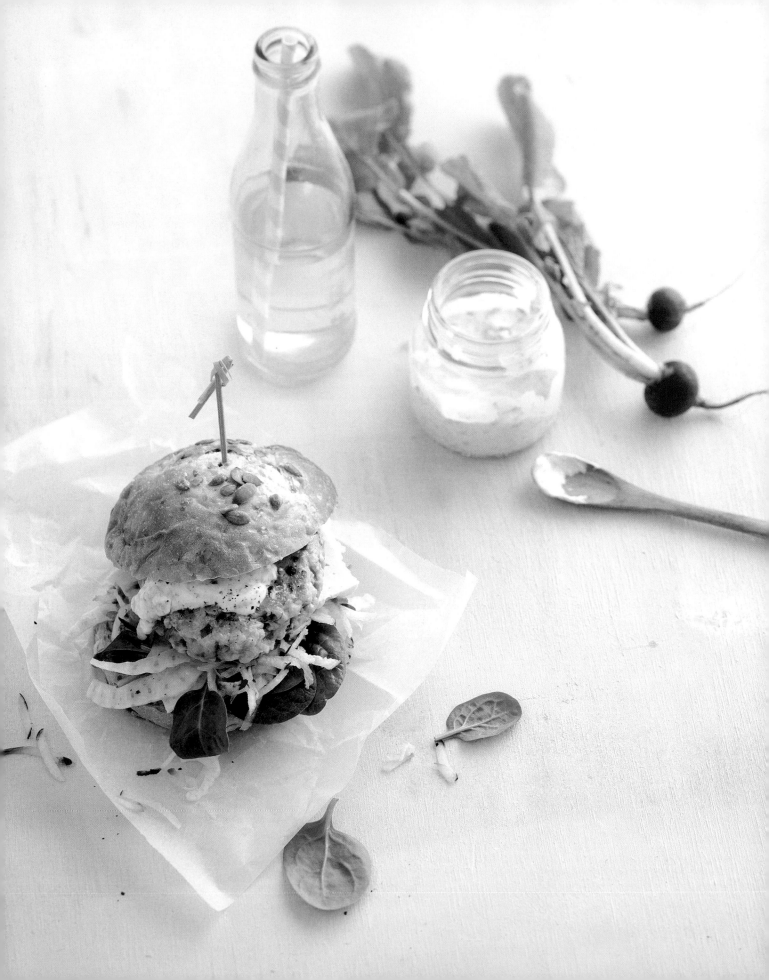

(B) FISH BURGER with CAPER YOGHURT

SERVES 2

PREP TIME 20 MINUTES +
30 MINUTES CHILLING TIME

COOKING TIME 15 MINUTES

DIFFICULTY EASY

Once you have a bite of this burger, you'll be hooked ;) The caper yoghurt adds a nice lemony flavour that complements not only the fish, but the salad too.

one 6-oz salmon fillet, skin removed, deboned and roughly chopped

1 scallion, finely chopped

2 teaspoons finely chopped fresh parsley

½ teaspoon Dijon mustard

sea salt and ground black pepper, to taste

oil spray

1 Lebanese cucumber, grated

4 radishes, grated

1 small fennel bulb, thinly sliced

2 whole wheat bread rolls

1 small handful baby spinach leaves

CAPER YOGHURT

3½ oz low-fat plain yoghurt

1 oz salt-reduced low-fat feta cheese, crumbled

2 tablespoon capers, rinsed, drained, and finely chopped

2 teaspoons chopped fresh dill

lemon juice, to taste

Place the salmon, scallion, parsley, mustard, salt, and pepper in a food processor and pulse briefly until the fish is roughly minced. Using wet hands, shape the mixture into two even patties. Place on a plate, cover with plastic wrap, and refrigerate for 30 minutes.

To make the caper yoghurt, whisk the yoghurt, feta, capers, dill, and lemon juice together in a small bowl.

Heat a large non-stick fry pan over medium heat and spray lightly with oil spray. Add the patties and cook for 4–5 minutes, then carefully turn and cook for a further 4–5 minutes or until cooked through.

Place the cucumber, radish, and fennel in a small bowl and toss gently to combine.

To serve, cut the bread rolls in half and toast lightly in a toaster or under a hot oven broiler. On one half of each roll, layer half of the spinach, cucumber mixture, and a salmon patty. Drizzle over the caper yoghurt and top with the other half of each roll.

CHICKEN & SWEET POTATO CURRY

SERVES 2
PREP TIME 10 MINUTES
COOKING TIME 40 MINUTES
DIFFICULTY EASY

This is such a hearty meal that will warm your insides. I love making this dish during the winter time!

4¼ oz brown rice

3 teaspoons olive oil

½ small brown onion, diced

7 oz boneless skinless chicken breast, cut into 1-in pieces

2 tablespoons korma curry paste

1 garlic clove, crushed

½ cup salt-reduced vegetable stock

5¼ oz tinned crushed tomatoes

1 medium sweet potato, peeled and cut into 1-in cubes

½ cup light coconut milk

1 small handful baby spinach leaves

fresh cilantro sprigs, to garnish

Place the rice and 1¼ cups of water in a small saucepan over high heat and bring to a boil, stirring occasionally. Cover and reduce the heat to medium–low. Simmer for 20–25 minutes or until the liquid is absorbed and the rice is tender. Remove from the heat and let stand, covered, for 5 minutes.

Meanwhile, heat the oil in a medium saucepan over medium heat. Add the onion and cook for 4–5 minutes or until soft and translucent, stirring frequently. Add the chicken and cook for 5 minutes or until lightly browned, stirring frequently.

Add the curry paste and garlic and cook for 2 minutes, stirring constantly. Stir in the stock, tomatoes, and sweet potato. Reduce the heat to medium–low and simmer for 20–25 minutes or until the chicken is cooked through and the sweet potato is tender.

Stir in the coconut milk and spinach and simmer for 5 minutes or until the spinach has wilted.

To serve, place the rice in two serving bowls and top with the chicken and sweet potato curry. Sprinkle over the cilantro.

Ⓑ VEGETABLE & BEAN TACOS

SERVES 2
PREP TIME 10 MINUTES
COOKING TIME 25 MINUTES
DIFFICULTY EASY

Looking for a quick dinner idea? These tacos are quick and easy to make. The filling also works for burritos, quesadillas, and enchiladas.

oil spray

½ small red onion, diced

1 garlic clove, crushed

1 teaspoon ground cumin

½ teaspoon sweet paprika

pinch of chilli powder

1 medium zucchini, diced

¼ medium red bell pepper, seeds removed and diced

2 oz frozen corn kernels

5¼ oz tinned crushed tomatoes

10¾ oz tinned kidney beans, drained and rinsed

1 tablespoon chopped fresh cilantro

lime juice, to taste

sea salt and ground black pepper, to taste

2 whole wheat wraps

4½ oz reduced-fat cheddar cheese, grated

Heat a non-stick fry pan over medium heat and spray lightly with oil spray. Add the onion and cook for 5 minutes or until soft and translucent, stirring occasionally. Add the garlic, cumin, paprika, and chilli powder and cook for 1 minute or until fragrant, stirring constantly.

Add the zucchini, bell pepper, and corn and cook for 5–7 minutes or until the vegetables are tender. Stir in the tomatoes and kidney beans. Reduce the heat to medium–low and simmer for 10 minutes, stirring occasionally.

Remove the pan from the heat. Add the cilantro and lime juice and stir to combine.

Warm the wraps in a large dry fry pan over medium–high heat for 30 seconds on each side. Remove from the heat and cut in half.

To serve, place the wrap halves on two serving plates. Top with the vegetable and bean mixture and sprinkle over the grated cheese. Fold in half.

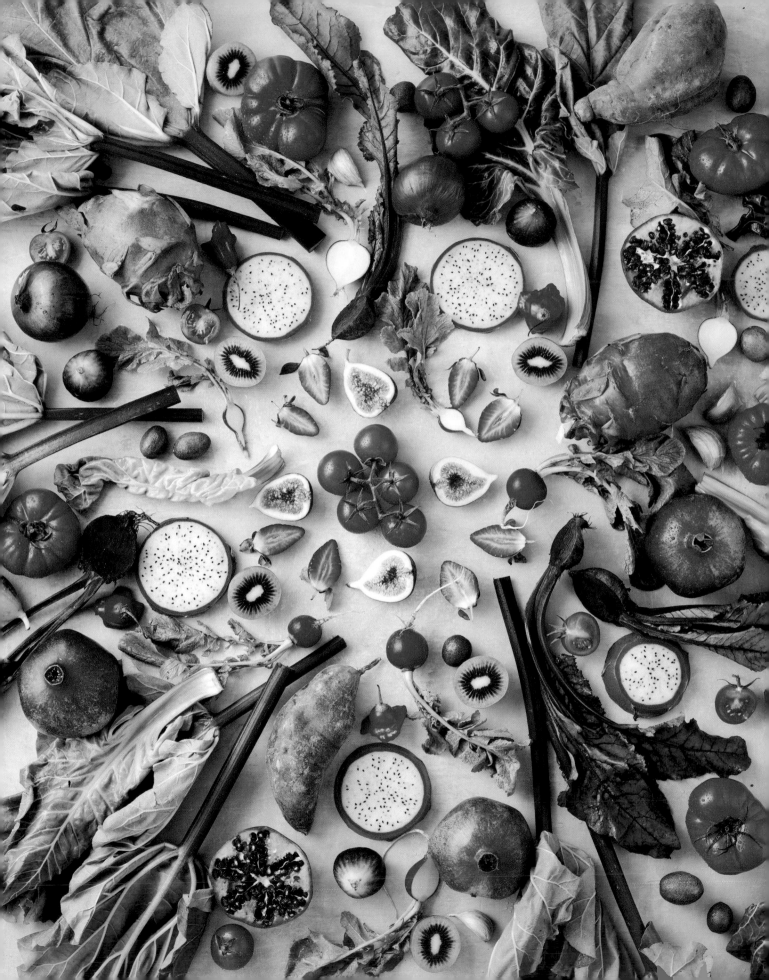

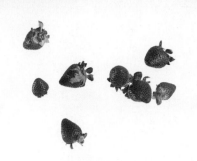

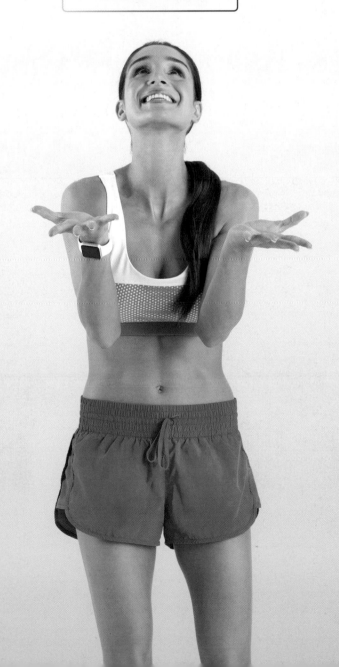

NAUGHTY
MADE NICE

CHOCOLATE BARK

MAKES ABOUT 10

PREP TIME 10 MINUTES +
2–3 HOURS OR OVERNIGHT
SETTING TIME

DIFFICULTY EASY

Here's your chance to get creative. Top your chocolate bark with your favourite nuts, seeds, or dried fruit. You can't go wrong!

17¾ oz dark chocolate, roughly chopped

TOPPINGS

⅔ oz coconut flakes

1¼ oz roast almonds, roughly chopped

1 tablespoon pumpkin seeds (pepitas)

2 tablespoons dried raspberries, strawberries, or goji berries

Line a baking sheet with parchment paper.

Fill a large saucepan with water over medium heat and bring to a simmer.

Place the chocolate in a heatproof bowl and place on top of the saucepan. Ensure that the bottom of the bowl is not touching the water.

Heat the chocolate until completely melted and smooth, stirring constantly.

Pour the melted chocolate onto the lined baking sheet. Use a spatula to ensure that it is spread evenly.

While the chocolate is still warm, sprinkle over the toppings.

Place the sheet in the refrigerator and let set for 2–3 hours or overnight.

To serve, peel off the parchment paper and break the chocolate into shards.

Store in an airtight container in the refrigerator for up to 2 weeks—if it lasts that long!

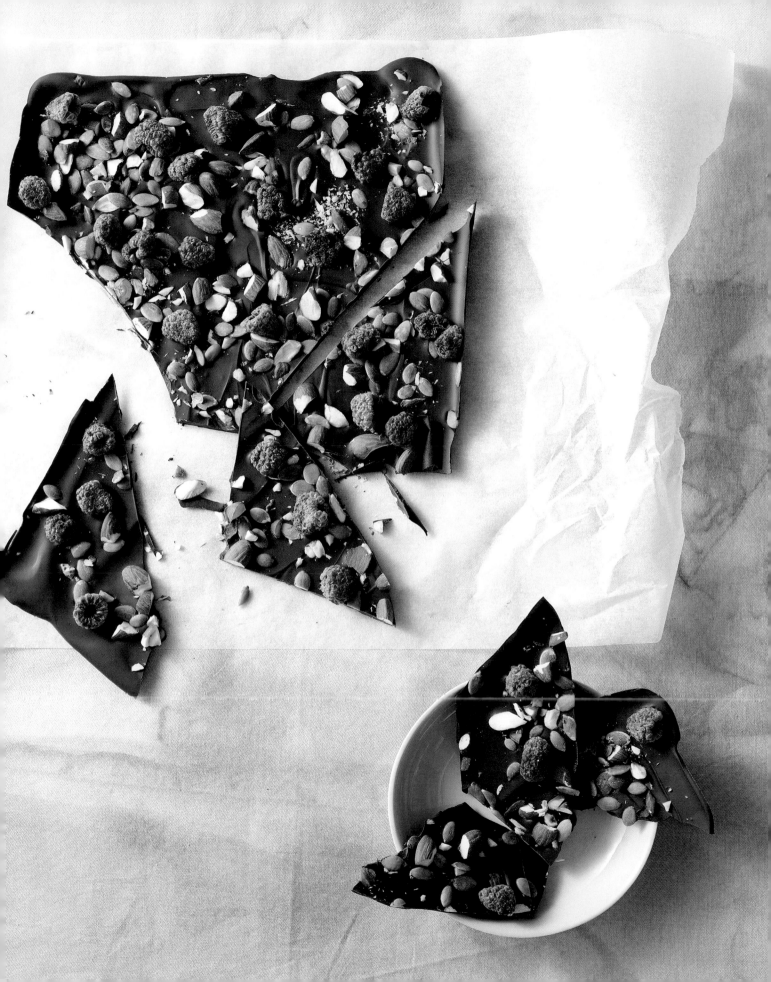

EPIC FRUIT PLATTER

SERVES 1
PREP TIME 15 MINUTES
DIFFICULTY EASY

When creating a fruit platter, I always try and select fruits that are in season—they are fresher and taste so much better!

My favourite fruit selection (subject to seasonal availability):

banana

blueberries

coconut flakes

dragonfruit

figs

kiwi fruit

mango

orange

passionfruit

pawpaw

pineapple

pomegranate

raspberries

strawberries

watermelon

To serve, place the fruit on a large serving platter and decorate with coconut flakes.

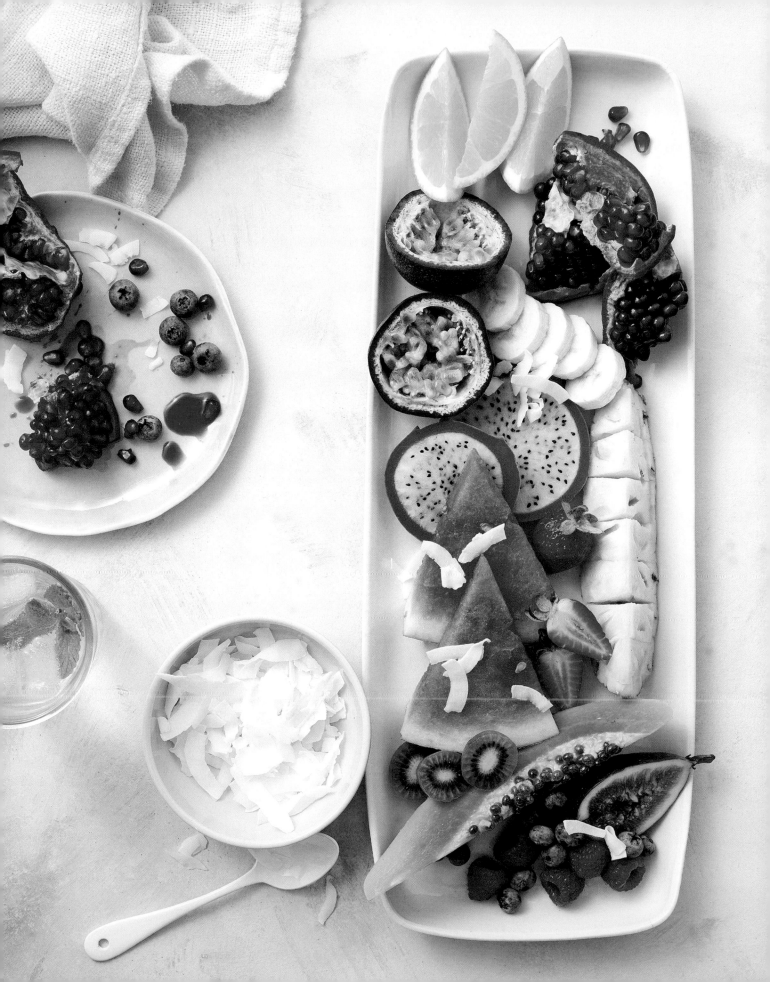

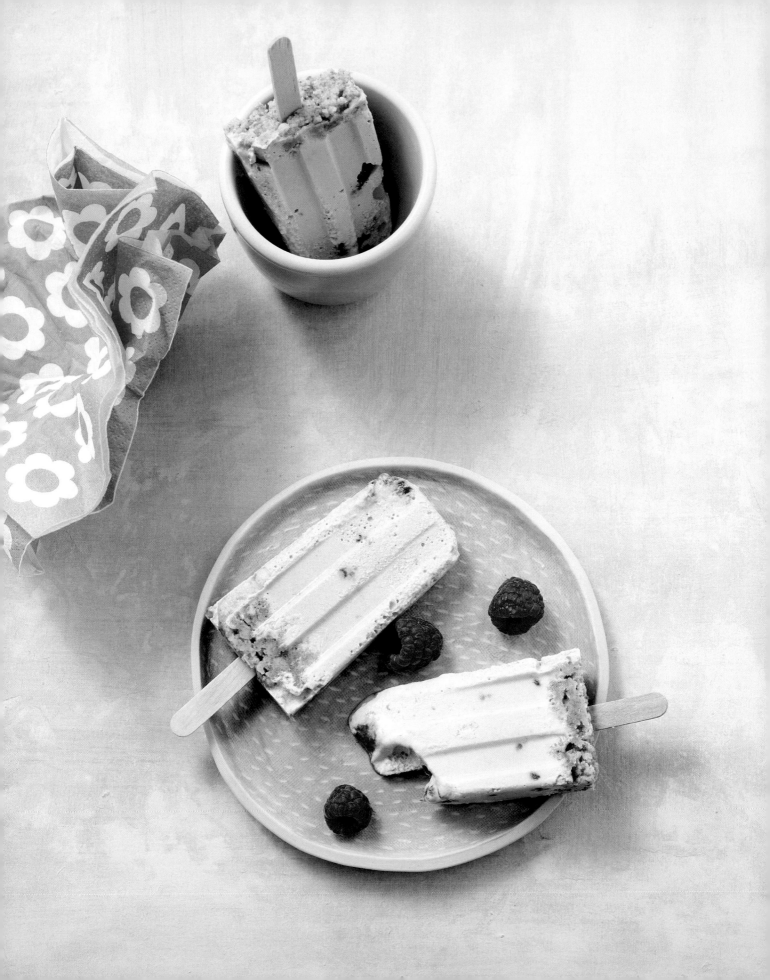

RASPBERRY CHEESECAKE POPSICLES

MAKES 6

PREP TIME 10 MINUTES +
OVERNIGHT FREEZING TIME

DIFFICULTY EASY

Question: What's better than raspberry cheesecake?
Answer: Raspberry cheesecake you can take on the go!

2⅓ oz raspberries, plus extra
for sprinkling

3 oz low-fat plain Greek-style yoghurt

4¼ oz light cream cheese

⅓ cup almond milk

1 teaspoon pure vanilla extract

NUTTY BASE

1¼ oz ground almonds

1 tablespoon coconut sugar

1 tablespoon coconut oil,
melted

To make the nutty base, place the almonds, coconut sugar, and coconut oil in a bowl and stir until the mixture becomes crumbly. Set aside.

Place the raspberries, yoghurt, cream cheese, almond milk, and vanilla in a food processor and process until smooth and creamy.

Evenly pour the cheesecake mixture into the popsicle moulds, sporadically adding some whole fresh raspberries as you go. Ensure that you do not fill the moulds completely, leaving a small gap at the top.

Spoon the nutty base into the top of the popsicle moulds, pressing down gently with the back of a spoon.

Insert the popsicle sticks and freeze overnight.

To remove the popsicles from the moulds, run under hot water for about 15 seconds and carefully pull out.

SWEET POTATO & CACAO BROWNIES

MAKES 16

PREP TIME 10 MINUTES +
10 MINUTES COOLING TIME

COOKING TIME 40 MINUTES

DIFFICULTY EASY

Yes, you heard me right! The idea of including sweet potato in a dessert might weird you out at first, but trust me, you are going to love it! It's chocolatey, gooey, and oh-so-delicious!

2 medium sweet potatoes, peeled and cut into chunks

2½ oz almond meal (about ¾ cup)

2 oz whole wheat flour

1 teaspoon ground cinnamon

10 medjool dates, pitted and chopped

⅓ cup raw cacao powder (see page 49), plus extra for dusting

¼ cup pure maple syrup

pinch of sea salt

Preheat the oven to 350°F (325°F convection) and line an 8-in square cake tin with parchment paper.

Fill a saucepan with water until 2 in deep and insert a steamer basket. Cover with a lid and bring the water to the boil over high heat, then reduce the heat to medium. Add the sweet potato and steam for 15 minutes or until very soft.

Place the sweet potato, almond meal, flour, cinnamon, dates, cacao powder, maple syrup, and salt in a food processor and process until a smooth batter has formed.

Pour the batter into the lined cake tin and bake in the oven for 20–25 minutes or until a skewer inserted into the centre comes out clean.

Leave to cool in the tin for 10 minutes. Remove from the tin and cut into even squares.

To serve, dust with extra cacao powder.

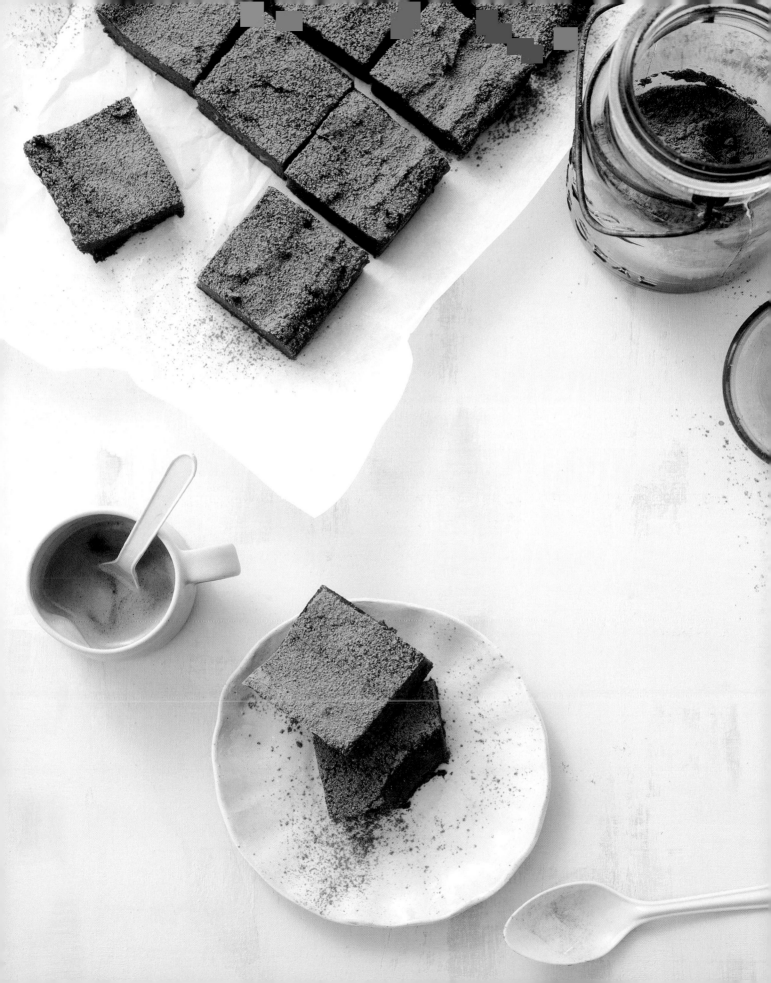

FROZEN CHOCOLATE BANANA BITES

SERVES 2

PREP TIME 5 MINUTES +
30 MINUTES FREEZING TIME

COOKING TIME 2 MINUTES

DIFFICULTY EASY

Got a spare 5 minutes? These are so easy to prepare and you only need three ingredients! Remember, you don't always need lots of expensive ingredients to create a delicious dessert.

5¾ oz dark chocolate chips

1 tablespoon coconut oil, melted

1 medium banana, peeled and cut into ¼-in thick slices

Line a baking sheet with parchment paper.

Place the chocolate in a microwave-safe bowl and warm in the microwave at medium heat for 30 seconds. Remove from the microwave and stir. Continue warming the chocolate for 30 seconds at a time until melted and smooth, stirring in between. Add the coconut oil and stir until well combined.

Using a fork, dip the banana slices into the chocolate mixture and place on the lined sheet.

Place the sheet in the freezer and allow to set for 30 minutes.

To serve, enjoy straight from the freezer.

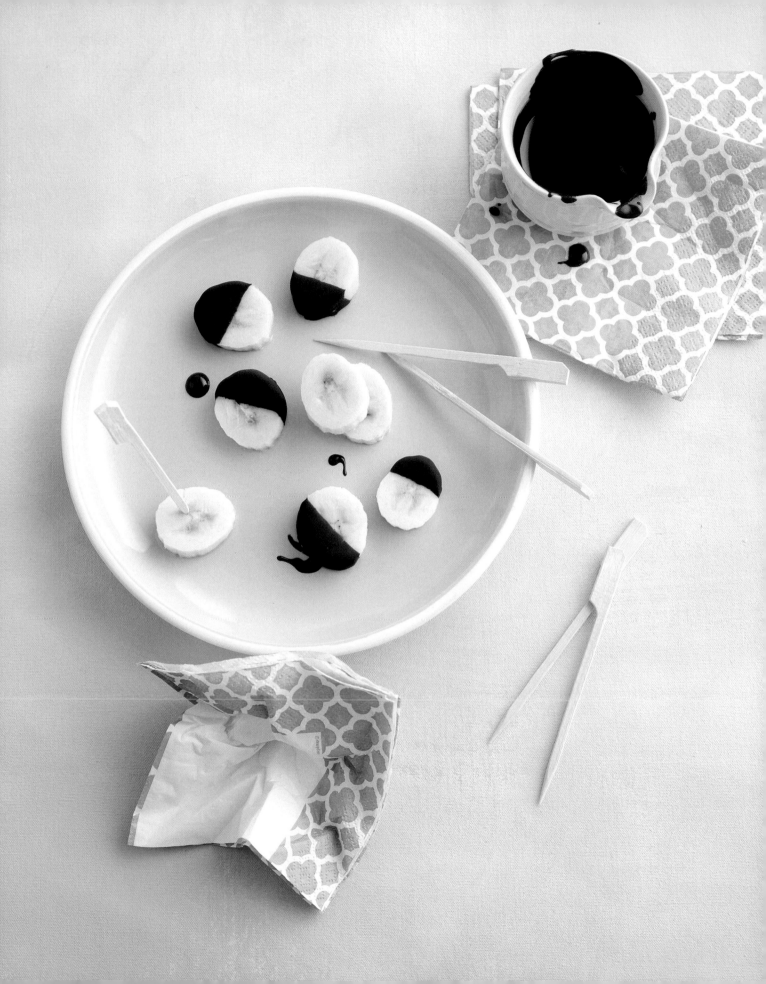

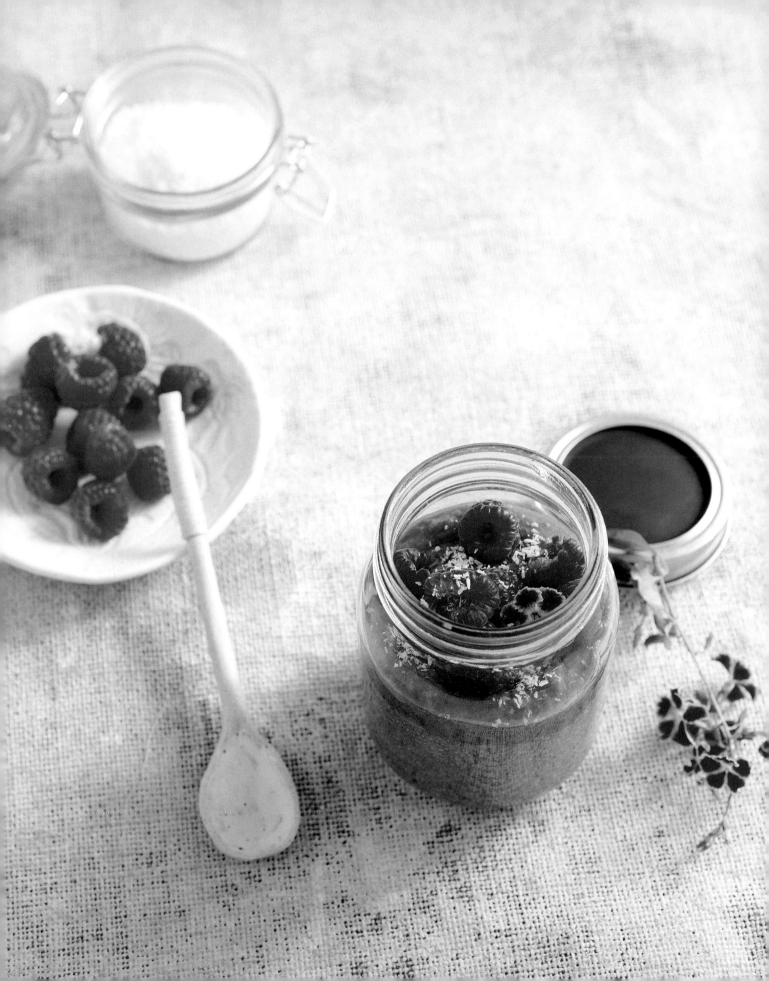

CHOCOLATE & RASPBERRY CHIA PUDDING

SERVES 1

PREP TIME 5 MINUTES +
20 MINUTES–1 HOUR OR
OVERNIGHT CHILLING TIME

DIFFICULTY EASY

You seriously can't go wrong with this combo. The tartness of the raspberries really helps to balance out the sweetness of the chocolate. Try experimenting with the topping by using blueberries, blackberries, or mixed berries to shake things up. Too good!

¼ cup chia seeds

1 cup milk of choice

½ teaspoon ground cinnamon

2 teaspoons raw cacao powder
(see page 49)

pinch of sea salt

TOPPING

2⅓ oz raspberries

2 tablespoons milk of choice

3 medjool dates, pitted
and roughly chopped

desiccated coconut, to garnish

Place the chia seeds, milk, cinnamon, cacao powder, and salt in a mixing bowl and stir until well combined. Pour into a 2-cup capacity jar and place in the refrigerator to set for 20 minutes to 1 hour or overnight.

Meanwhile, to make the topping, place 1¾ oz of the raspberries, milk, and dates in a high-powered blender and blend until smooth.

To serve, top the chocolate chia pudding with the raspberry sauce and sprinkle over the remaining raspberries and coconut.

SNICKERS SLICE

MAKES 12
PREP TIME 15 MINUTES +
1 HOUR 30 MINUTES
CHILLING TIME
DIFFICULTY EASY

Chocolate + peanut butter = enough said! This healthier version of a Snickers bar is to die for!

BASE

1 cup unsalted cashew nuts

8 medjool dates, pitted and chopped

1 teaspoon vanilla bean paste or pure vanilla extract

1 tablespoon coconut oil

pinch of sea salt

PEANUT FILLING

2¾ oz roasted unsalted peanuts

2 tablespoons 100% natural peanut butter

8 medjool dates, pitted and chopped

½ cup almond milk (or milk of choice)

CHOCOLATE LAYER

1 oz raw cacao powder (see page 49)

1¾ oz coconut oil, melted

2 tablespoons pure maple syrup

crushed peanuts, to garnish (optional)

Line a 10 in x 6 in slice tin with plastic film.

To make the base, place the cashews in a food processor and process until crumbly. Add the dates, vanilla, coconut oil, and salt and process until well combined. The mixture should be a little sticky. If it's too thick, add 1–2 tablespoons of water.

Using wet hands, press the mixture into the lined slice tin and place in the freezer while you make the peanut filling.

To make the peanut filling, place the peanuts in a food processor and process until crumbly. Add the peanut butter, dates, almond milk, and 3 tablespoons of water and process until smooth. Ensure that you scrape down the sides of the processor bowl occasionally.

Pour the peanut filling over the base and place in the refrigerator to set for 1 hour.

To make the chocolate layer, whisk the cacao powder, coconut oil, and maple syrup together in a bowl. Pour the chocolate layer over the peanut filling and sprinkle over the peanuts (if using).

Place the slice in the refrigerator for 30 minutes to set, then cut into bars and serve.

Store in an airtight container in the refrigerator for up to 10 days.

THREE-INGREDIENT CHOCOLATE NUT BUTTER CUPS

MAKES 24
PREP TIME 10 MINUTES +
45 MINUTES FREEZING TIME
COOKING TIME 2 MINUTES
DIFFICULTY EASY

Almond butter? Cashew butter? Or how about peanut butter? The choice is yours! You can also sprinkle the nut butter cups with a few sea salt flakes, if you like.

8½ oz dark chocolate chips
⅓ cup coconut oil, melted

8½ oz 100% natural nut butter of choice

Place 24 mini-cupcake liners in a 24-cup muffin tin.

Place the chocolate in a microwave-safe bowl and warm in the microwave on medium heat for 30 seconds. Remove from the microwave and stir. Continue warming the chocolate in the microwave for 30 seconds at a time until melted and smooth, stirring in between. Add 2 tablespoons of coconut oil and stir until well combined.

Spoon 1 teaspoon of the chocolate mixture into each paper liner. Use the spoon to push the chocolate up the sides of each paper liner slightly. This will help to hold the filling in.

Place the tin in the freezer for 10 minutes to set.

Meanwhile, place the remaining coconut oil and nut butter in a small bowl and mix until well combined.

Remove the tin from the freezer and spoon about 2 teaspoons of the nut butter mixture into each of the paper liners. Place back into the freezer to set for 5 minutes.

If the remaining chocolate mixture has begun to set, microwave for 15 seconds and stir until smooth.

Remove the tin from the freezer and spoon the remaining chocolate mixture evenly over the nut butter. Ensure that there is no nut butter visible.

Place the tin in the freezer for 30 minutes or until the nut butter cups have set. Peel off the paper liners and serve.

Store in an airtight container in the refrigerator for up to a week.

DESSERT PIZZA

SERVES 2
PREP TIME 10 MINUTES
COOKING TIME 15 MINUTES
DIFFICULTY EASY

Pizza night with friends? This recipe is sure to be a crowd favourite! If you use frozen berries rather than fresh ones, make sure that you let them thaw completely before topping your pizza.

BROWNIE BASE

1¾ oz almond meal

1¾ oz all-purpose flour

2 tablespoons cornstarch

1 egg

2 tablespoons raw cacao powder (see page 49)

2 tablespoons coconut sugar

½ teaspoon baking powder

½ cup milk of choice

1 teaspoon coconut oil, melted

TOPPING

4¼ oz low-fat cream cheese

4½ oz low-fat plain Greek-style yoghurt

½ teaspoon pure vanilla extract

strawberries, hulled and sliced, to serve

raspberries, to serve

coconut flakes, to serve

mint leaves, to serve

Preheat the oven to 350°F (325°F convection) and line a pizza pan with parchment paper.

To make the brownie base, place the almond meal, flour, and cornstarch in a mixing bowl and stir until well combined. Add the egg, cacao powder, coconut sugar, baking powder, and milk and stir until well combined.

Pour the mixture into the centre of the lined pan and bake in the oven for 10 minutes. Brush with the coconut oil and bake for a further 5 minutes. Set aside to cool slightly.

Meanwhile, to make the topping, place the cream cheese, yoghurt, and vanilla in a bowl and stir until well combined. Spread onto the brownie base using a spatula.

To serve, top with the strawberries, raspberries, coconut flakes, and mint. Cut the pizza into smaller pieces using a sharp knife.

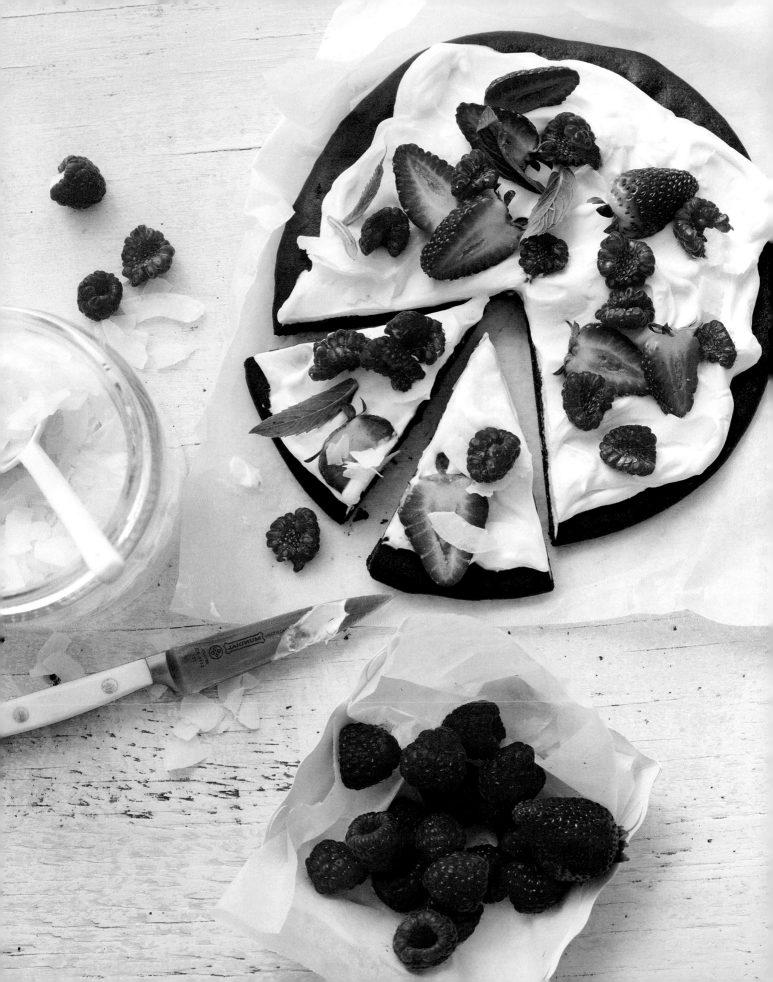

HEALTHIER TIRAMISU

SERVES 6–8

PREP TIME 20 MINUTES +
10 MINUTES RESTING TIME +
20 MINUTES COOLING TIME +
OVERNIGHT CHILLING TIME

COOKING TIME 25 MINUTES

DIFFICULTY MEDIUM

When I go out for dinner with my family, I can't say no to a delicious tiramisu. It would have to be my favourite dessert by far! If you're a tiramisu lover like me, then you've got to try this (healthier) recipe!

raw cacao powder
(see page 49), for dusting

LADYFINGERS

2 large eggs

½ cup almond milk

2 teaspoons pure
maple syrup

1 teaspoon vanilla bean
paste or pure vanilla extract

6 oz apple sauce

7 oz coconut sugar

2 cups oat flour

1 tablespoon baking powder

1 teaspoon sea salt

VANILLA BEAN CREAM

2 large eggs

2½ tablespoons

1 tablespoon vanilla bean
paste or pure vanilla extract

1 teaspoon pure maple syrup

1 cup almond milk

7 oz mascarpone,
at room temperature

COFFEE SAUCE

½ cup strong coffee, at room
temperature

½ cup apple juice

Preheat the oven to 350°F (325°F convection) and line two baking sheets with parchment paper.

To make the ladyfingers, whisk the eggs, almond milk, maple syrup, and vanilla together in a large bowl. Add the apple sauce and the coconut sugar and whisk to combine again. Place the oat flour, baking powder, and salt in a separate bowl and mix until well combined. Add the oat mixture to the egg mixture, then fold together until a light and fluffy batter forms. Let the batter to rest for 10 minutes.

Scoop the batter into a large piping bag and pipe 3-in long lines onto the lined baking sheets until all of the mixture has been used. Leave a bit less than an inch in between each line to allow room for spreading during baking. Bake in the oven for 15 minutes or until firm when tapped. Transfer to a wire rack and set aside to cool.

To make the vanilla bean cream, fill a large saucepan with water over medium heat and bring to a simmer. Place a heatproof bowl on top of the saucepan. Add the eggs and cornstarch and whisk to combine. Add the vanilla, maple syrup, and almond milk and whisk to combine again. Cook for a further 10 minutes or until thickened, whisking constantly. Ensure that you do not overcook the mixture as this will cause the eggs to curdle.

Pour the egg mixture into a bowl and set aside to cool. Once completely cooled, add the mascarpone and mix until well combined.

Line a 6½ in x 4 in loaf tin with plastic wrap, leaving some overhanging on each side. Set aside.

To make the coffee sauce, whisk the coffee and apple juice together in a shallow bowl.

To assemble, dunk both sides of the ladyfingers into the coffee sauce and layer on the bottom of the loaf tin. Spread an even layer of vanilla cream over the ladyfingers. Repeat the layers again until the tin is filled and all of the ladyfingers and vanilla cream have been used. Cover with plastic wrap and place in the refrigerator to set overnight.

Use the overhanging plastic wrap to remove the tiramisu from the tin, then flip it over onto a serving dish. Gently peel off the remaining plastic wrap and dust with cacao powder. Cut into slices and serve.

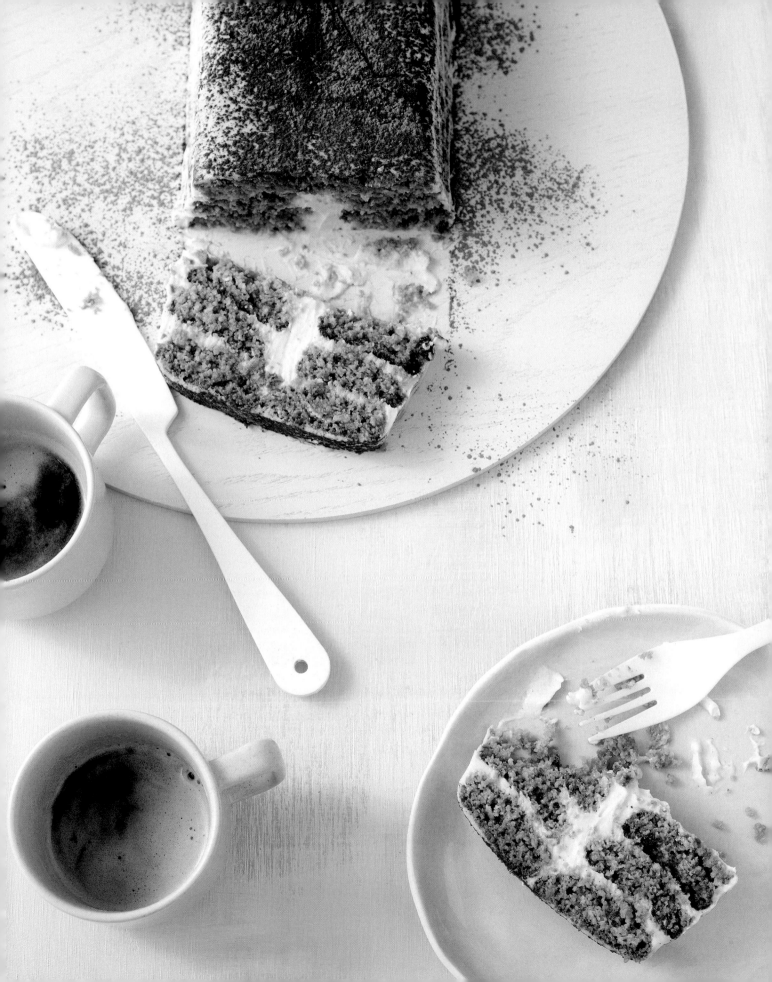

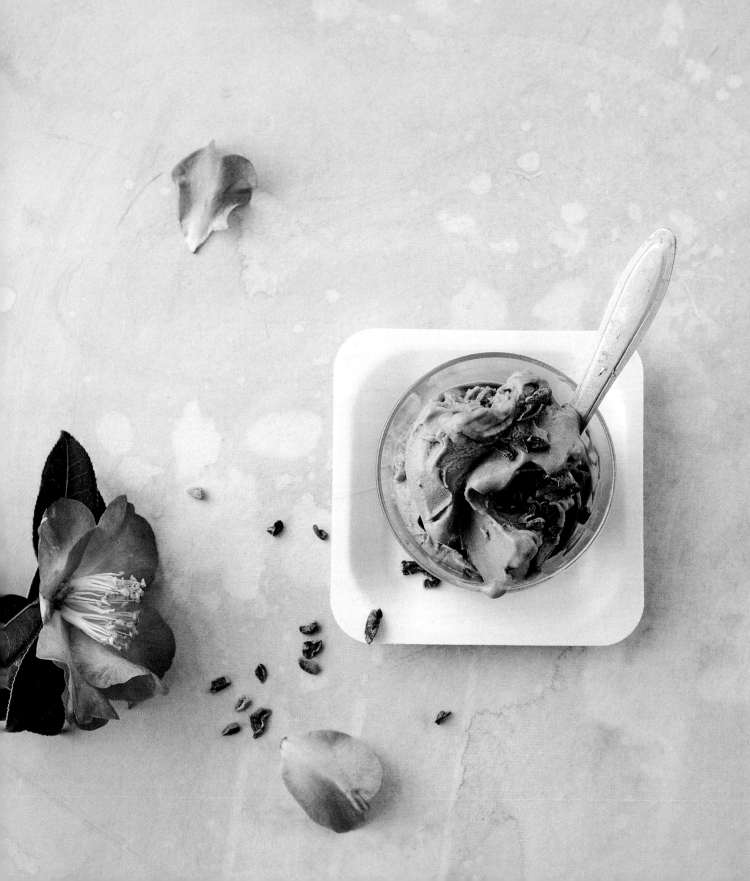

CHOCOLATE & BANANA "SOFT SERVE" NICE CREAM

SERVES 2
PREP TIME 5 MINUTES
DIFFICULTY EASY

The trick to a delicious nice cream is ripe bananas—the riper, the better! Just peel, slice, and place in the freezer and you're halfway there!

2 frozen medium bananas, chopped
½ cup almond milk or low-fat milk
1 tablespoon 100% natural almond butter

1 tablespoon raw cacao powder (see page 49)
1 tablespoon raw cacao nibs

Place the banana, milk, almond butter, and cacao powder in a food processor and process until smooth and creamy.

To serve, place the nice cream in two serving bowls and sprinkle over the cacao nibs.

HEALTHY HOT CHOCOLATE

SERVES 1
PREP TIME 5 MINUTES
COOKING TIME 2 MINUTES
DIFFICULTY EASY

Best served on a cold winter's night with friends.

2 oz raw cacao powder (see page 49)
1 tablespoon coconut sugar
½ teaspoon ground cinnamon

½ teaspoon ground cardamom
1 cup milk of choice

Mix the cacao powder, coconut sugar, cinnamon, and cardamom together in a small bowl. You can store this mixture in an airtight container for future use.

Place a heaped tablespoon of the hot chocolate mixture in a large mug and pour over a dash of boiling water. Stir to combine.

Heat the milk in a small saucepan over high heat until hot, but not boiling. Pour into the mug and stir until well combined.

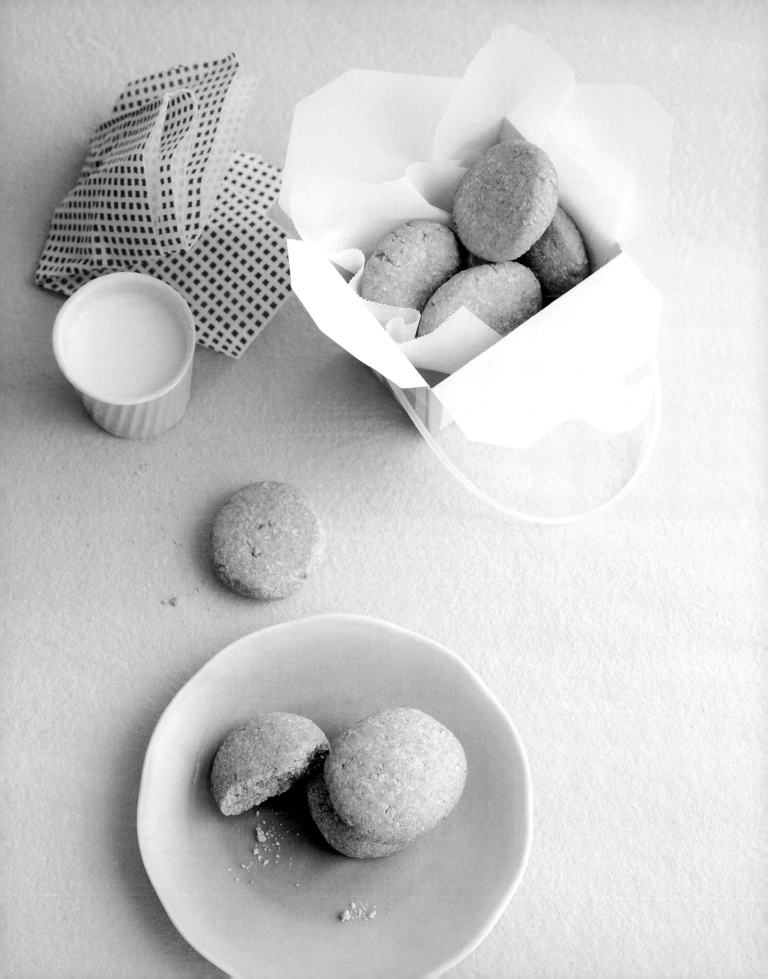

COCONUT & LIME COOKIES

MAKES ABOUT 10
PREP TIME 10 MINUTES
COOKING TIME 12 MINUTES
DIFFICULTY EASY

The sweet and tangy flavours in this recipe will take your mind to a tropical island! These cookies make a great summer treat.

4¼ oz spelt flour
⅔ oz desiccated coconut
3 oz honey

2 tablespoons coconut oil, melted
finely grated zest and juice of 1 lime
pinch of sea salt

Preheat the oven to 350°F (325°F convection) and line a baking sheet with baking paper.

Place the flour, coconut, honey, coconut oil, lime zest and juice, and salt in a large mixing bowl and stir until well combined and a dough forms.

Scoop out 1 heaped tablespoon of the mixture and roll into a ball using wet hands. Place on the prepared baking sheet and flatten slightly using the back of a spoon. Repeat with the remaining mixture. Ensure that you leave ¾ in between each ball to allow room for spreading during baking.

Bake for 10–12 minutes or until the edges of the cookies are slightly brown. Leave to cool for 2–3 minutes on the sheet before moving to a cooling rack to cool completely before serving.

Store in an airtight container for up to 10 days.

MANGO & PASSIONFRUIT NICE CREAM

SERVES 2
PREP TIME 10 MINUTES
DIFFICULTY EASY

Mangoes are my absolute FAVOURITE. I'm obsessed! This dessert is perfect in summertime when they are in season.

1 medium mango, peeled, chopped and frozen
1 passionfruit, pulp removed

½ cup light coconut milk
finely grated zest and juice of ½ lime

Place the mango, half of the passionfruit pulp, coconut milk, lime zest, and juice in a food processor and process until smooth and creamy.

To serve, place the nice cream in two serving bowls and top with the remaining passionfruit pulp.

BLUEBERRY & CASHEW MINI TARTS

MAKES 12

PREP TIME 25 MINUTES +
1–2 HOURS SOAKING TIME +
1–2 HOURS FREEZING TIME

DIFFICULTY EASY

A great little dessert to bring along to a dinner party with friends. Sweet, decadent, and healthy—it really hits the spot!

BASE

1¾ oz walnuts

1¾ oz almond meal

8 medjool dates, pitted

1 tablespoon coconut oil, melted

CASHEW FILLING

4¾ oz unsalted cashew nuts, soaked in water for 1–2 hours

¼ cup milk of choice

2 teaspoons coconut oil, melted

1 tablespoon pure maple syrup

¼ teaspoon vanilla bean paste or pure vanilla extract

BLUEBERRY FILLING

2⅓ oz unsalted cashew nuts, soaked in water for 1–2 hours

1½ tablespoons milk of choice

3 oz frozen blueberries, lightly thawed

2 teaspoons coconut oil, melted

2 teaspoons pure maple syrup

finely grated zest and juice of 1 small orange

extra blueberries and finely grated orange zest, for sprinkling (optional)

Place 12 cupcake liners in a 12-cup muffin tin.

To make the base, place the walnuts, almond meal, dates, and coconut oil in a food processor and process until crumbly. The mixture should stick together when pressed. If too dry, add up to 2 tablespoons of melted coconut oil until the mixture sticks together.

Press the base mixture evenly into the bottom of the lined muffin cups. Place in the refrigerator to set while you make the cashew filling.

To make the cashew filling, place the drained cashews, milk, coconut oil, maple syrup, and vanilla in a food processor and process until smooth. Spoon evenly over the base, leaving space for the blueberry filling. Place in the refrigerator while you make the blueberry filling.

To make the blueberry filling, place the drained cashews, milk, blueberries, coconut oil, maple syrup, orange zest, and juice in a food processor and process until smooth. Spoon evenly over the cashew filling.

Place the muffin tin in the freezer to set for 1–2 hours or overnight.

Remove the mini tarts from the freezer 20 minutes before serving. Top with the extra blueberries and orange zest, if desired. Store in the refrigerator for 1–2 days or in the freezer for up to 2 months.

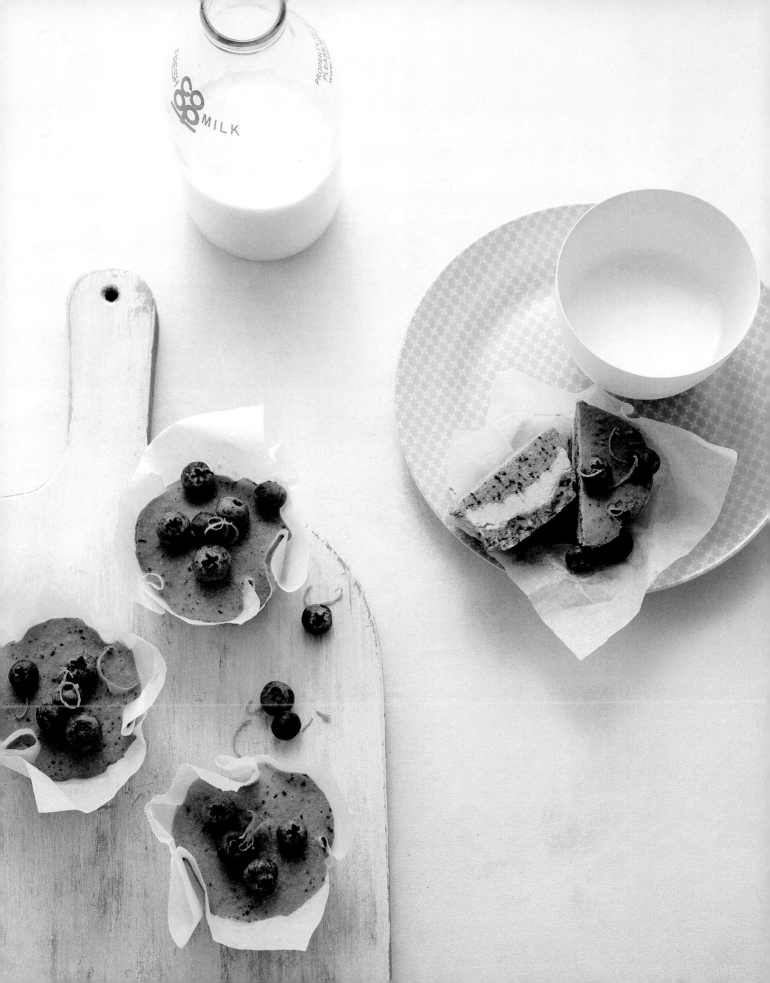

FUDGY BROWNIES

MAKES 12
PREP TIME 10 MINUTES
COOKING TIME 35 MINUTES
DIFFICULTY EASY

These brownies are the ultimate comfort food. Enjoy with a dollop of coconut ice cream for an extra special treat!

4½ oz whole wheat flour

2¾ oz raw cacao powder (see page 49)

pinch of sea salt

¾ cup coconut oil, melted and cooled

1 tablespoon pure maple syrup

7 oz coconut sugar

1 tablespoon pure vanilla extract

3 large eggs

4½ oz dark chocolate chips (about 1¼ cups), plus extra for sprinkling (optional)

Preheat the oven to 350°F (325°F convection) and line an 8-in square cake tin with parchment paper.

Place the flour, cacao powder, and salt in a mixing bowl and mix until well combined. Set aside.

Place the coconut oil, maple syrup, coconut sugar, and vanilla in another large mixing bowl and mix until well combined. Add 1 egg and stir until just combined. Repeat with the remaining eggs.

Add the flour mixture to the egg mixture and gently stir to combine. Stir until there are no streaks of flour left, but avoid over-mixing. Gently fold in the chocolate chips.

Pour the brownie mixture into the lined cake tin and sprinkle with extra chocolate chips, if desired.

Bake in the oven for 30–35 minutes or until the brownie feels set and a thin crust has formed on the top. A skewer or toothpick inserted into the centre should be a little wet, but have some moist crumbs on it. The brownie will continue to cook as it cools in the tin.

Leave the brownie to cool completely in the tin, then cut into 12 even squares. Store in an airtight container at room temperature for up to 4 days or refrigerate for a fudgier texture.

CHOC CHIA COOKIES

MAKES 24
PREP TIME 10 MINUTES
COOKING TIME 15 MINUTES
DIFFICULTY EASY

The cookies are a perfect accompaniment to your favourite herbal tea. They're super rich, so you'll only need one or two to satisfy your sweet tooth.

2 tablespoons chia seeds

5 oz blanched almonds

1 cup plus 2 tablespoons walnuts

1 tablespoon raw cacao powder (see page 49)

¼ cup light coconut cream

1¾ oz coconut sugar

1 egg

1 teaspoon pure vanilla extract

5¾ oz dark chocolate chips

Preheat the oven to 350°F (325°F convection) and line a baking sheet with parchment paper.

Soak the chia seeds in 2½ tablespoons of hot water and let sit while you prepare the cookie mixture. This will create a "gel."

Place the almonds and walnuts in a food processor and process until crumbly.

Add the cacao powder, coconut cream, and coconut sugar and pulse until well combined. Add the chia-seed gel, egg, vanilla, and chocolate chips and pulse until well combined.

Scoop out 1 heaped tablespoon of the mixture and roll into a ball using wet hands. Place on the prepared baking sheet and flatten slightly using the back of a spoon. Repeat with the remaining mixture. Ensure that you leave ¾ in between each ball to allow room for spreading during baking.

Bake in the oven for 15 minutes. The cookies should still be soft to touch, but will harden upon cooling. Leave to cool on the tray before serving.

Store in an airtight container for up to 10 days.

CHOC-MINT BLISS BALLS

MAKES ABOUT 8
PREP TIME 5 MINUTES +
30 MINUTES CHILLING TIME
DIFFICULTY EASY

After-dinner mint, anybody? These little babies are a great palate cleanser!

3½ oz almond meal

2 tablespoons raw cacao powder
(see page 49), plus extra for dusting

½ teaspoon pure vanilla extract

1 teaspoon peppermint extract

2 tablespoons pure maple syrup

Line a baking sheet with parchment paper.

Place the almond meal, cacao powder, vanilla, peppermint, and maple syrup in a mixing bowl and mix until well combined. The mixture should be a little sticky. If it is too thick, add 1–2 tablespoons of water.

Scoop out 1 heaped tablespoon of the mixture and roll into a ball using wet hands.

Place the balls on the lined baking sheet and refrigerate for 30 minutes.

To serve, lightly dust with extra cacao powder. Store in an airtight container in the refrigerator for up to a week.

LEMON PIE BLISS BALLS

MAKES ABOUT 8
PREP TIME 5 MINUTES +
30 MINUTES CHILLING TIME
DIFFICULTY EASY

These remind me of lemon meringue pie, but a bite-sized version. So delicious!

3½ oz almond meal

1¾ oz desiccated coconut,
plus extra for rolling

finely grated zest and juice of ½ lemon

½ teaspoon pure vanilla extract

2 tablespoons honey

Line a baking sheet with parchment paper.

Place the almond meal, coconut, lemon zest and juice, vanilla, and honey in a bowl and mix until well combined. The mixture should be a little sticky. If it is too thick, add 1–2 tablespoons of water.

Scoop out 1 heaped tablespoon of the mixture and roll into a ball using wet hands.

Place the balls on the lined baking sheet and refrigerate for 30 minutes.

To serve, roll through some extra coconut to coat. Store in an airtight container in the refrigerator for up to a week.

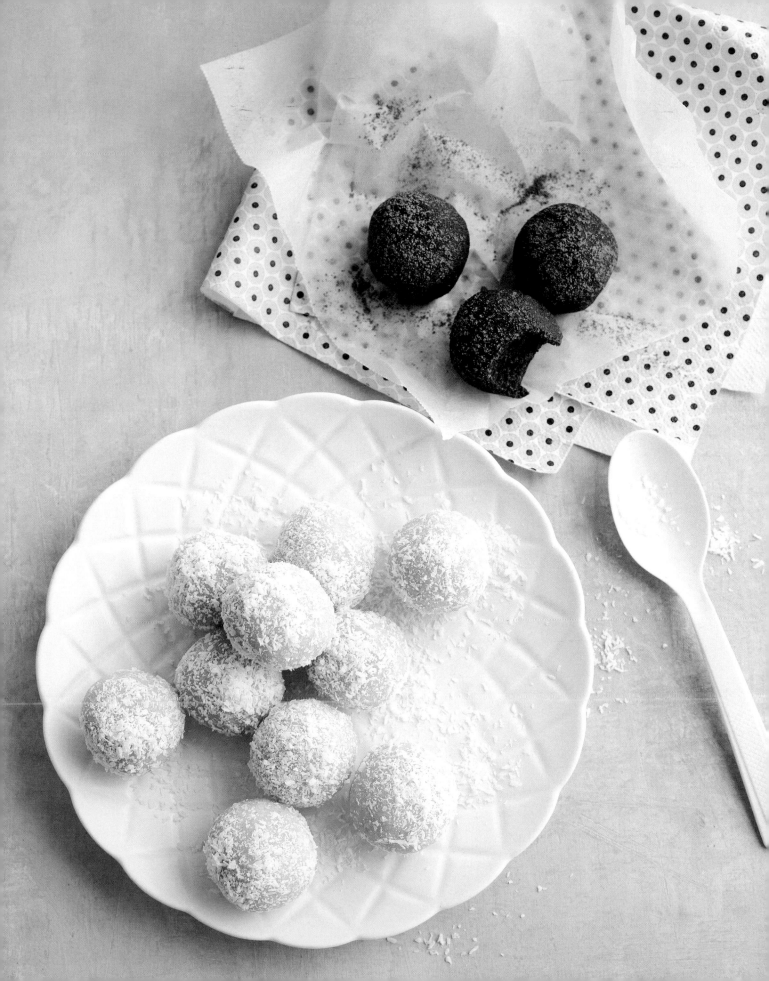

RASPBERRY COCONUT BLISS BALLS

MAKES ABOUT 8

PREP TIME 5 MINUTES +
30 MINUTES CHILLING TIME

DIFFICULTY EASY

Sometimes I'll have one or two of these after dinner with a big mug of peppermint tea. Best!

3½ oz unsalted cashew nuts

2⅓ oz raspberries

1¾ oz desiccated coconut, plus extra for rolling

2 tablespoons 100% natural cashew butter

½ teaspoon pure vanilla extract

2 tablespoons pure maple syrup

Line a baking sheet with parchment paper.

Place the cashews in a food processor and process until crumbly.

Add the raspberries, coconut, cashew butter, vanilla, and maple syrup and process until well combined. The mixture should be a little sticky. If it is too thick, add 1–2 tablespoons of water.

Scoop out 1 heaped tablespoon of the mixture and roll into a ball using wet hands.

Place the balls on the lined baking sheet and refrigerate for 30 minutes.

To serve, roll through extra coconut to coat. Store in an airtight container in the refrigerator for up to a week.

SALTED CARAMEL BLISS BALLS

MAKES ABOUT 8

PREP TIME 5 MINUTES +
30 MINUTES CHILLING TIME

DIFFICULTY EASY

Feel like something sweet? Or maybe a little salty? These bliss balls give you the best of both worlds!

3½ oz unsalted cashew nuts

10 medjool dates, pitted

½ teaspoon pure vanilla extract

generous pinch of sea salt

Line a baking sheet with parchment paper.

Place the cashews in a food processor and process until crumbly.

Add the dates, vanilla, and salt and process until well combined. The mixture should be a little sticky. If it is too thick, add 1–2 tablespoons of water.

Scoop out 1 heaped tablespoon of the mixture and roll into a ball using wet hands.

Place the balls on the lined baking tray and refrigerate for 30 minutes.

Serve. Store in an airtight container in the refrigerator for up to a week.

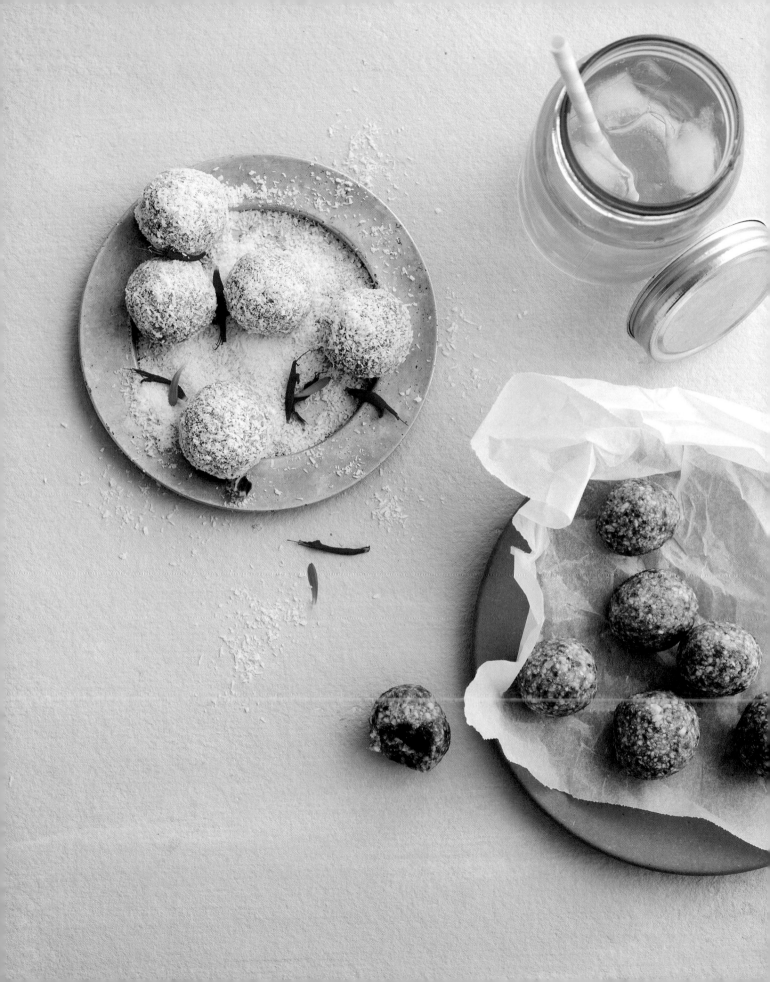

CHERRY RIPE SLICE

MAKES 20

PREP TIME 15 MINUTES +
1 HOUR CHILLING TIME

DIFFICULTY EASY

Make sure that you thaw the frozen cherries completely for this slice. You can do this on a plate with some paper towel to help soak up the excess water.

BASE

1 cup unsalted cashew nuts

8 medjool dates, pitted and chopped

1 teaspoon vanilla bean paste or pure vanilla extract

1 tablespoon coconut oil, melted

2 tablespoons raw cacao nibs

CHERRY FILLING

4¾ oz unsalted cashew nuts

3½ oz desiccated coconut

½ cup light coconut milk

5¾ oz frozen cherries, thawed

2 tablespoons pure maple syrup

CHOCOLATE LAYER

1¾ oz raw cacao powder (see page 49) (about ½ cup)

2¾ oz coconut oil, melted

⅓ cup pure maple syrup

shredded or desiccated coconut, to garnish

Line a 10 in x 6 in slice tin with plastic film.

To make the base, place the cashews in a food processor and process until crumbly. Add the dates, vanilla, coconut oil, and cacao nibs and process until well combined. The mixture should be a little sticky. If it is too thick, add 1–2 tablespoons of water.

Using wet hands, press the mixture into the lined tin and place in the freezer to set while you make the cherry filling.

To make the cherry filling, place the cashews in a food processor and process until crumbly. With the motor running, gradually add the coconut, coconut milk, cherries, and maple syrup and process until smooth. Ensure that you scrape down the side of the bowl occasionally.

Pour the cherry filling over the base and return to the freezer for 30 minutes while you make the chocolate layer.

To make the chocolate layer, whisk the cacao powder, coconut oil, and maple syrup together in a bowl.

Pour the chocolate layer over the cherry filling and sprinkle over the coconut.

Place the tin in the freezer for 30 minutes to set, then cut into bars and serve.

Store in an airtight container in the refrigerator for up to 10 days.

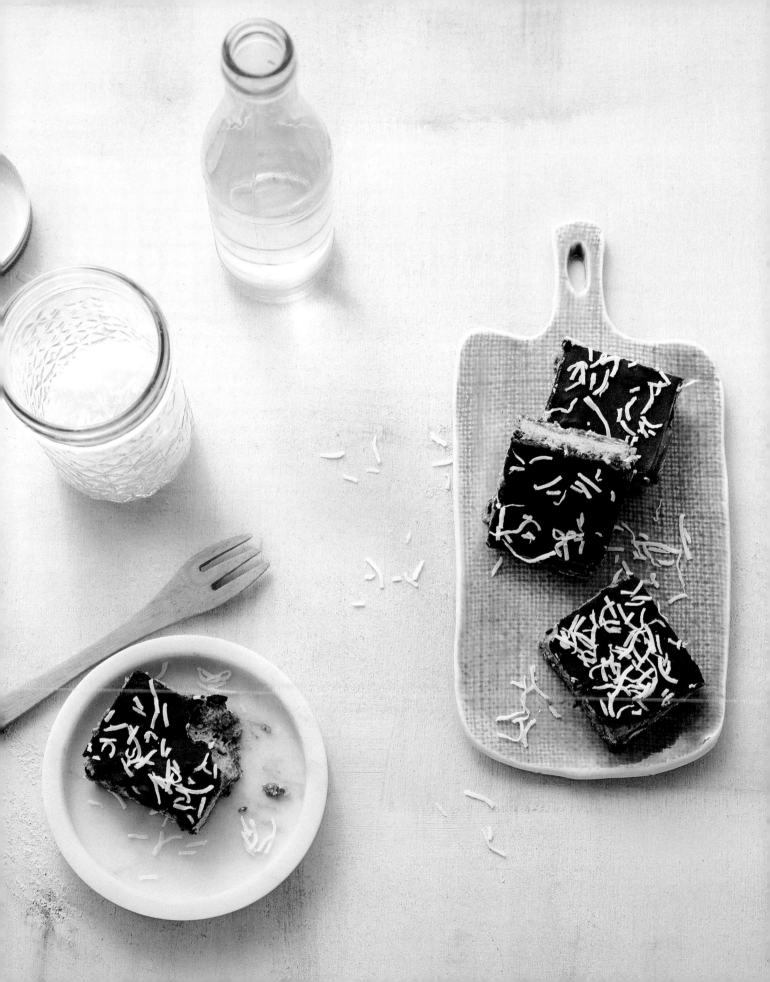

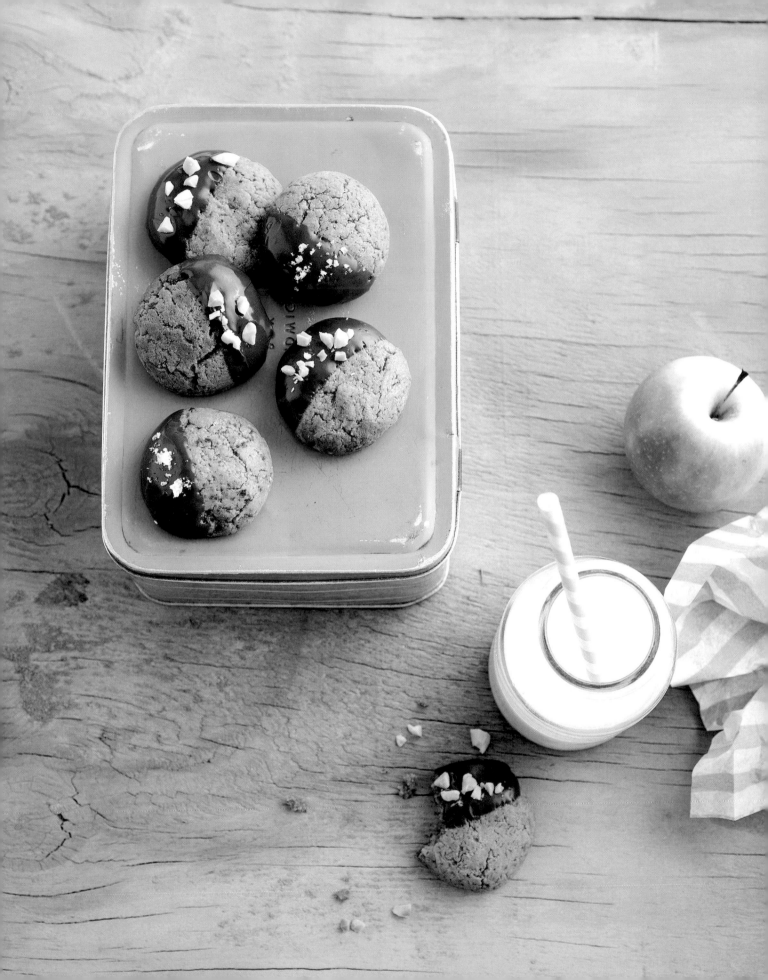

PEANUT BUTTER PROTEIN COOKIES

MAKES ABOUT 10
PREP TIME 10 MINUTES
COOKING TIME 15 MINUTES
DIFFICULTY EASY

One for all the peanut butter lovers . . .

7 oz 100% natural peanut butter

3½ oz coconut sugar

2 scoops vanilla protein powder (optional)

½ teaspoon vanilla bean paste or pure vanilla extract

2 large eggs

CHOCOLATE DIP

5¾ oz dark chocolate chips

sea salt or crushed unsalted peanuts, for sprinkling

Preheat the oven to 350°F (325°F convection) and line a baking sheet with parchment paper.

Place the peanut butter, coconut sugar, protein powder (if using), vanilla, and eggs in a bowl and stir until well combined. The mixture should be a little sticky. If it is too thick, add 1–2 tablespoons of water.

Scoop out 1 heaped tablespoon of the mixture and roll into a ball using wet hands. Place on the lined baking sheet and flatten slightly using the back of a spoon. Repeat with the remaining mixture. Ensure that you leave ¾ in between each ball to allow room for spreading during baking.

Bake for 10–12 minutes or until the edges of the cookies are slightly brown. Leave to cool for 2–3 minutes on the tray before moving to a cooling rack to cool completely.

To make the chocolate dip, place the chocolate in a microwave-safe bowl and warm in the microwave on medium heat for 30 seconds. Remove from the microwave and stir. Continue warming the chocolate in the microwave for 30 seconds at a time until melted and smooth, stirring in between.

Dip half of each cookie into the chocolate dip. Return to the baking sheet and sprinkle the chocolate side with salt or crushed peanuts.

Store in an airtight container for up to 10 days.

FOOD GROUP SAMPLE SERVING SIZES

FOOD GROUP	SAMPLE SERVINGS
GRAINS	**BREADS** ½ medium bread roll ½ medium whole wheat lavash ½ medium whole wheat pita ½ medium whole wheat wrap 1 slice whole wheat bread **CEREALS** 1 oz muesli 1 oz rolled oats **GRAINS** 3 oz cooked brown rice 3½ oz cooked couscous 3½ oz cooked hokkien noodles 3 oz cooked pearl couscous 4¼ oz cooked polenta 3 oz cooked quinoa 3½ oz cooked rice vermicelli noodles 3½ oz cooked spelt 3 oz cooked whole wheat pasta 8 small rice paper wraps
FRUIT	1 medium apple 5 small apricots 1 medium banana 7 oz frozen berries 7 oz blackberries 5½ oz blueberries 20 cherries 3 medjool dates 2 medium figs ½ cup fruit juice (no added sugar) 5¼ oz mixed fruit salad 1 medium grapefruit 25 grapes 3 guava 2 kiwifruit 3 lemons 2 small mandarins 1 medium mango 2 medium nectarines 1 medium orange 5 passionfruit 1 large peach 1 small pear 6 oz pineapple 3 small plums 1 pomegranate 5¾ oz raspberries 9 oz cantaloupe 14 oz rhubarb 1 medium tangelo 9 oz watermelon

FOOD GROUP	SAMPLE SERVINGS
VEGETABLES & LEGUMES	**STARCHY** 2 oz corn kernels (frozen or tinned) ½ medium ear sweet corn 1 oz frozen or fresh peas ½ medium potato ½ medium sweet potato **NON-STARCHY** 1 large handful alfalfa sprouts 1 large handful baby spinach leaves 15 green beans 1 large handful bean sprouts 1 small beetroot 4¼ oz bok choy 3 oz broccoli florets 4 Brussels sprouts 3½ oz cabbage (white or red) ½ medium capsicum 1 medium carrot 3½ oz cauliflower florets 2 celery stalks 10 cherry tomatoes 1 medium cucumber ½ medium eggplant 1 small fennel bulb 1 large handful kale ½ large leek 1 large handful lettuce leaves 3½ oz button/white mushrooms 1 portobello mushroom (100 g) 8 kalamata olives 1 small red or brown onion 1 small parsnip 4¼ oz pumpkin 4 medium radishes 1 large handful arugula leaves 2 large scallions 3 oz snow peas 5¼ oz tinned crushed tomatoes 1 medium tomato 5 pieces semi-dried tomato 1 medium zucchini **LEGUMES** 2¾ oz cooked or tinned bean mixes 2¾ oz cooked or tinned black beans 2¾ oz cooked or tinned butter beans 2¾ oz cooked or tinned cannellini beans 2¾ oz cooked or tinned chickpeas 2¾ oz cooked or tinned kidney beans 2¾ oz cooked or tinned lentils 2¾ oz cooked or tinned split peas

FOOD GROUP	SAMPLE SERVINGS
LEAN MEAT, SEAFOOD, EGGS & MEAT ALTERNATIVES	**RED MEAT (lean cuts)** 2⅓ oz cooked beef 2½ oz cooked kangaroo 2⅓ oz cooked lamb 1 medium lamb chop 2½ oz cooked pork 2⅓ oz cooked veal 2⅓ oz cooked venison **POULTRY** 2½ oz cooked chicken breast or thigh 3 oz cooked turkey breast **SEAFOOD** 4¼ oz cooked squid 3½ oz cooked white fish fillet 8 medium mussels 4¼ oz cooked octopus 10 medium prawns 2½ oz cooked, tinned or smoked salmon 3½ oz cooked or tinned tuna **ALTERNATIVES** 2 large eggs 5¼ oz cooked or tinned bean mixes 5¼ oz cooked or tinned black beans 5¼ oz cooked or tinned butter beans 5¼ oz cooked or tinned cannellini beans 5¼ oz cooked or tinned chickpeas 5¼ oz cooked or tinned kidney beans 5¼ oz cooked or tinned lentils 5¼ oz cooked or tinned split peas 6 oz plain tofu
DAIRY PRODUCTS & ALTERNATIVES	**MILK** 1¼ cups calcium-fortified almond milk 1 cup calcium-fortified milk alternatives 1 cup low-fat (cow's) milk **YOGHURT** 7 oz low-fat plain yoghurt 7 oz calcium-fortified soy yoghurt **CHEESE** 1½ oz bocconcini cheese 1½ oz reduced-fat cheddar cheese 4¼ oz low-fat cottage cheese 1¾ oz light cream cheese 2 oz salt-reduced low-fat feta cheese 1¾ oz soft goat's cheese 1¾ oz haloumi cheese 1½ oz mozzarella cheese 1½ oz parmesan cheese 3½ oz low-fat ricotta cheese 1½ oz soy cheese

FOOD GROUP	SAMPLE SERVINGS
HEALTHY FATS	**NUTS & SEEDS** ⅓ oz almonds (1 tablespoon) ⅓ oz brazil nuts ⅓ oz cashew nuts ⅓ oz chestnuts ⅓ oz chia seeds (2 teaspoons) ⅓ oz hazelnuts ⅓ oz macadamia nuts ⅓ oz peanuts ⅓ oz pecan nuts ⅓ oz pine nuts (2 teaspoons) ⅓ oz pistachio nuts ⅓ oz sesame seeds (2 teaspoons) ⅓ oz sunflower seeds ⅓ oz walnuts (1 tablespoon) **OIL** 1½ teaspoons almond oil 1½ teaspoons avocado oil 1½ teaspoons canola oil 1½ teaspoons coconut oil 1½ teaspoons corn oil 1½ teaspoons linseed oil 1½ teaspoons macadamia oil 1½ teaspoons olive oil 1½ teaspoons peanut oil 1½ teaspoons rice bran oil 1½ teaspoons safflower oil 1½ teaspoons sesame oil 1½ teaspoons sunflower oil 1½ teaspoons walnut oil **NUT BUTTER/SPREADS** 2 teaspoons nut butter 2 teaspoons peanut butter 2 teaspoons tahini **OTHER** 1 oz avocado 2 teaspoons margarine/spreads ¼ cup light coconut milk

UNCOOKED TO COOKED FOOD WEIGHTS

Throughout the book, I have used the raw or uncooked weights for the majority of the grain and protein foods. If you are tailoring any of my recipes to suit your preferences, or creating your own recipes using the serving recommendations, it is important that you consider the change in weight of these ingredients once cooked. To help you with this, these handy charts provide the uncooked and (approximate) cooked weights for many common foods.

PROTEINS

LEAN RED MEATS (beef, lamb, kangaroo, pork, veal and venison)

Uncooked	Cooked	Number of servings
1¾ oz	1¼ oz	½
3 oz	2⅓ oz	1
4¾ oz	3½ oz	1½
6 oz	4¾ oz	2
12 oz	9 oz	4

POULTRY (chicken breasts, chicken thighs)

Uncooked	Cooked	Number of servings
1¾ oz	1½ oz	½
4 oz	3 oz	1
5¼ oz	4¼ oz	1½
7 oz	5½ oz	2
14 oz	11¼ oz	4

POULTRY (turkey breast)

Uncooked	Cooked	Number of servings
2 oz	1¾ oz	½
4 oz	3 oz	1
6 oz	4¾ oz	1½
8 oz	6⅓ oz	2
15 oz	12⅔ oz	4

WHITE FISH FILLET

Uncooked	Cooked	Number of servings
2⅓ oz	1¾ oz	½
4½ oz	3½ oz	1
6⅔ oz	5¼ oz	1½
9 oz	7 oz	2
17¾ oz	14 oz	4

SALMON FILLET

Uncooked	Cooked	Number of servings
1¾ oz	1¼ oz	½
3 oz	2½ oz	1
4½ oz	3⅔ oz	1½
6 oz	5 oz	2
12 oz	10 oz	4

SQUID, OCTOPUS

Uncooked	Cooked	Number of servings
2½ oz	2 oz	½
5¼ oz	4¼ oz	1
8 oz	6⅓ oz	1½
10¾ oz	8½ oz	2
21 oz	17 oz	4

DRIED BEANS

Uncooked	Cooked	Number of servings
1¼ oz	2½ oz	½
2½ oz	5¼ oz	1
3⅔ oz	8 oz	1½
5 oz	10¾ oz	2
10 oz	21 oz	4

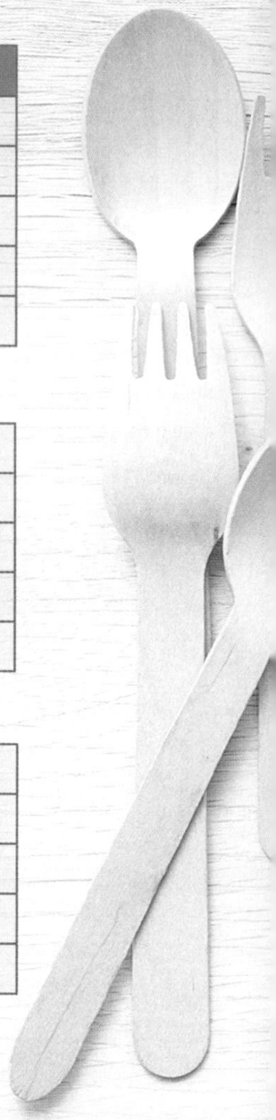

GRAINS

QUINOA

Uncooked	Water needed	Cooked	Number of serves
1 oz	½ cup	3 oz	1
2 oz	⅔ cup	6⅓ oz	2
3 oz	¾ cup	9½ oz	3
4¼ oz	1⅓ cups	12⅔ oz	4

BROWN RICE

Uncooked	Water needed	Cooked	Number of serves
1 oz	½ cup	3 oz	1
2 oz	1 cup	6⅓ oz	2
3 oz	1 cup	9½ oz	3
4¼ oz		12⅔ oz	4

COUSCOUS

Uncooked	Water needed	Cooked	Number of serves
1¼ oz	½ cup	3½ oz	1
2½ oz	¾ cup	7 oz	2
3½ oz	1 oz	10¾ oz	3
4¾ oz	1⅔ cups	14 oz	4

PEARL COUSCOUS

Uncooked	Water needed	Cooked	Number of serves
1 oz	1 cup	3 oz	1
2 oz	1⅔ cups	5¾ oz	2
3 oz	3⅓ cups	9½ oz	3
4¼ oz	5 cups	12⅔ oz	4

PASTA

Uncooked	Water needed	Cooked	Number of serves
1½ oz	2 cups	3 oz	1
2 oz	3 cups	4¼ oz	1½
3 oz	4¼ cups	5¾ oz	2
4¼ oz	6⅓ cups	8½ oz	2½
5¾ oz	8½ cups	11¼ oz	4

RICE VERMICELLI NOODLES

Uncooked	Water needed	Cooked	Number of serves
1 oz	1 cup	1¾ oz	½
1¾ oz	2 cups	3½ oz	1
2¾ oz	3 cups	5¼ oz	1½
3½ oz	4¼ cups	7 oz	2
7 oz	9½ cups	14 oz	4

28-DAY BEGINNER WORKOUT GUIDE

This workout guide consists of two weeks of workouts to be completed twice. Step-by-step instructions (the Exercise Glossary) can be found on pages 375–379. The exercises are shown on pages 380–385.

Each week includes: **(1) Three resistance workouts that focus on different areas—legs, arms & abs, and full body** (shown on pages 380–385); **(2) Two to three low-intensity steady state (LISS) cardio sessions** (examples include walking, swimming, or cycling for 30–45 minutes); and **(3) One rehabilitation (active recovery) session** (a brief 5–10 minute walk followed by some foam-rolling and stretching).

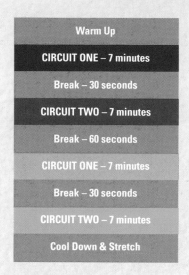

Warm Up
CIRCUIT ONE – 7 minutes
Break – 30 seconds
CIRCUIT TWO – 7 minutes
Break – 60 seconds
CIRCUIT ONE – 7 minutes
Break – 30 seconds
CIRCUIT TWO – 7 minutes
Cool Down & Stretch

Each resistance workout is 28 minutes. The workout consists of two circuits that are completed twice. In each circuit you will need to repeat the four given exercises as many times as possible within seven minutes. You stop when the timer stops!

Take 30–60 seconds rest between circuits. Alternate between circuits. And remember, while you are trying to complete the circuits as fast as you can, it's also important that you maintain proper technique—in this case, quality is better than quantity.

Here is a suggested timetable that incorporates all these elements into a 4-week period:

WEEK 1

Monday	Tuesday	Wednesday	Thursday	Friday	Saturday	Sunday
Legs	LISS	Arms & Abs	LISS	Full Body	Rehabilitation	Rest

WEEK 2

Monday	Tuesday	Wednesday	Thursday	Friday	Saturday	Sunday
Legs	LISS	Arms & Abs	LISS	Full Body	Rehabilitation	Rest

WEEK 3 Repeat Week 1, but for Saturday add an LISS cardio session to your rehabilitation.

WEEK 4 Repeat Week 2, but for Saturday add an LISS cardio session to your rehabilitation.

This plan is **flexible** and can easily be adapted to suit any lifestyle. Just Follow these guidelines when arranging your own schedule:

- Do not complete more than two workouts in any given day.
- If you choose to complete two workouts in the same day, avoid doing them back-to-back—do one in the morning and one in the evening.
- Rehabilitation is a low-intensity form of exercise and can be done after any resistance or cardio workout.

EXERCISE GLOSSARY

Here are step-by-step instructions for each of the exercises featured on pages 380–385.

AB BIKE

1 Start by lying flat on your back on a yoga mat with your feet extended out in front of you.

2 Bend your elbows and place your hands behind your earlobes.

3 Gently raise both feet, your head and shoulder blades off the floor. This is your starting position.

4 At the same time, extend your left leg so that it is just slightly off the floor and bring your right knee into your chest.

5 Extend your right leg completely so that it is just slightly off the floor and bring your left knee into your chest. This creates a "pedalling/bike-like" motion.

6 Once you have grasped this movement, incorporate a twist with your upper body by bringing the knee to meet the opposite elbow. For example, as you bring the right knee into the chest, twist your upper body over to the right so that your right knee can meet your left elbow.

7 Continue alternating between left and right for the specified number of repetitions.

BENT LEG RAISE

1 Start by lying flat on your back on a yoga mat and place both hands underneath your coccyx.

2 Extend both legs and engage your abdominal muscles by drawing your belly button in towards your spine. This is your starting position.

3 Keeping your feet together, contract your abdominal muscles, and bend your legs to bring your knees in to your chest.

4 Slowly extend your legs until they are slightly off of the floor.

5 Repeat for the specified number of repetitions.

BROAD JUMP

1 Plant both feet on the floor slightly further than shoulder-width apart.

2 Bend at both the hips and knees, ensuring that your knees remain in line with your toes.

3 Continue bending your knees until your upper legs are parallel with the floor. Ensure that your back remains at a 45–90 degree angle to your hips. This is called squat position.

4 Propel your body upwards and forwards into the air.

5 Land back into squat position. When landing, ensure that you maintain "soft" knees to prevent injury.

6 Repeat for the specified number of repetitions.

BURPEE

1 Plant both feet on the floor slightly further than shoulder-width apart. Bend at both the hips and knees, and place your hands on the floor directly in front of your feet.

2 Keeping your body weight on your hands, kick both of your feet backwards so that your legs are completely extended behind you, resting on the balls of your feet. Your body should be in one straight line from head to toe.

3 Jump both of your feet back in towards your hands, ensuring that your feet remain shoulder-width apart.

4 Propel your body upwards into the air. Extend your legs below you and your arms above your head.

5 Land in a neutral standing position, ensuring that you maintain "soft" knees to prevent injury.

6 Repeat for the specified number of repetitions.

COMMANDO

1 Start by placing your forearms on the floor and extending both legs behind you, resting on the balls of your feet. This is called plank position.

2 Release your right forearm and place your right hand firmly on the floor directly below your right shoulder.

3 Push up onto your right hand, followed immediately by your left in the same pattern. Ensure that you brace through your abdominals to prevent your hips from swaying.

4 Return to plank position by releasing your right hand and lowering onto your forearm, before doing the same with your left hand.

5 Repeat this exercise, starting with your left hand. Continue alternating between right and left for the specified number of repetitions.

DUMBBELL CURL & PRESS

1 Holding one dumbbell in each hand on either side of your body, plant both feet on the floor slightly further than shoulder-width apart.

2 Bend your elbows to bring both dumbbells into your chest. Ensure that the heads of the dumbbells are facing forwards.

3 Extend your arms and press both dumbbells up above your head.

4 Gently lower the dumbbells into your chest and then extend your arms down by your sides.

5 Repeat for the specified number of repetitions.

DUMBBELL SQUAT & PRESS

1. Holding one dumbbell in each hand on either side of your body, plant both feet on the floor slightly further than shoulder-width apart.

2. Bend at both the hips and knees, ensuring that your knees remain in line with your toes. Allow the dumbbells to gently run down the outside of your legs.

3. Continue bending your knees until your upper legs are parallel with the floor. Ensure that your back remains at a 45–90 degree angle to your hips.

4. Push through your heels to extend your legs and bend your elbows to bring both dumbbells into your chest. Ensure that the heads of the dumbbells are facing forwards.

5. Extend your arms and press both dumbbells up above your head.

6. Gently lower the dumbbells into your chest and then extend your arms down by your sides.

7. Repeat for the specified number of repetitions.

HIGH KNEES

1. Plant both feet on the floor slightly further than shoulder-width apart.

2. Keeping your weight on your left foot, bend your right leg to bring your knee into your chest.

3. Lower your right leg and plant your foot on the floor.

4. Keeping your weight on your right leg, bend your left leg to bring your knee into your chest. Once you are comfortable with this movement, increase your speed so that you are hopping from one foot to the other.

5. Continue alternating between right and left for the specified number of repetitions. Each knee lift is equivalent to one repetition.

INCLINE PUSH-UP

1. Place a bench horizontally in front of you.

2. Place both hands on the bench slightly further than shoulder-width apart, and both feet together on the floor behind you, resting on the balls of your feet. This is your starting position.

3. Keeping a straight back and stabilising through your abdominals, bend your elbows and lower your torso towards the bench.

4. Push through your chest and extend your arms to lift your body back into starting position.

5. Repeat for the specified number of repetitions.

JUMP SQUAT

1. Plant both feet on the floor slightly further than shoulder-width apart.

2. Bend at both the hips and knees, ensuring that your knees remain in line with your toes.

3. Continue bending your knees until your upper legs are parallel with the floor. Ensure that your back remains at a 45–90 degree angle to your hips. This is called squat position.

4. Propel your body upwards into the air. Extend both your legs and your hips before landing back into squat position. When landing, ensure that you maintain "soft" knees to prevent injury.

5. Repeat for the specified number of repetitions.

KNEE-UP

1. Place a bench horizontally in front of you and plant both feet on the floor slightly further than shoulder-width apart.

2. Firmly plant your entire right foot on the bench, making sure your knee is in line with your toes.

3. Push through the heel of your right foot to extend your right leg. Avoid pushing through your toe to prevent placing additional pressure on your shins, knees, and quadriceps.

4. As you straighten your right leg, bend your left leg and bring your knee in towards your chest.

5. Release your left knee from your chest and place your foot back on the floor.

6. Repeat half of the specified number of repetitions on the same leg before completing the remaining repetitions on the other leg.

LATERAL LUNGE

1. Plant both feet on the floor slightly further than shoulder-width apart. This is your starting position.

2. Keeping your left foot on the floor, release your right foot, and take a big step to your right.

3. As you plant your foot on the floor, bend your right knee, ensuring that your left leg remains straight.

4. Push through the heel of your right foot to bring your feet back into starting position.

5. Repeat this movement by stepping out to your left side with your left leg. Continue alternating between right and left for the specified number of repetitions.

LAY DOWN PUSH-UP

1 Start by lying flat on your stomach, with arms extended out in front of you and both legs straight behind you. Position your toes facing down towards the floor.

2 Bring your arms into your body and place your hands on the floor on either side of your chest.

3 Push through your chest and extend your arms to lift your body up into push-up position, resting on the balls of your feet.

4 Ensure that you maintain a straight back and stabilise through your abdominal muscles.

5 Slowly lower your body completely to the floor and extend your arms out in front of you.

6 Repeat for the specified number of repetitions.

MOUNTAIN CLIMBER

1 Place both hands on the floor shoulder-width apart and both feet together behind you, resting on the balls of your feet. This is your starting position.

2 Keeping your left foot on the floor, bend your right leg and bring your knee in towards your chest.

3 Extend your right leg and return to starting position.

4 Keeping your right foot on the floor, bend your left leg and bring your knee in towards your chest.

5 Extend your left leg and return to starting position.

6 Continue alternating between right and left for the specified number of repetitions. Gradually increase your speed, ensuring that the leg that is moving does not touch the floor.

OUTWARD SNAP JUMP

1 Place both hands on the floor slightly further than shoulder-width apart and both feet together behind you, resting on the balls of your feet. This is your starting position.

2 Quickly jump both feet outwards so that they are wider than your hips.

3 Quickly jump both feet inwards to bring them back together into starting position.

4 Continue alternating between feet together and feet apart for the specified number of repetitions.

PLANK

1 Start by placing your forearms firmly on the floor.

2 Extend both legs behind you, resting on the balls of your feet.

3 Brace your abdominals and maintain a straight back, ensuring that your elbows are directly below your shoulders.

4 Hold this position for the specified amount of time.

PUSH-UP

1 Place both hands on the floor slightly further than shoulder-width apart and both feet together behind you, resting on the balls of your feet. This is your starting position.

2 Keeping a straight back and stabilising through your abdominals, bend your elbows and lower your torso towards the floor until your arms form a 90 degree angle.

3 Push through your chest and extend your arms to lift your body back into starting position.

4 Repeat for the specified number of repetitions.

REVERSE LUNGE & KNEE LIFT

1 Plant both feet on the floor slightly further than shoulder-width apart. Carefully take a big step backwards with your left foot.

2 As you plant your left foot on the floor, bend both knees to approximately 90 degrees, ensuring that your weight is evenly distributed between both legs. If done correctly, your front knee should be aligned with your ankle and your back knee should be hovering just off the floor.

3 Extend both knees and transfer your weight completely onto your right foot.

4 At the same time, lift up your left foot and bring your knee into your chest.

5 Release your left knee from your chest and place your foot back on the floor behind you.

6 Complete half of the specified number of repetitions on the same leg, before completing the remaining repetitions on the other leg.

RUSSIAN TWIST

1 Start seated on a yoga mat with your hands clasped in front of your chest.

2 Bend your knees and position your feet firmly on the floor. Keeping your feet together, raise your feet off the floor and extend your legs so that they are almost straight. This is your starting position.

3 Twist your torso to the right so that your right hand touches the floor immediately beside you.

4 Untwist your torso to return to starting position.

5 Twist your torso to the left so that your left hand touches the floor immediately beside you.

6 Untwist your torso to return to starting position.

7 Continue alternating between right and left for the specified number of repetitions.

SIDE CRUNCH (ON BACK)

1 Start by lying flat on your back on a yoga mat.

2 Bend your knees and position your feet firmly on the floor, then turn out your left leg so that your ankle is resting on your right leg just below your knee.

3 Place your hands behind your earlobes and slowly lift your head and shoulder blades off the floor. Engage your abdominal muscles by drawing your belly button in towards your spine.

4 Twist your torso to the right so that your right elbow touches the floor immediately beside you. This is your starting position.

5 Twist your torso to the left to bring your right elbow across your body to your left knee (or as far as you can). Try to keep your knee still so that you only bring your elbow to your knee, and not your knee to your elbow.

6 Slowly release your torso and return to starting position.

7 Complete half of the specified number of repetitions on the same side, before completing the remaining repetitions on the other side.

SKIPPING

1 Standing on the balls of your feet, hold one skipping-rope handle in your right hand and the other in your left.

2 Step your feet in front of the skipping rope to begin.

3 Swing the rope over your head through a small rotation in your wrist.

4 As the rope is about to touch the floor, quickly jump upwards to allow it to swing under your feet and behind your body.

5 Repeat for the specified number of repetitions.

SNAP JUMP

1 Plant both feet on the floor slightly further than shoulder-width apart. Bend at both the hips and knees, and place your hands on the floor directly in front of your feet.

2 Keeping your body weight on your hands, kick both of your feet backwards so that your legs are completely extended behind you, resting on the balls of your feet.

3 Jump both of your feet back in towards your hands, ensuring that your feet remain shoulder-width apart.

4 Repeat for the specified number of repetitions.

SPLIT SQUAT

1 Plant both feet together on the floor. This is your starting position.

2 Bend your knees slightly and propel your body upwards into the air.

3 Reposition your legs so that your feet land in sumo (wide) squat position.

4 Continue bending your knees until your upper legs are parallel with the floor, ensuring that your back remains at an angle of 45–90 degrees to your hips.

5 Propel your body upwards into the air again.

6 Reposition your legs to bring your feet together into starting position, ensuring that you maintain "soft" knees to prevent injury.

7 Repeat for the specified number of repetitions.

SQUAT

1 Plant both feet on the floor slightly further than shoulder-width apart. This is your starting position.

2 Looking straight ahead, bend at both the hips and knees, ensuring that your knees remain in line with your toes.

3 Continue bending your knees until your upper legs are parallel with the floor. Ensure that your back remains at a 45–90 degree angle to your hips.

4 Push through the heels of your feet and extend your legs to return to starting position.

5 Repeat for the specified number of repetitions.

STATIC LUNGE

1 Plant both feet on the floor slightly further than shoulder-width apart.

2 Take a big step forward with your left foot. As you plant your foot on the floor, bend both knees to approximately 90 degrees. If done correctly, your front knee should be aligned with your ankle and your back knee should be hovering just off the floor.

3 Gently touch your right knee on the floor before extending both knees.

4 Complete half of the specified number of repetitions on the same leg, before completing the remaining repetitions on the other leg.

STEP UP

1 Place a bench horizontally in front of you.

2 Plant both feet on the floor slightly further than shoulder-width apart.

3 Firmly plant your entire left foot on the bench, making sure your knees are in line with your toes.

4 Push through the heel of your left foot to extend your left leg. Avoid pushing through your toes to prevent placing additional pressure on your shins, knees and quadriceps.

5 As you straighten your left leg, release your right leg and step up on to the bench.

6 Reverse this pattern back to the floor, starting with your left leg.

7 Repeat this exercise, starting with your right foot. Continue alternating between left and right for the specified number of repetitions.

STRAIGHT LEG RAISE

1 Start by lying straight on your back on a yoga mat and place both hands underneath your coccyx.

2 Engage your abdominal muscles by drawing your belly button in towards your spine.

3 Keeping your feet together, slowly raise your legs off the floor.

4 Continue raising your legs until they form a 90 degree angle with your hips.

5 Slowly lower your legs until they are just slightly off the floor.

6 Repeat for the specified number of repetitions.

STRAIGHT LEG SIT-UP

1 Start by lying straight on your back on a yoga mat, with your hands behind your earlobes.

2 Engage your abdominal muscles by drawing your belly button in towards your spine. This is your starting position.

3 Keeping your heels firmly planted on the floor, slowly lift your head, shoulder blades and torso off the floor. Ensure your abdominals initiate the movement, and you do not use your arms to "swing" your torso up.

4 As you sit up, reach forwards with your hands and touch your toes (or go as far as you can).

5 Slowly release your arms and torso to return to starting position.

6 Repeat for the specified number of repetitions.

SUMO SQUAT

1 Plant both feet on the floor wider than shoulder-width apart. Point both feet slightly outward. This is your starting position.

2 Looking straight ahead, bend at both the hips and knees, ensuring that your knees point toward your toes.

3 Continue bending your knees until your upper legs are parallel with the floor, ensuring that your back remains at a 45–90 degree angle to your hips.

4 Push through your heels of your feet and extend your legs to return to starting position.

5 Repeat for the specified number of repetitions.

TRICEP DIP

1 Start seated on a bench.

2 Position your hands on the edge of the bench under your glutes and directly below your shoulders. Ensure that your fingers are facing forwards.

3 Shift your glutes forwards off the bench. This is your starting position.

4 Lower your body by bending at the elbows to create a 90 degree angle. Ensure that your shoulders, elbows, and wrists remain in line with one another at all times.

5 Push through the heels of your hands and extend your arms to return to starting position. Avoid using your legs to assist you and always try and maintain an upright position.

6 Repeat for the specified number of repetitions.

X JUMP

1 Plant both feet on the floor slightly further than shoulder-width apart.

2 Looking straight ahead, bend at both the hips and knees, ensuring that your knees remain in line with your toes.

3 Continue bending your knees until your upper legs are parallel with the floor. Lean your body forward slightly so that you are able to touch your left foot with your right hand.

4 Propel your body upwards into the air. Extend both your legs and your hips before landing back into squat position. When landing, ensure that you maintain "soft" knees to prevent injury.

5 Lean your body forward slightly so that you are able to touch your right foot with your left hand.

6 Propel your body upwards into the air. Extend both your legs and your hips before landing back into squat position.

7 Continue alternating between left and right for the specified number of repetitions.

WEEKS 1 & 3

Monday   LEGS

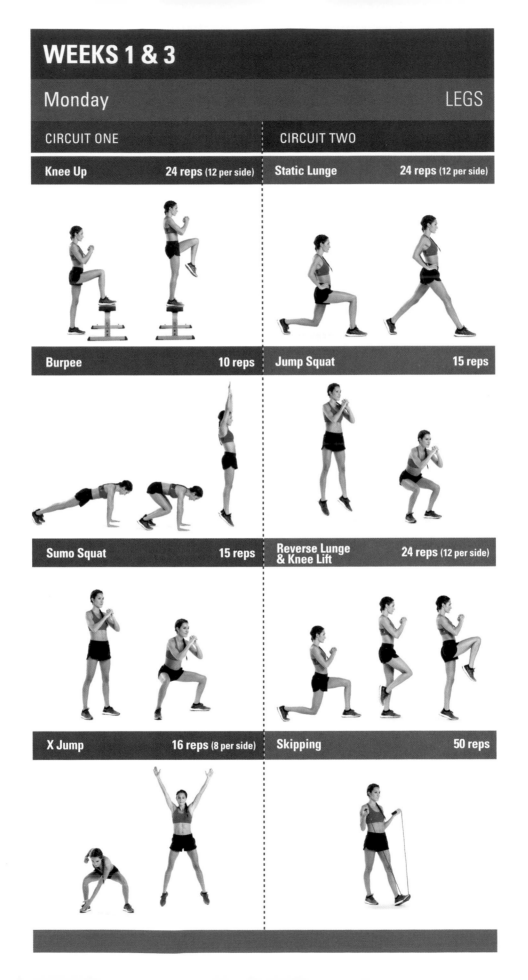

CIRCUIT ONE		CIRCUIT TWO	
Knee Up	24 reps (12 per side)	**Static Lunge**	24 reps (12 per side)
Burpee	10 reps	**Jump Squat**	15 reps
Sumo Squat	15 reps	**Reverse Lunge & Knee Lift**	24 reps (12 per side)
X Jump	16 reps (8 per side)	**Skipping**	50 reps

WEEKS 1 & 3

Wednesday   ARMS & ABS

CIRCUIT ONE		CIRCUIT TWO	
Mountain Climber	30 reps (15 per side)	**Snap Jump**	15 reps
Bent Leg Raise	15 reps	**Russian Twist**	24 reps (12 per side)
Lay Down Push Up	10 reps	**Incline Push Up**	15 reps
Ab Bike	30 reps (15 per side)	**Tricep Dip**	15 reps

Friday

FULL BODY

CIRCUIT ONE		CIRCUIT TWO	
X Jump	**16 reps** (8 per side)	**Russian Twist**	**24 reps** (12 per side)

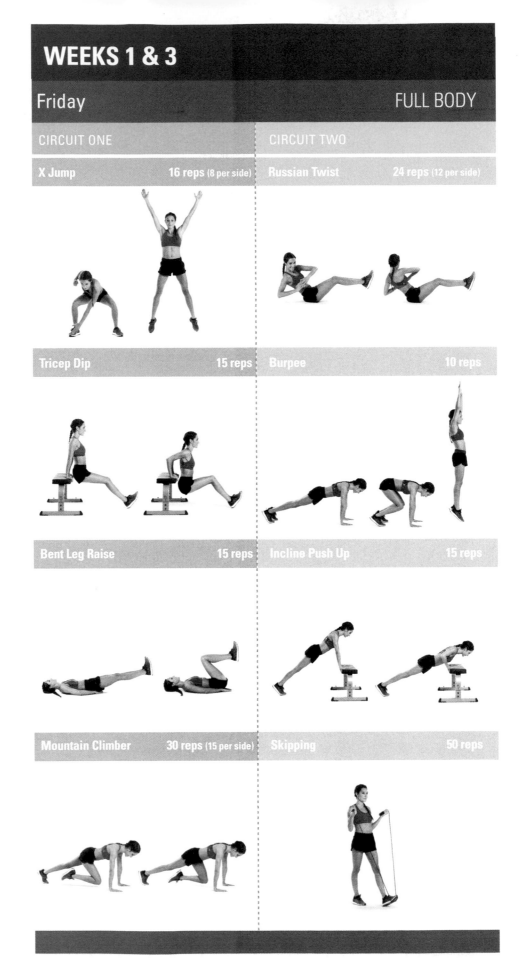

Tricep Dip	**15 reps**	**Burpee**	**10 reps**
Bent Leg Raise	**15 reps**	**Incline Push Up**	**15 reps**
Mountain Climber	**30 reps** (15 per side)	**Skipping**	**50 reps**

WEEKS 2 & 4

Monday | LEGS

CIRCUIT ONE		CIRCUIT TWO	
Static Lunge	**24 reps** (12 per side)	**High Knees**	**50 reps** (25 per side)

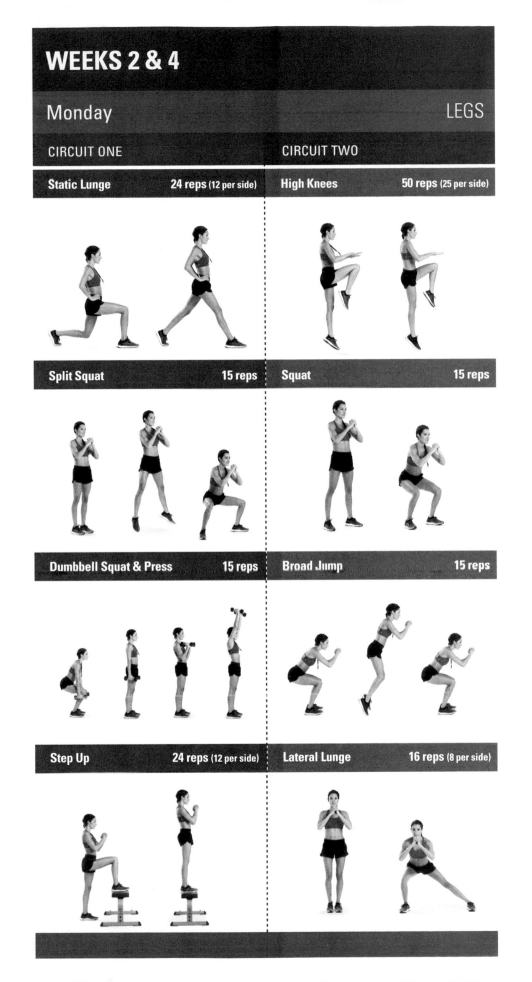

Split Squat	**15 reps**	**Squat**	**15 reps**
Dumbbell Squat & Press	**15 reps**	**Broad Jump**	**15 reps**
Step Up	**24 reps** (12 per side)	**Lateral Lunge**	**16 reps** (8 per side)

WEEKS 2 & 4

Wednesday   ARMS & ABS

CIRCUIT ONE		CIRCUIT TWO	
Straight Leg Sit Up	15 reps	**Outward Snap Jump**	15 reps
Push Up	10 reps	**Side Crunch** (On Back)	20 reps (10 per side)
Dumbbell Curl & Press	10 reps	**Commando**	16 reps (8 per side)
Plank	30 secs	**Straight Leg Raise**	15 reps

384

WEEKS 2 & 4

Friday   FULL BODY

CIRCUIT ONE		CIRCUIT TWO	
Commando	16 reps (8 per side)	**Dumbbell Curl & Press**	10 reps

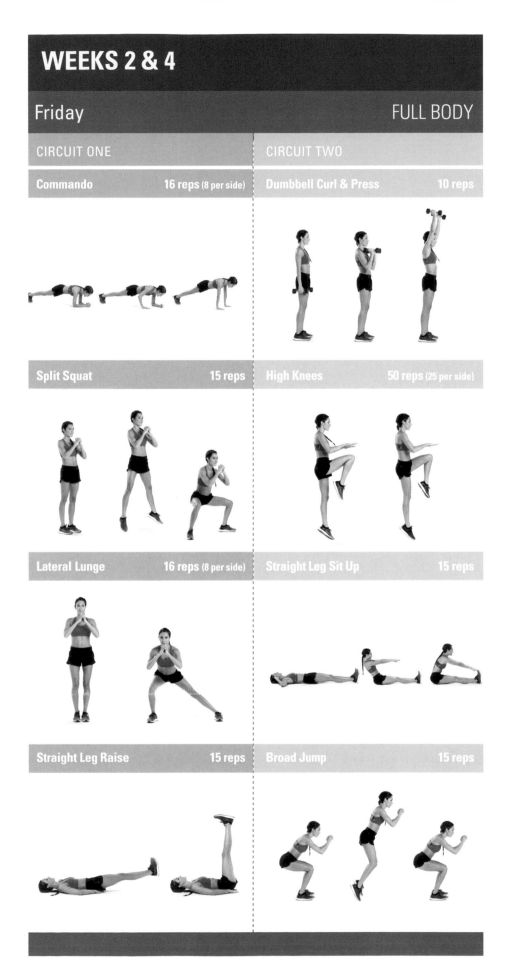

CIRCUIT ONE		CIRCUIT TWO	
Split Squat	15 reps	**High Knees**	50 reps (25 per side)
Lateral Lunge	16 reps (8 per side)	**Straight Leg Sit Up**	15 reps
Straight Leg Raise	15 reps	**Broad Jump**	15 reps

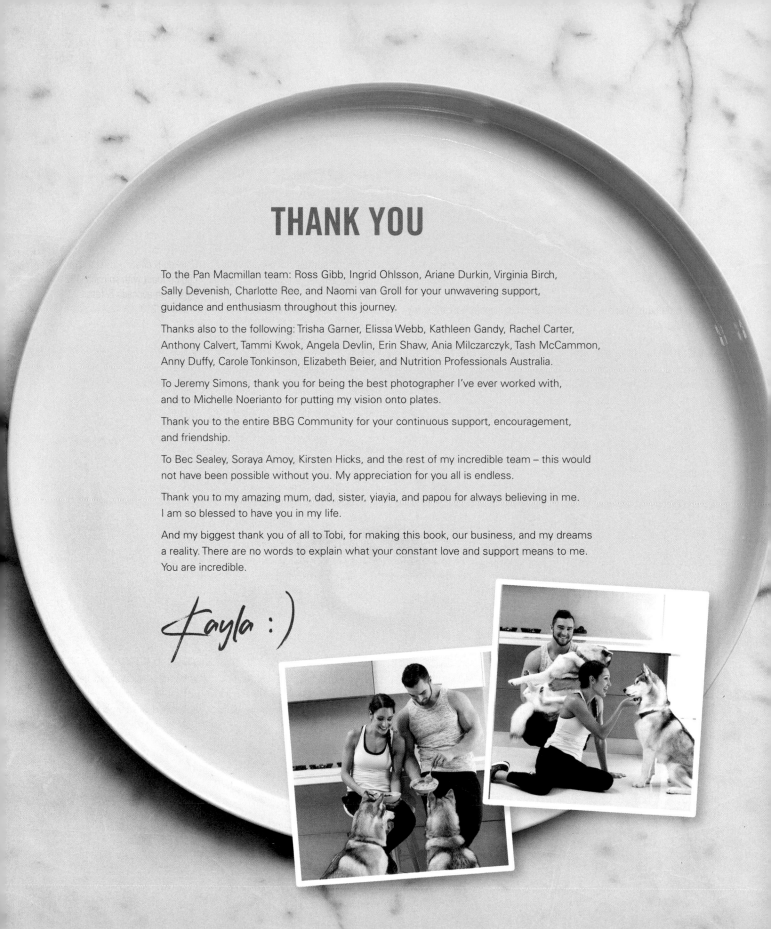

THANK YOU

To the Pan Macmillan team: Ross Gibb, Ingrid Ohlsson, Ariane Durkin, Virginia Birch, Sally Devenish, Charlotte Ree, and Naomi van Groll for your unwavering support, guidance and enthusiasm throughout this journey.

Thanks also to the following: Trisha Garner, Elissa Webb, Kathleen Gandy, Rachel Carter, Anthony Calvert, Tammi Kwok, Angela Devlin, Erin Shaw, Ania Milczarczyk, Tash McCammon, Anny Duffy, Carole Tonkinson, Elizabeth Beier, and Nutrition Professionals Australia.

To Jeremy Simons, thank you for being the best photographer I've ever worked with, and to Michelle Noerianto for putting my vision onto plates.

Thank you to the entire BBG Community for your continuous support, encouragement, and friendship.

To Bec Sealey, Soraya Amoy, Kirsten Hicks, and the rest of my incredible team – this would not have been possible without you. My appreciation for you all is endless.

Thank you to my amazing mum, dad, sister, yiayia, and papou for always believing in me. I am so blessed to have you in my life.

And my biggest thank you of all to Tobi, for making this book, our business, and my dreams a reality. There are no words to explain what your constant love and support means to me. You are incredible.

Kayla :)

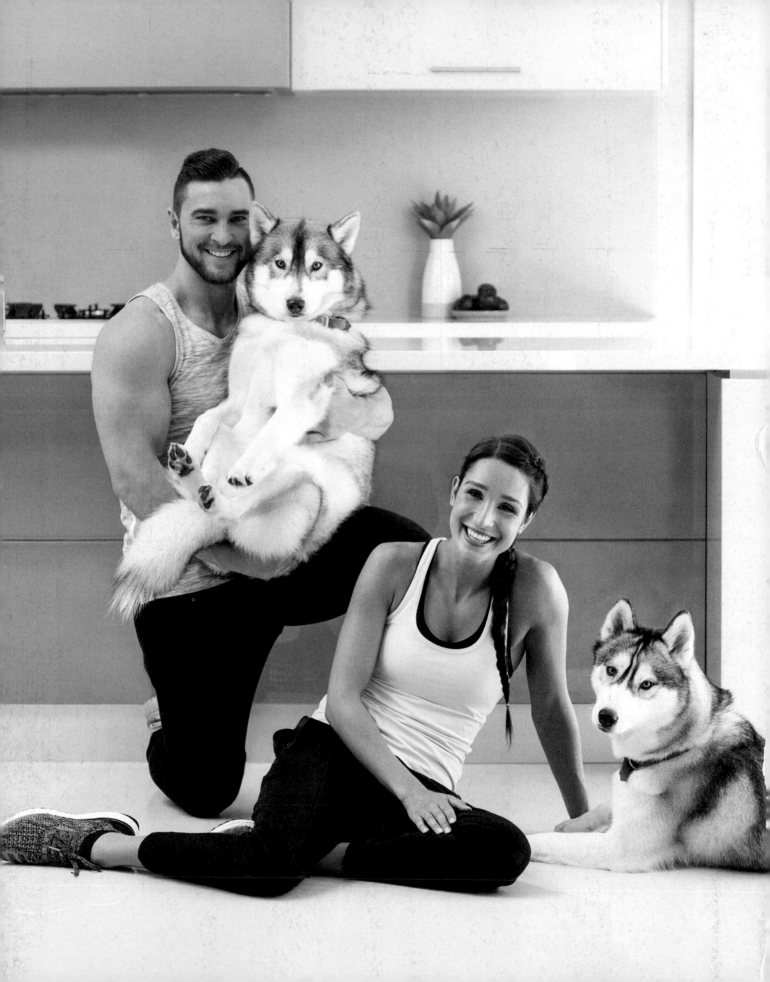